OXFORD MEDICAL PUBLICATIONS

An Introduction to the
Psychotherapies

THIRD EDITION

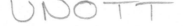

An Introduction to the Psychotherapies

EDITED BY

SIDNEY BLOCH

Department of Psychiatry
St Vincent's Hospital
University of Melbourne
Melbourne
Australia

THIRD EDITION

Oxford   New York   Melbourne

OXFORD UNIVERSITY PRESS

1996

Oxford University Press, Walton Street, Oxford OX2 6DP
Oxford New York
Athens Auckland Bangkok Bombay
Calcutta Cape Town Dar es Salaam Delhi
Florence Hong Kong Istanbul Karachi
Kuala Lumpur Madras Madrid Melbourne
Mexico City Nairobi Paris Singapore
Taipei Tokyo Toronto
and associated companies in
Berlin Ibadan

Oxford is a trade mark of Oxford University Press

Published in the United States
by Oxford University Press Inc., New York

© Oxford University Press 1979, 1986, 1996

First edition published 1979
Second edition 1986
Third edition 1996

A catalogue for this book is available from the British Library

Library of Congress Cataloging in Publication Data

An introduction to the psychotherapies / edited by Sidney Bloch. - -
3rd ed.
    p.   cm. - - (Oxford medical publications)
Includes bibliographical references and index.
    ISBN 0-19-262710-4 hbk.). - - ISBN 0-19-262709-0 (pbk.)
    1. Psychotherapy.   I. Bloch, Sidney.   II. Series.
    [DNLM: 1. Psychotherapy.   WM 240 I61 1996]
RC480.I59   1996
616.89'14 - - dc20
DNLM/DLC
for Library of Congress   95-39062
                                                                CIP

Typeset by Dobbie Typesetting Limited, Tavistock, Devon
Printed in Great Britain by Biddles Ltd, Guildford & King's Lynn

Preface to the first edition

The most striking memory I have of my first few months in psychotherapy training was how bewildering it all seemed. No one could define it, controversy raged over the question of its effectiveness, different schools engaged in constant warfare with one another, and the training programme itself lacked goals and a coherent structure. I realized later when I continued my training in the United States and Britain that this sense of bewilderment was not indigenous to my native Antipodes. The 'acute confusional state' was universal! In recent years I have noted, as a teacher of psychotherapy, that contemporary trainees still undergo a similar type of experience to the one I had.

This situation is not at all surprising. Psychotherapy after all *is* a nebulous term with widely differing connotations; the controversy over its value is still with us; dozens of psychotherapy schools, each with its own theories on psychopathology (often contradictory) and particular set of techniques, compete for the trainee's attention; and there is no apparent link between research and clinical practice—psychotherapists are influenced only occasionally by the results of research.[1] Overwhelmingly, theory determines practice and works vigorously to protect itself from forces that might lead to change.

I hope that this book, mainly an introduction for students in the mental health professions, will help to remove at least some of the hurdles that commonly obstruct them in approaching the complex and demanding subject of psychotherapy. The general objectives of the book are: (1) To make the concept of psychotherapy more understandable. To this end I have used the term *psychotherapies* in the sense that there are several forms of psychotherapeutic treatment which can be distinguished from one another according to their goals, techniques, and target of intervention. We can therefore differentiate, for example, between crisis intervention, supportive psychotherapy for chronically disabled psychiatric patients, family therapy, sex therapy, long-term intensive individual psychotherapy, and so forth. The clinician's task is to match the needs of the patient, couple, or family

---

[1]Malan, D. H. (1973). The outcome problem in psychotherapy research. A historical review. *Archives of General Psychiatry*, **29**, 719–29.

with the appropriate psychotherapy rather than the converse of fitting the patient to the treatment. By using this approach psychotherapy as a generic term may fade into oblivion. (2) To minimize the differences between schools of psychotherapy and to emphasize the features they have in common. Alongside this aim, the book attempts to eschew the dogmatism and doctrinaire attitudes that have tended to permeate the field. Jerome Frank, who has made such a valuable contribution in bringing the issue of 'shared factors' to our attention, considers it in his introductory chapter and the other contributors have been guided by it. A central focus in this book is on what Yalom refers to as 'core' factors (in contrast to 'front' factors).[2] The significance of theory is not denied; trainees must ultimately familiarize themselves with various models for each of the psychotherapies but they should not be swamped by them before they have grasped basic common principles. Each contributor therefore comments on theoretical aspects and provides a guide to further reading. (3) To draw a relationship between research and clinical practice. Although psychotherapy research is still in its infancy, the therapist needs to keep abreast of it in order to maximize his effectiveness. For example, the value of preparing the patient for psychotherapy has been replicated in several studies and the procedure should logically be incorporated into clinical work. When appropriate, reference is made to the contribution of such investigations on clinical practice. By taking cognizance of research findings, I hope that the heat will also be removed from the lingering debate over whether psychotherapy works or not. This debate is futile because we have no way as yet of even attempting to answer the basic questions. In any event, a more suitable question is whether each of the psychotherapies is of value, for whom and in what circumstance. Limitations of space do not allow more than a superficial examination of pertinent research but references are recommended for the interested reader at the end of each chapter. (4) To guide the trainee in his reading. A common problem in psychotherapy education is the bombardment of the novice with references. Inevitably, he wonders how to get into the material, and once having entered, often how to extricate himself. Since the literature is voluminous, reading must of necessity be done rationally. The contributors hope that the recommended reading lists following each chapter will help the trainee to reconnoitre without injury.

---

[2]Yalom, I. D. (1975). *The theory and practice of group psychotherapy*. Basic Books, New York.

I hope that the book comes some way in meeting these objectives.

The presentation of eight different psychotherapies does not mean that the reader should be able to master them all. Presumably, he will select therapies which are intrinsic to his particular work and those which he finds interesting. However, he should also be in a better position to refer appropriately patients who require one of the treatments in which he has not trained.

The masculine pronoun is used, where appropriate, to represent both sexes so as to avoid clumsiness and unnecessary repetition.

Oxford   S. B.
April 1978

Preface to the second edition

For the second edition, coverage of the psychotherapies has been broadened by the inclusion of new chapters on brief, focal psychotherapy and child psychotherapy. In addition, the existing chapters have been updated by their authors to take into account recent developments in each particular field.

I hope the book will continue to prove helpful to students seeking an introduction to what remains a most complex subject.

Oxford   S. B.
April 1985

Preface to the third edition

An Introduction to the Psychotherapies has carved a niche for itself in the training in the psychotherapies of mental health professionals since 1979. It has been a great pleasure to edit this new edition, which I hope will prove as useful as its predecessors to students who need a 'gentle' guide to what is commonly experienced as a bewildering subject.

Both content and the team of contributors have undergone some changes since the second edition. Firstly, cognitive psychotherapy and behavioural psychotherapy have been uncoupled, with each now having a chapter to itself, written by Nicholas Allen and Lynne Drummond respectively. A new chapter, authored by Byram Karasu, has been included to cover the important topic of the ethical dimension of psychotherapy practice. Previous chapters have been updated by the authors, in some cases with the collaboration of new co-authors, namely Mark Aveline on group psychotherapy, Jeremy Holmes on individual long-term psychotherapy, and Cynthia Graham on crisis intervention.

The original objectives set out in the preface to the first edition remain as pertinent as ever. I hope this new edition succeeds in fulfilling those aims.

Melbourne   S. B.
November 1995

Acknowledgements

First edition

I have been helped by many colleagues in editing this book. To the contributors, with whom collaboration proved smooth and pleasant, my thanks. I am grateful to several colleagues who reviewed sections of the manuscript and offered valuable suggestions—Derek Bergel, Pepe Catalan, Michael Gelder, Dave Kennard, Michael Orr, William Parry-Jones, Bob Potter, and Nick Rose. Professor Gelder was helpful in many ways and I thank him for his support.

I would like to pay special tribute to the late Dr Phyllis Shaw. She not only provided the encouragement I needed to initiate the project but also agreed to contribute the chapter on supportive psychotherapy. Many ideas contained in this chapter come from her preparatory notes.

I am grateful to several secretaries in the Oxford University Department of Psychiatry who helped to prepare the manuscript. Finally, I thank my wife, Felicity, for her constant support and editorial suggestions.

Second edition

Again it is a pleasure to thank the contributors for their helpful collaboration. Gillian Forrest, Ian Goodyer, Keith Hawton, and David Mushin reviewed sections of the manuscript—to them my gratitude. My secretary Ann Robinson was most obliging in helping to prepare the final typescript.

Third edition

My gratitude to the contributors is boundless; their colleagueship has been a source of much pleasure. I thank Nicholas Allen, George Halasz, and Edwin Harari who provided valuable advice on parts of the manuscript. Julie Larke has proved time and time again through the editing process how blessed one is when assisted by a bright and congenial secretary; I am most grateful to her. I would like to thank Sandra Russell and Gillian Hiscock and their respective staff in the Mental Health Library of Victoria and St. Vincent's Hospital Library for their unstinting assistance in tracking down references. The Victorian branch of the Australian and New Zealand Association of Psychotherapy has generously permitted the use of its logo for the cover—a wonderful representation of the therapeutic process. Finally, I thank Felicity, Leah, David, and Aaron for putting up with a husband and father who has not always been accessible in recent months, especially as nasty deadlines loomed!

Contents

List of contributors

NICHOLAS B. ALLEN, M.Sc., Ph.D.
Lecturer in Psychology, Department of Psychology, University of
Melbourne and Department of Psychiatry, St Vincent's Hospital,
Melbourne

MARK AVELINE, M.D., F.R.C.Psych., D.P.M.
Consultant Psychotherapist, Nottingham Psychotherapy Unit,
Nottingham

JOHN BANCROFT, M.D., F.R.C.P., F.R.C.Psych.
Director, Kinsey Institute for Research in Sex, Gender and
Reproduction, Indiana University, Bloomington, Indiana

ARNON BENTOVIM, M.B., B.S., F.R.C.Psych.
Formerly Consultant Psychiatrist, The Hospital for Sick Children,
London

SIDNEY BLOCH, M.B., Ch.B., Ph.D., F.R.C.Psych.,
F.R.A.N.Z.C.Psych.
Associate Professor and Reader, Department of Psychiatry,
University of Melbourne, St Vincent's Hospital, Melbourne

MICHAEL CROWE, D.M., F.R.C.P., F.R.C.Psych.
Consultant Psychiatrist, Bethlem Maudsley NHS Trust and Honorary
Senior Lecturer, Institute of Psychiatry, London

SIDNEY CROWN, Ph.D., F.R.C.P., F.R.C.Psych.
Formerly Consultant Psychotherapist, The London Hospital, London

LYNNE DRUMMOND, M.R.C.P., M.R.C.Psych.
Consultant Psychiatrist and Senior Lecturer in Behavioural
Psychotherapy, St George's Hospital Medical School, London

JEROME D. FRANK, M.D., Ph.D.
Emeritus Professor of Psychiatry, Johns Hopkins University,
Baltimore, Maryland

CYNTHIA GRAHAM, M.Appl.Sci., Ph.D.
Department of Psychology, Indiana University, Bloomington, Indiana

MICHAEL HOBBS, M.A., M.B., B.Chir., M.Sc.,
F.R.C.Psych.
Honorary Senior Lecturer in Psychotherapy, University of Oxford and
Consultant Psychotherapist, Warneford Hospital, Oxford

JEREMY HOLMES, M.R.C.P., F.R.C.Psych.
Consultant Psychotherapist, North Devon District Hospital,
Barnstaple, Devon

T. BYRAM KARASU, M.D.
Silverman Professor and Chairman, Department of Psychiatry, Albert
Einstein College of Medicine, New York

SULA WOLFF, B.M., B.Ch., F.R.C.P., F.R.C.Psych.
Honorary Fellow, Department of Psychiatry, University of
Edinburgh, Edinburgh

1

What is psychotherapy?

JEROME D. FRANK

In this introductory, now classic chapter, Jerome Frank attempts to answer the complex question 'what is psychotherapy?' by approaching the subject in historical and cultural contexts. After describing psychotherapy's practitioners, the kinds of treatment they offer, and the patients who receive it, he pays particular attention to the common therapeutic functions of the rationales and procedures of all psychotherapies. The chapter ends with general principles and guidelines for the trainee setting out to practise psychotherapy.

As social beings, humans are totally dependent on each other for maintenance of their biological and psychological well-being. When this is threatened in any way, they typically turn to each other for help, whether this be protection against a physical danger such as an enemy group, protection of a food supply endangered by drought, or for assuagement of distress created by the vicissitudes of life.

This book is concerned with the attempt of one person to relieve another's psychological distress and disability by psychological means. These are typically words, but include other communicative or symbolic behaviours, ranging from laying a reassuring hand on someone's shoulder to elaborate exercises aimed at combating noxious emotions and promoting inner tranquillity.

Informal psychological help in the form of solace, guidance, advice, and the like is frequently sought and received from family members and other intimates. Other sources may sometimes be casual acquaintances and even strangers, especially if they occupy roles like that of the bartender, for example, that create the expectation that they will be good listeners.

Psychotherapy, the form of help-giving with which we are here concerned, differs from such informal help in two significant ways.

First, the practitioners are specially trained to conduct this activity and they are sanctioned by their society or by a subgroup to which they and the patients belong. Secondly, their activity is systematically guided by an articulated theory that explains the sources of the patients' distress and disability and prescribes methods for alleviating them. Psychotherapy differs from medical and surgical procedures in its major reliance on symbolic communications as contrasted with bodily interventions. This implies that it is concerned with the content of the symptoms and their meaning for the patient's life, e.g. what the hallucinated voices are saying, or what the patient is depressed about, or what he fears when anxious. Drugs, when used, are regarded as facilitative adjuncts, and their choice is determined by the form and severity of the patient's symptomatology, such as auditory hallucinations and depressed mood.

An important consequence of the primacy of communication as the medium of healing is that the success of all forms of psychotherapy depends more on the personal influence of the therapist than do medical and surgical procedures. Even when the success of psychotherapeutic procedures is believed to depend solely on their objective properties, as some behaviour therapists maintain, the personal influence of the therapist determines whether the patient carries out the prescribed treatment in the first place, as well as having healing effects in itself. While important in all medical treatment, the personal impact of the therapist is crucial to psychotherapy (Frank and Frank 1991; Greben 1983).

AN HISTORICAL-CULTURAL PERSPECTIVE

Although there are a bewildering number of schools of psychotherapy, each proclaiming its own special virtues, viewed from a historical-cultural standpoint, all can be subsumed under two categories: the religio-magical and the empirical-scientific (Frank 1977; Zilboorg and Henry 1941). The former is as old as human culture and continues to predominate in most non-industrialized societies. Although viewed askance by many persons in industrialized societies, healing cults continue to have large followings in them as well.

Religio-magical therapies are grounded in what has been termed the perennial philosophy (Huxley 1941). This underlies all major religions and avers that humans are manifestations of the 'Divine Ground' which links us into a kind of seamless web. Each individual, as it were, contains the universe. The conventional or sensory reality in which we live is only one of reality. Health is a harmonious integration of forces within the person coupled with a corresponding harmony in his relations with other persons and the spirit world. Illness is a sign that he has transgressed the rules of nature or society, thereby disrupting his internal harmony and creating vulnerability to harmful influences from other persons and spirits.

Such a conceptualization takes for granted that mental states can powerfully affect bodily functions and that the state of bodily health, conversely, can affect mental functions. The therapist's goal is to restore the patient's harmony within himself, with his group, and with the spirit world through special rituals requiring the participation of the patient and, usually, those important to him, the purpose of which is to intercede with the spirit world on the patient's behalf. The religio-magical healer is as well trained in special techniques as his scientific colleague but attributes his healing powers to supernatural sources which are linked to a religious system that he and the patient share. Healing involves a special state of consciousness of both healer and patient, in which both temporarily enter another reality characterized by such phenomena as clairvoyance, communion with the spirit world, and out-of-the-body experiences.

Empirical-scientific psychotherapy was foreshadowed by Hippocrates. It has been practised continuously in the West since the mid-eighteenth century, beginning with the charismatic physician Anton Mesmer, who viewed his treatment as the scientific application of animal magnetism. Although his theories and he himself were discredited, empirical-scientific psychotherapy continued as hypnosis and then experienced a sharp rise in popularity and influence thanks to the genius of Freud (see Chapter 2). More recently empirical-scientific psychotherapy has been expanded by therapies based on the theories of Pavlov and Skinner (see Chapter 7), and therapies that seek to help the patient correct pathogenic cognitions (Beck 1976).

The empirical-scientific approach is conducted with the patient in an unaltered state of consciousness but may involve hypnotic states, fantasies, dreams, and the state of reverie which may accompany free association in psychoanalysis. The therapies which appear most scientific, however, notably cognitive therapy and behaviour therapy, depend on full utilization of the patient's waking intellect. Healers in the scientific tradition, instead of basing their powers on supernatural sources, invoke science as the sanction for their methods.

Despite striking differences in their underlying world views, religio-magical and empirical-scientific therapies have much in common. They share the aim of restoring the patient's harmony with himself and with his group. Both approaches, furthermore, depend on a belief system shared by the patient and the therapist that the treatment has been empirically validated. This is as true for the religio-magical systems of pre-scientific cultures as for the supposedly scientifically based systems in our own. The therapeutic procedures express the belief system in tangible form, thereby reinforcing it. In both, a trained healer derives his power from the belief system—whether it be as scientifically grounded Western practitioner or a supernaturally inspired shaman—and in both he serves as an intermediary between the patient and his group. Finally, empirical-scientific healers, no less than shamans, expend considerable effort to mobilize the patient's faith in their procedures.

PRACTITIONERS OF PSYCHOTHERAPY

Starting with Mesmer and until the middle of the twentieth century, empirical-scientific psychotherapy was conducted by physicians, initially neurologists, later psychiatrists. In recent decades they have been joined by psychiatric social workers and later by clinical psychologists and psychiatric nurses. These mental health professionals often work under medical supervision but some have achieved virtually complete autonomy. To these must be added clergymen, for whom psychotherapy is a natural extension of pastoral counselling.

In addition, especially in the United States, the excess of demand for help over the supply of trained practitioners has led to a proliferation of self-appointed healers and cult leaders, with or without training, who work not only in conventional settings but in ones specially designated as 'growth centres' as well as in hotel rooms, meeting halls, and private homes. Most utilize group approaches, some of which are similar to those of healing religious cults such as 'scientology'. Although many do not set themselves up as therapists, the great majority of their clientele have had previous psychotherapy or are currently in treatment.

Also important are groups composed of fellow sufferers. These 'peer self-help psychotherapy groups' function autonomously and maintain various degrees of rapport with the medical profession. Some welcome all comers, but most, such as Alcoholics Anonymous, are offered only for those suffering from a specific common problem.

KINDS OF PSYCHOTHERAPY

The goal of all forms of psychotherapy is to enable a person to satisfy his legitimate needs for affection, recognition and sense of mastery through helping him to correct the maladaptive attitudes, emotions, and behaviour that impede the attainment of such satisfactions. In so doing, psychotherapy seeks to improve his social interactions and reduce his distress, while at the same time helping him to accept the suffering that is an inevitable aspect of life and, when possible, to utilize it in the service of personal growth.

Although all psychotherapies take into account all aspects of personal life, different schools vary considerably in emphasis. They can be roughly ordered in accord with their primary target, their temporal orientation, and whether they seek primarily to modify thoughts and attitudes, emotional states, or behaviour.

To over-simplify vastly, insight-therapies focus on the individual patient and see distress as arising primarily from unresolved internal conflicts. Some, such as psychoanalysis, focus on the past. They see the internal conflicts as caused by traumatic experiences of early life and seek to unearth their sources and thereby resolve them. Behaviour therapies also are primarily concerned with counteracting the effects of previous damaging experiences.

Other behaviour therapists who emphasize modelling or operant conditioning view the primary difficulties as located at the interface between the patient and his immediate social environment and are oriented to the present; that is, they try to help the patient identify and modify the proximate causes and consequences of behaviour that create distress. Existentially oriented therapists are apt to emphasize helping the patient to open up the future, that is, to discover new potentialities for personal satisfaction and growth.

Therapists who regard the primary focus of treatment as the patient in his family (see Chapters 8 and 10) or in an artificially composed group (see Chapter 4) pay particular attention to the patient's reactions to other family or group members as casting light on the sources of their symptoms and seek to mobilize therapeutic group or family forces. Family and group therapists differ in the extent to which they search in the patient's past for sources of current problems, and in whether they focus on the individual patient or on the pathogenic or healing potentials of the family or group as a system.

For psychoanalytically derived therapies, the kind of treatment the patient receives depends primarily on the therapeutic school of the therapist to whom he is referred. That is, these therapists tend to apply their particular method to all their patients, and justify this on the grounds that their goal is to enhance the patient's general integration or to foster personality growth. Relief of specific symptoms is assumed to follow automatically. Cognitive and behaviour therapists reverse this. They believe that the patient's success in correcting faulty cognitions or overcoming specific symptoms will promote more general improvement by enhancing social competence and self-confidence. Hence, they attempt to tailor their methods to combat the patient's specific complaints. As is reported in Chapter 6, behaviour therapists have succeeded to some extent with complaints that are fairly circumscribed. Unfortunately, patients whose chief complaints are of this kind represent a very small proportion of those seeking help. Most feel a pervasive distress or sense of incompetence or alienation, and evidence is still lacking that they respond better to one approach than another, a point to be considered more fully below.

RECEIVERS OF PSYCHOTHERAPY

Since psychotherapy is a cultural institution, those who are considered suitable candidates for it vary among different societies. In the West, psychotherapy is believed to be appropriate for all persons in whom psychological factors are perceived as causing or contributing significantly to distress and disability. Although this criterion is more generously applied in the United States than elsewhere, by and large, individuals are selected from the following categories in Western societies:

(1) *The psychotically disturbed*, such as schizophrenic patients,whose symptoms in all likelihood stem predominantly from an organic source. The aim of psychotherapy for these patients is to help them to recognize and try to deal more effectively with life stresses to which they are particularly vulnerable (see Chapter 12).

(2) *The neurotically and personality disordered*, who suffer from persistent faulty strategies for dealing with the vicissitudes of life, based presumably on important early experiences that were either damaging or lacking, thereby distorting the processes of maturation

and learning. These patients and those in the next category constitute the vast majority of individuals in psychotherapy.

(3) *The psychologically shaken*, who are temporarily overwhelmed by current life stresses such as bereavement (see Chapter 5). Relatively brief help usually suffices to restore their emotional equilibrium. Since such individuals can manifest the entire gamut of clinical symptoms and respond gratifyingly to any form of help, they fan the competitiveness between different schools of psychotherapy.

(4) *The unruly*, whose behaviour upsets other people but is attributed to illness rather then wickedness. This category includes 'acting-out' children and adolescents, spouses whose heedless or self-indulgent behaviour distresses their partners, as well as antisocial personalities and substance abusers. Some could be classified under the preceding categories. The distinguishing feature is, perhaps, the degree of motivation for help; the unruly are brought to it by others, which makes them, by and large, poor candidates.

Two additional categories of persons receiving psychotherapy exist in affluent or intellectual circles: the discontented, struggling with boredom or existential problems; and professionals who undergo training in psychotherapy as a prerequisite to offering it to others.

HOW EFFECTIVE IS PSYCHOTHERAPY?

This is an easy question to ask but a surprisingly hard one to answer. Evaluation of therapies bristles with methodological problems of which two important ones are how to measure improvement and how to disentangle the effects of psychotherapy from those of other concurrent life experiences.

Criteria of improvement, to the extent that they depend on the conceptualizations of therapeutic schools, are not readily comparable. Thus, psychoanalysts define improvement in part as being able to experience consciously previously unconscious feelings and thoughts, while behaviour therapists look for overcoming of symptoms elicited by particular situations. They are interested in whether the agoraphobic patient can leave the house or the socially inhibited one can enjoy a party, not in the relationship of unconscious to conscious experiences.

Moreover, improvement is not unitary, and so can change in different directions on different criteria. If a husband's chronic abdominal pain disappears after he takes to mistreating his wife instead of submitting to her, is he better or worse? Another problem of evaluation arises from the fact that psychotherapeutic sessions constitute only a small proportion of a person's waking life and he may well be seeking informal help at the same time. Hence, improvement during therapy may primarily reflect this outside help or beneficial changes in his life situation. To complicate matters further, these changes may be the result of shifts in the patient's attitudes and behaviour resulting from psychotherapy.

These and other problems present more difficulties for the evaluation of long-term psychotherapies with loosely defined, open-ended goals, such as increased personality integration than of short-term therapies focused on the relief of particular target complaints.

Nevertheless, findings from many studies have consistently found that all the types of psychotherapy that have been studied produce greater beneficial change than 'spontaneous improvement'; that is improvement occurring over the same time interval in the absence of psychotherapy (Smith *et al.* 1980, p. 183): 'Psychotherapy is beneficial, consistently so and in many different ways. Its benefits are on a par with other expensive and ambitious interventions, such as schooling and medicine.' Findings are less clear with regard to the relative effectiveness of various types of therapy for different conditions.

It must be emphasized that failure to demonstrate significant differences between various therapies by no means excludes the possibility that such differences exist; failure may be due to the lack of criteria for classifying patients with respect to their relative response to various therapeutic approaches. As a result, if a cohort of patients, selected by any criterion, are divided into two groups, one receiving therapy A and one receiving therapy B, each may contain some patients who respond to neither and some who do well with both, and those who respond differentially may get lost in the statistical shuffle.

Improvement in methods of diagnosis and evaluation of change may yet reveal some differences in effectiveness of different therapies that present methods fail to detect. In the meanwhile, a reasonable conclusion is that, whatever their specific symptoms, most patients share a source of distress that responds to the common features of all forms of psychotherapy (Frank and Frank 1991).

THE DEMORALIZATION HYPOTHESIS

A common source of distress may be termed 'demoralization'—a state of mind that ensues when a person feels subjectively incompetent, that is, unable to cope with a problem that he and those about him expect him to be able to handle (DeFigueiredo and Frank 1982; Frank 1974). Demoralization can vary widely in duration and severity, but the full-blown form includes the following manifestations, not all of which need be present in any one person. The individual suffers a loss of confidence in himself and in his ability to master not only external circumstances but his own feelings and thoughts. The resulting sense of failure typically engenders feelings of guilt and shame. The demoralized person frequently feels alienated or isolated, as well as resentful because others whom he expects to help him seem unable or unwilling to do so. Their behaviour in turn may reflect their own irritation with him, thus creating a vicious circle. With the weakening of his ties often goes a loss of faith in the group's values and beliefs, which have formerly helped to give him a sense of security and significance. The psychological world of the demoralized person is constricted in space and time. He becomes self-absorbed, loses sight of his long-term goals, and is preoccupied with avoiding further failure. His dominant moods are usually anxiety, ranging from mild apprehension to panic, and depression, ranging in severity from being mildly dispirited to feeling utterly hopeless.

Most episodes of demoralization are self-limiting. These responses to crisis can enhance a person's mental health by stimulating him to seek better solutions to his problems, strengthening his emotional ties with others, and demonstrating to himself that he can overcome obstacles. Prolonged states of demoralization, however, are self-perpetuating and self-aggravating, since they lead to increasing discouragement which impedes recovery. Those who seek psychotherapeutic help are usually in the middle range of demoralization. Mild forms are relieved by advice or reassurance from family or friends, or changes in life situation, such as a change of job, as a result of which the person regains his sense of mastery and links with his group. At the other extreme, if demoralization is sufficiently severe, the person believes he is beyond help and simply withdraws into a shell. Such individuals do not seek help and some, such as derelicts, seem unable to use it.

In order to come to psychotherapy, the patient must experience certain symptoms, which are viewed as especially amenable to this form of treatment. Many of these, such as anxiety, depression, and feelings of guilt, seem to be direct expressions of demoralization. Others, such as obsessions, dissociative phenomena and hallucinations have a variety of causes, many of which are still not understood. Sometimes, they seem to be symbolic ways through which the patient expresses or attempts to resolve the problems which demoralize him.

Whatever their ultimate aetiology, symptoms interact in two ways with the degree of demoralization. First, the more demoralized the person is, the more severe these symptoms tend to be; thus patients troubled with obsessions find them becoming worse when they are depressed. Secondly, by crippling the person to some degree, symptoms reduce his coping capacity, thereby aggravating his demoralization. The demoralization hypothesis asserts that the shared features of psychotherapies, which account for much of their effectiveness, combat demoralization, as a result of which symptoms diminish or disappear.

Features of all psychotherapies that combat demoralization are:

(1) An intense, emotionally charged, confiding *relationship* with a helping person, often with the participation of a group. In this relationship the patient allows himself to become dependent on the therapist for help because of his confidence in the latter's competence and goodwill. The patient's dependence is reinforced by his knowledge of the therapist's training, the setting of treatment (see below), and by the congruence of his approach with the patient's expectations. While these factors determine the therapist's ascendancy initially, after they are face to face the main source of the therapist's power increasingly becomes his personal qualities, especially his ability to convince the patient that he can understand and help him; that is, his ability to establish what has been termed 'a therapeutic alliance'.

(2) A *healing setting* which reinforces the relationship by heightening the therapist's prestige through the presence of symbols of healing: a clinic in a prestigious hospital, or an office complete with bookshelves, impressive desk, couch, and easy chair. The setting often contains evidence of the therapist's training such as diplomas and pictures of his teachers.

Furthermore, the setting is a place of safety; that is, the patient is secure in the knowledge that his self-revelation will have no consequences beyond the walls of the office. As a result, he can dare to let into awareness of, and come to terms with, thoughts and feelings that had been avoided or repressed.

(3) A *rationale* or conceptual scheme that explains the cause of the patient's symptoms and prescribes a ritual or procedure for resolving them. The rationale must be convincing to the patient and the therapist; hence it is validated by being linked to the dominant world view of their culture and cannot be shaken by therapeutic failures. In the Middle Ages, the belief system underlying what we today call psychotherapy was demonology. In many primitive societies it is witchcraft. In the Western world today it is science.

(4) Linked to the rationale is a *procedure* that requires active participation of both patient and therapist and which is believed by both to be the means for restoring the patient's health. Proponents of all schools of psychotherapy agree that they offer essentially the same kind of therapeutic relationship, but each claims special virtues for their particular rationales and procedures.

SHARED THERAPEUTIC FUNCTIONS OF THE RATIONALES AND PROCEDURES OF PSYCHOTHERAPY

Despite marked differences in content, all rationales and procedures in psychotherapy, reinforced by the setting, share six therapeutic functions:

(1) *They strengthen the therapeutic relationship.* Since the therapist represents society, his mere acceptance of the patient as worthy of help reduces the latter's sense of isolation and re-establishes his sense of contact with his group. This is further reinforced by the fact that therapist and patient adhere to the same belief system, a powerful unifying force in all groups. Explanations of the patient's symptoms or problems in terms of a theory of therapy, moreover, implicitly convey to him that he is not unique, since the rationale obviously must have developed out of experiences with many patients. The treatment procedure also serves as a vehicle for maintaining the therapist–patient relationship over stretches when little seems to be happening, by giving both participants work to do.

(2) The rationales and procedures of all therapies inspire and maintain the patient's *hope for help*, which not only keeps him coming but is a powerful healing force in itself. Hope is sustained by being translated

into concrete expectations. Thus, experienced therapists spend considerable time early in treatment teaching the patient their particular therapeutic 'game' and shaping his expectations to coincide with what he will actually experience.

(3) The rationales and procedures provide the patient with opportunities for both *cognitive and experiential learning* by offering him new information about his problems and possible ways of dealing with them, or new ways of conceptualizing what he already knows. All schools of psychotherapy agree that intellectual insight is not sufficient to produce change. The patient must also have a new experience, whether this be related to reliving the past, discovering symptom-reinforcing contingencies in the environment, or becoming aware of distortions in interpersonal communications. Experiential learning occurs through, for example, emotionally charged self-discovery, transference reactions, and the feelings aroused by attempts to change the contingencies governing behaviour. It is facilitated by the therapist and, in therapy groups, by the group members, both of whom the patient uses as models and as sources of knowledge.

(4) Experiential learning implies *emotional arousal*; this supplies the motive power for change in attitudes and behaviour (Frank *et al.* 1978, Chapter 3). The revelations emerging in psychotherapy may be pleasant surprises, but more often they are unsettling shocks, as the patient discovers features of himself he had previously not let himself face. Some therapists deliberately cultivate emotional arousal, since they see it as central to treatment.

(5) Perhaps the chief therapeutic effect of the rationales and procedures is enhancement of the patient's sense of *mastery*, self-control, competence, or effectiveness. Ability to control one's environment starts with the ability to accept and master one's own impulses and feelings, an achievement which in itself overcomes anxiety and strengthens self-confidence. Nothing is more frightening than feeling oneself to be at the mercy of inchoate and mysterious forces. A powerful source of a sense of mastery is being able to name and conceptualize one's experiences, an activity facilitated by each of the therapeutic rationales. That naming a phenomenon is a means for gaining dominance over it is a frequent theme in folklore and religion as in the fairy tale of Rumpelstiltskin, and the book of Genesis in which the first task God assigns Adam is to name the animals, thereby asserting his dominion over them.

The sense of mastery is reinforced by *success experiences*, which all therapeutic procedures provide in one form or another. These successes maintain the patient's hopes, increase his sense of mastery over his feelings and behaviour, and reduce his fear of failure. The role of success experiences is most obvious in behaviour therapy, which is structured to provide continual evidence of progress and aims to have every session end with a sense of attainment. For example, exposure, by showing the patient that he can survive the full impact of feelings he feared would destroy him, powerfully enhances his sense of self-mastery. Psychoanalytically and existentially oriented therapies, being less clearly structured, yield more subtle but equally potent successes. Patients who respond well to these approaches master problems through verbalization and conceptualization, so that the achievement of a new insight or ability to formulate clearly previously muddled thoughts can powerfully raise their self-confidence.

(6) Finally, all therapies tacitly or openly encourage the patient to digest or '*work through*' and practise what he has learned in his daily living, thereby fostering generalization of the therapeutic gains beyond the psychotherapy situation itself. Some therapies assign homework and require the patient to report back how well he has carried out his assignment. For others, this remains an implicit, but nevertheless strong, expectation.

Differences in the length of therapy used by different schools depend in part on the expectations implicit in their rationales. Behaviour therapies are expected to be brief, those that are psychoanalytically oriented long. Within each school, differences in duration may depend primarily on how long it takes to establish a genuine therapeutic alliance (i.e. win the patient's trust), and how much practice he needs to unlearn old attitudes and habits and develop new, healthier ones.

In short, evidence available to date strongly suggests that in treating most conditions for which persons come or are brought into psychotherapy, the shared functions of different rationales and procedures, not their differing content, contribute most of their therapeutic power. These functions, which are interwoven, all help to re-establish the patient's morale by combating his sense of isolation, reawakening his hopes, supplying him with new information as a basis for both cognitive and experiential learning, stirring him emotionally, providing experiences of mastery and success, and encouraging him to apply what he has learned.

IMPLICATIONS FOR PSYCHOTHERAPY PRACTICE

The probability that the rationales and procedures of all psychotherapies differ little in their effectiveness for most patients by no means implies that familiarity with a particular psychotherapeutic rationale and procedure is unnecessary. Most psychotherapists need a conceptual framework to guide their activities, maintain self confidence, and provide adherents of similar orientation to whom they can turn for support.

The demoralization hypothesis does imply, however, that a therapist will probably do best with the method most congenial to his personality. Some therapists are effective hypnotists, others are not; some welcome emotional outbursts, others avoid them; some work best with groups, others with an individual patient; some enjoy exploring the psyche, others prefer to try to change behaviour. As far as possible, therefore, the trainee therapist would do well to look into a variety of approaches with the aim of mastering one or more that best accord with his own personal predilection and, if he can handle several, selecting the one most appropriate for a given patient. Criteria that could help guide his choice, as well as the procedures themselves, are described in the remainder of this volume.

This chapter concludes with some general principles and guidelines on which almost all schools of psychotherapy agree, and which therefore can be put to immediate use while the student is learning to master a particular approach. The suggestions concern primarily the first encounter with the patient but apply in varying degrees throughout treatment.

Most patients enter therapy with more or less covert conflicts and doubts that distort or impede free communication with the therapist. Your success in overcoming these obstacles in the initial interview may determine whether the patient returns for a second visit as well as the course of therapy thereafter. Hence, from the very beginning, cultivate sensitivity to patients' attitudes that may be blocking the interview. They can be grouped into three classes: (1) those arising from the patient's internal state; (2) those reflecting his attitude toward the interview situation; and (3) those springing from his feelings towards you.

With respect to patients' internal states, most are more or less demoralized; their self-esteem damaged. They may also experience a conflict between wanting to change and unwillingness to surrender their habitual ways of dealing with life, especially since change usually entails the distress felt in confronting their own repressed feelings and the anxiety of venturing into new, uncharted territory. Like Hamlet, many prefer to bear the ills they have than fly to others they know not of.

As to the interview situation, patients have a wide range of sophistication concerning psychotherapy. Some are fully informed; others are bewildered, even frightened, and do not know what to expect. They may suspect that referral to a psychotherapist means that others regard them as crazy, and they may fear what you may discover about their less admirable qualities. The route by which they have arrived at your office influences their initial attitude. A self-referred patient usually feels differently than one who has been referred by his physician in such a way that he experiences it as a brush-off, or one who faces criminal charges or has been referred by his probation officer.

Finally, many patients have doubts about your competence and trustworthiness, especially if you are young and inexperienced. It is prudent to assume that the patient is covertly forming an impression of you at the same time that you are evaluating him. Hence your initial aim is to help the patient to overcome these blocks to open communication. Central to this is your ability to convince the patient that you desire to help him and are competent to do so. To this end, try to act in such a way as to show that you are trustworthy, concerned about his welfare, and seeking to understand him. Try to elicit hidden doubts and misgivings and respond appropriately. The sense that one's message is being received and understood by someone who cares is a powerful reliever of anxiety.

This implies suggestions as to some general attitudes and specific procedures that facilitate patient–therapist communication, thereby supplying the necessary basis for the success of all forms of psychotherapy:

(1) *Be yourself* within the boundaries of the professional role. A stiff, artificial therapist discourages communication. Accordingly, you should not fear being spontaneous within wide limits, expressing pleasure, concern, sorrow, or even anger, admitting when you are sleepy or uncertain as to what is going on, and the like. If humour is within your repertoire, it can be a great help in enabling the patient to achieve some detachment from his troubles, as long as he feels that you are laughing with him and not at him (Bloch and McNab 1987).

By being open with the patient you make it easier for him to be open with you and also to use you as a model. While relying on spontaneity increases the likelihood of making errors, if the patient is convinced that you genuinely care about his welfare, he will forgive and forget almost any blunder you may commit.

(2) *Maintain an attitude of respectful, serious attention*. For many patients, especially socially disadvantaged ones, the psychotherapist may be the first person with status who is willing to hear them out. You should keep in mind that, especially in early interviews, the patient is covertly testing you to see how understanding and trustworthy you are. The best way to pass the test is to maintain an attitude of respectful attention no matter how shocking, trivial, or ridiculous the patient's productions are. This does not mean that the patient should be allowed to ramble. It is possible, tactfully, to guide the patient while preserving a respectful attitude.

(3) Throughout the interview *emphasize the positive*. It is necessary, of course, to explore what is going.wrong in the patient's life. After all, it is because of this that he has come for help. Exclusive pursuit of this goal, however, can increase the patient's demoralization by turning the interview into what has been aptly described as a degradation ceremonial. Remember that patients would not have survived to be in your office today unless they had some assets and coping skills. So be sure to listen for these and remind the patient of them, especially after particularly damaging self-disclosures. This must be done with care. Nothing is more harmful to the progress of an interview than unwarranted or empty reassurance, because the patient hears it as evidence that you do not take his troubles seriously or have not understood their gravity. It is always reassuring, however, after listening to a patient's worst misgivings without implying that you share them, to utilize every appropriate opportunity to remind him of what is going well, or of latent abilities that he is not fully utilizing.

In prolonged therapy, a patient's goals often seem to become more ambitious as he improves. Because the goals keep receding in this way, he may feel he is making no progress. If you sense this, a reminder of the patient's state when he first entered therapy and the gain he has made since can be powerfully reassuring.

(4) *Make sure the patient understands the interview situation*. Depending on the patient's sophistication, take sufficient time to find out his understanding of the nature and purpose of the interview and, to the degree necessary, explain them to him. Let him know how much, if any, of what he reveals will be reported back to the referring

agent. Usually the patient can be reassured that information he reveals will be given to others only with his explicit permission. In the rare cases where complete confidentiality in this sense cannot be guaranteed, as in some court referrals, the patient should be so informed at the start.

(5) *Pay attention to physical arrangements*. The chairs should not be separated by a desk, and be so placed that you and the patient can comfortably maintain or avoid eye contact. It may be facilitative sometimes, for example, for you to avert your gaze when the patient embarks on an acutely embarrassing topic. The lighting should be arranged so that illumination is equal for both parties, or more on you than the patient, to avoid the impression that the patient is being interrogated.

(6) *Be alert to the patient's non-verbal behaviour*. These include tone of voice, hesitancies of speech, facial expression, as well as gestures and bodily postures. Is the patient's manner ingratiating, challenging, tense? Does he maintain eye contact? Are his responses forthright or defensive and evasive? Such clues as to covert attitudes may help you to evaluate what the patient is saying.

Evidence of autonomic activity like sweating or flushing may signal that the topic under discussion is emotionally significant. If a patient indicates that he has non-visible autonomic responses such as heart-pounding, abdominal pain, or headache during the interview, he should be asked to report when they occur.

Since commenting on non-verbal communication may increase the patient's uneasiness, you should reserve comment until you are sure that his trust in you is sufficiently strong to enable him to hear and use the information. Then you may offer immediate feedback of your own reactions, so as to clarify for the patient responses of others that have disturbed him in the past. This is most apt to happen when the patient is unaware of aspects of his communicative behaviour that upsets others. In this connection, a useful manoeuvre is to call the patient's attention to discrepancies between his verbal and non-verbal communications (e.g. that he states he is angry in a sweet tone of voice while smiling). Video-tape playback, by sharply confronting a patient with the way he presents himself to others, can enhance this aspect of therapy.

(7) *Focus on the present*. The patient comes to therapy for help in resolving current problems, however long-standing they may be. He

wants to talk about the here and now, and encouraging this helps to establish rapport. It is also the most direct route towards understanding the patient's characteristic ways of coping. Another reason for focusing primarily on the present is that, although maladaptive patterns of perceiving, feeling, and behaving are rooted in the past, they are sustained by present forces and, therefore, it is these that must be changed.

(8) *Take a history.* Emphasis on the present must not preclude taking a history, especially in the first interview, and returning to aspects of it periodically when relevant. Irrespective of its contents, and therapists of different persuasions emphasize different aspects, taking a full history is the best way to get acquainted with someone. Moreover, it is essential to a full understanding of the patient's current reactions, for we perceive events and react to them not as they exist objectively but in terms of what they mean to us. The same objective event, such as the death of a close relative, may be experienced as a tragedy or a relief. Since the meaning of present events is largely determined by past experiences, considerable review of the latter may be needed to understand the patient's predicament today.

   Sometimes a review of the past serves to enhance rapport: a patient may be able to reveal embarrassing or anxiety-provoking features of his history before he can discuss his current difficulties, and may need to test the therapist's reactions to remote material before he can bring up present feelings. As the patient progresses in therapy, moreover, changes in his interpretations of past events may be important clues as to his progress.

(9) *Repeat what you have heard.* Repeating back what the patient has said, either precisely or with modifications to emphasize a point, is evidence that you are listening attentively and are not angered, frightened, or otherwise disturbed by what you have heard. This implicitly encourages the patient to continue.

(10) *Interpret, but sparingly.* Calling attention to points a patient has overlooked, bringing together statements he had not realized were linked, or offering explanations for his feeling and actions, if skilfully done, shows that you not only heard him but can make sense of what you have heard in ways he had not considered, thereby demonstrating your competence. Premature or implausible interpretations, however, may have the opposite effect, so it is well to be sure of one's ground before offering them.

(11) *Ending the interview*. At the close of the first interview offer the patient an opportunity to make comments and ask questions. He may need encouragement to bring up matters of concern that were not adequately dealt with, seek additional information, ask for further clarification of some of your comments, and the like. Review the mundane aspects of therapy with the patient including the fee (if appropriate), frequency of interviews, and tentative duration. If possible, try to establish with the patient preliminary goals of therapy, recognizing that they might require subsequent revision. At the close of every interview, it is well to sum up the major topics and call attention to significant points. Sometimes it is also possible to offer a formulation in terms of a theme that links the topics together. Finally, when appropriate, suggest homework. This may be to think more about a certain issue, to record dreams, to keep a diary noting when certain symptoms occur, or to try to put into action what has been learned. At the next interview ask the patient to report on the assignment. This helps to preserve the continuity of psychotherapy during the intervals between sessions.

SUMMARY

This chapter has attempted to answer the question: what is psychotherapy? by considering it in an historical-cultural perspective and by discussing its practitioners, the kinds of therapies they offer, and to whom. Particular emphasis has been placed on the shared therapeutic functions of the rationales and procedures of all psychotherapy. Finally, some general principles and guidelines common to all the psychotherapies covered in this book are briefly dealt with.

REFERENCES

Beck, A. (1976). *Cognitive therapy and the emotional disorders*. International Universities Press, New York.

Bloch, S. and McNab, D. (1987). Humour in psychotherapy. *British Journal of Psychotherapy*, **3**, 216–25.

Defigueiredo, J. M. and Frank, J. D. (1982). Subjective incompetence, the clinical hallmark of demoralization. *Comprehensive Psychiatry*, **23**, 353–63.

Frank, J. D. (1974). The restoration of morale. *American Journal of Psychiatry*, **131**, 271–4.

Frank, J. D. (1977). The two faces of psychotherapy. *Journal of Nervous and Mental Disease*, **164**, 3–7.

Frank, J. D. and Frank, J. (1991). *Persuasion and healing: a comparative study of psychotherapy*, 3rd edn. Johns Hopkins University Press, Baltimore.

Frank, J. D., Hoehn-Saric, R., Imber, S. D., Liberman, B. L., and Stone, A. R. (1978). *Effective ingredients of successful psychotherapy*. Brunner/Mazel, New York.

Greben, S. E. (1983). *Love's labor: twenty-five years in the practice of psychotherapy*. Schocken, New York.

Huxley, A. (1941). *Introduction to Bhagavad-Gita*, (trans. by Swami Prabhavananda and C. Isherwood). New American Library, New York.

Smith, M. L., Glass, G. V., and Miller, T. I. (1980). *The benefits of psychotherapy*. Johns Hopkins University Press, Baltimore.

Zilboorg, C. and Henry, G. W. (1941). *History of medical psychology*. Norton, New York.

2

Individual long-term psychotherapy

JEREMY HOLMES and SIDNEY CROWN

In this chapter Jeremy Holmes and Sidney Crown describe that form of individual long-term psychotherapy whose aims are symptom relief and personality change. Following a comprehensive outline of its psychoanalytic basis, they describe the practical aspects of treatment: patient selection, assessment, preparation, the therapeutic contract, setting goals, and termination. Detailed attention is paid to the techniques used and to the problems that may arise in the course of therapy. The chapter ends with a section on the training necessary for long-term treatment.

The psychotherapies are a broad family of 'talking treatments' that can be classified by model (psychoanalytic, cognitive-behavioural, systemic, etc.), mode (individual, group, family), and duration (brief, time-limited, long-term) (Holmes 1991). Although the term 'individual long-term psychotherapy' could, if taken literally, be applied to supportive therapy or prolonged cognitive therapy, it is generally thought of as synonymous with psychoanalytic psychotherapy, which forms the subject matter of this chapter. Psychoanalytic psychotherapy is a modified form of psychoanalysis in which the patient is seen over a prolonged period lasting months or even years, at a frequency of between one and three times per week.

PSYCHOANALYSIS AND PSYCHOANALYTIC PSYCHOTHERAPY

Psychoanalysis (Freud 1922) was the first systematic attempt to use a psychological method to alleviate psychological symptoms and to modify aspects of the personality. It also attempted to link abnormal mental states, particularily hysteria, with a psychological theory with its own models of the mind, how the personality develops and such everyday phenomena as dreaming, slips of the tongue, and memory-lapses.

The defining characteristics of psychoanalysis as currently practised include:

- Seeing the patient four or five times per week.
- Use of the couch.
- An emphasis on dreams, and free association in which the patient is encouraged to say whatever comes into their mind, however absurd, irrelevant or embarrassing it may appear.
- The use of interpretations, linking statements that relate the patient's current troublesome symptoms with past difficulties especially those in early childhood.
- An expressive rather than a supportive pattern, in which the patient's defences are challenged and the experiencing and verbal expression of child-like irrational feelings are encouraged.
- Therapeutic reticence, passivity, and opacity in which, compared with other therapies, the analyst responds rather than initiates dialogue, and reveals little about himself.
- According central importance to transference and counter-transference. The notion of transference/counter-transference has widened from Freud's original idea of past patterns of relationship repeated in the present with the therapist, to refer now to the totality of the unconscious aspects of the therapist–patient relationship (Sandler and Sandler 1984). The transference is held to reveal the fundamental constellation of the patient's inner world, and determines the assumptions and preconceptions which he brings into relationships.
- Effecting psychological change through a combination of insight or self-understanding derived from interpretation, and new experience in which the encounter with a neutral but empathic therapist disconfirms previous assumptions about the world.

This list is heterogeneous, referring partly to the arrangements of therapy, partly to the stance of the therapist, partly to theoretical conceptions about what may or may not be effective in bringing about change. In psychoanalytic psychotherapy the patient is usually seen one to three times per week, most often 'sitting up' (especially in the early phase of therapy), and yet the basis of the therapy is the use of interpretations and working in the transference. Much debate and some research has taken place in an attempt to define the unique elements of psychoanalysis as opposed to less intense forms of psychotherapy. The Menninger Project, a long-term study looking at process and outcome in a group of 42 severely ill patients who received either psychoanalysis or a modified form of psychoanalysis classified as 'supportive psychotherapy' but akin to psychoanalytic psychotherapy, revealed no significant differences in outcome between the two treatments (Wallerstein 1986). Kantrowitz *et al.* (1990) similarly found that only about half of a group of patients in analysis were judged by their analysts to have developed an 'analytic process', that is, a transference neurosis which was worked through in the course of treatment, and that outcome was in any case unrelated to the development of such a process. These results suggest that analytic intensity and the use of the couch are not in themselves a guarantee that 'analysis' will take place, and, conversely, that transference-based treatment is feasible even if the patient is seen less frequently.

Individual long-term treatments are therefore best seen as a spectrum ranging from full psychoanalysis, through psychoanalytic psychotherapy, which may be 'expressive-supportive' or supportive-expressive' according to emphasis, to overtly supportive therapy and long-term counselling. Psychoanalytic psychotherapy can be distinguished as a dimension but not a category from psychoanalysis in its reduced intensity and greater 'impurity', containing more supportive and cognitive elements alongside a still predominantly transference-based therapeutic slant. The emphasis in psychoanalytic psychotherapy is also often more interpersonal and social, and thus 'existential' in the sense of considering man and his relationships in their entirety, compared with some traditional intrapsychic psychoanalytic approaches.

The justification for psychoanalytic psychotherapy is essentially pragmatic: being perhaps less demanding of time and training and certainly less expensive than full psychoanalysis, it is suitable for publicly-funded therapy, and for those whose resources are limited. More importantly, it is particularly suitable for two contrasting groups of patients: those whose difficulties are not severe enough to justify full analysis, and those with severe personality disturbance who need long-term therapy at an intensity sufficient to produce progress, but not so great that it results in regression and further breakdown.

THE THEORETICAL BASIS OF
PSYCHOANALYTIC PSYCHOTHERAPY

Contributions from psychoanalysis

The majority of the concepts used by psychoanalytic psychotherapists today had been established by Freud in the early 1920s. These include the idea of unconscious mental life as manifest in dreams and transference, a model of psychosexual development based around the Oedipus complex, the importance of defences against anxiety, the tripartite model of the mind divided into ego, id, and super-ego (conscience), and the use of free association and interpretation as basic therapeutic methods (Freud 1900, 1923).

Since Freud there have been many important theoretical developments within psychoanalysis. Freud's daughter Anna (A. Freud 1937) systematized the idea of defence mechanisms, and her ideas were further developed in the United States by Hartmann into ego psychology, an approach which emphasizes the central role of the ego in adaptation to the environment and the importance of defences to protect it both from the disruptive effects of failure of the supportive environment and from powerful inner feelings in need of mastery (Erikson 1965). Vaillant (1977) has further developed this work in his longitudinal studies of mental health in men, showing that the use of 'primitive' defences such as splitting are associated with psychopathology, while 'mature' ones like humour and sublimation, are linked with physical and mental health.

British psychoanalytic thought has, since the 1930s, been dominated by object relations theory (ORT), which emerged from the ideas of Klein, Fairbairn, Balint, Bion, and Winnicott (Greenberg and Mitchell 1983; Kohon 1986) all of whom were, in different ways, reacting against the emphasis in Freud's early work on 'drive theory', and picking up on his later concept of internal psychic representations of significant figures and relationships.

Melanie Klein's psychoanalytic work with children convinced her that Freud's model of the unconscious as a 'seething cauldron' of untamed sexual and aggressive drives needed to recognize that these drives were directed towards significant figures (or 'objects') in the child's environment. Balint postulated a 'primary clinging' in the human infant who is a relationship-seeking being from birth, while Fairbairn similarly maintained that 'drives are a signpost to the object', rather than vice versa. Klein (Mitchell 1985; Segal 1964;

Hinshelwood 1989) detected internal representations of parents, siblings, the self, and parts of the body ('part-objects') such as the breast, mouth, penis, faeces and urine in various relationships in the child's mind. She postulated a primitive moral universe in which, in the early months of life, 'good' objects (built up from satisfying experiences) must be kept separate from 'bad' objects (derived from experiences of frustration and pain). She called this the 'paranoid-schizoid position' (PSP) which she believed formed the basis of the splitting and emotional lability of patients with borderline personality disorder. An important aspect of the PSP is the use of the obscurely named 'projective identification', a defence in which the infant is presumed to deal with unbearable feelings of pain and hatred by projecting them into suitable 'objects' around him, who are then perceived as, and may actually be induced to behave in accordance with whatever is projected. The apparently unaccountable feelings of impotence, hostility, or sometimes inappropriate protectiveness which therapists treating borderline patients may feel, can be understood in terms of projective identification—they are unconsciously embodying and enacting aspects of the patient's inner world (Kernberg 1977).

In normal development, 'good' and 'bad' come together in the 'depressive position' (DP), so called because Klein imagined primitive feelings of guilt in the developing child when he discovers that the mother whom he has hated (the 'bad breast') is one and the same as his good object (the 'good breast'). For Bion (1978) this movement from PSP to DP is based on the mother's 'containment', the capacity to tolerate and 'detoxify' the infant's rage so that, at the appropriate moment it can be reunited with love, and so transformed into healthy aggression and self-assertion. The therapist similarly provides 'containment' in order to help the patient progress from splitting to integration.

Although a product of a Kleinian analysis, Donald Winnicott (1971; Phillips 1988) differed from Klein in that he had a much more benign view of the mother–infant interaction. Winnicott is best known for his description of transitional space, an intermediate and overlapping zone between the unconscious of the infant and mother (and therapist and patient), within which emotional development, play and creativity occurs. He saw the use of 'transitional objects' (teddy-bears, comfort blankets etc.) as a continuation of this process.

Since the 1980s, American psychoanalysis has been influenced by the ideas of Heinz Kohut (1977) who developed a model of self-psychology, derived from Freud's distinction between self-preservative drives (which he called narcissistic) and those which led to relationships with others (which he saw as 'leaning on' the narcissistic drives and were therefore 'anaclitic'). In contrast to Freud however, Kohut saw what he called 'self-object' (i.e. narcissistic) needs not as primitive precursors of relationship needs, but as coexisting with them from birth, continuing throughout life, and as healthy rather than otherwise. He viewed the idealization of the therapist which so often takes place in therapy as a positive manifestation of self-object needs, similar to the idealization of parents by their children, only gradually to be replaced with a more realistic view through 'optimal disillusion'. He saw psychopathology as arising from environmental failure, mainly the lack of maternal empathy, rather than, as in the Kleinian model (espoused by the Klein-influenced American psychoanalyst Kernberg 1984), being the result of intrapsychic factors such as a superabundance of aggression. Psychotherapists influenced by Kohut therefore tend to emphasize empathy as a central therapeutic tool.

Contributions from psychoanalytic heretics

The history of psychoanalysis is littered with controversy and schism, and the ideas of several outstanding figures who disagreed with Freud continue to influence psychoanalytic psychotherapy. Jung felt that Freud neglected the importance of man's spiritual aspirations and overemphasized sex as the source of human misery (Stevens 1991). The Jungian approach in therapy is perhaps more holistic than the strictly Freudian, with an emphasis on self-actualization and integration of the personality. Adler introduced a social dimension into therapy, seeing 'organ inferiority' and the 'inferiority complex' in sociological as well as psychological terms. Therapists such as Karen Horney, one of the forerunners of feminist psychoanalysis (Chodorow 1978; Sayers 1992), extended this to a view of man (and woman) in a cultural context of patriarchy.

    John Bowlby (1988; Holmes 1993) similarly felt that psychoanalysis tended to underemphasize the impact of environmental failure as a cause of neurosis. Bowlby's theory of attachment, a mixture of psychoanalytic and ethological concepts, placed the need for a 'secure base' both in reality and in the inner world, at the heart of psychic health. Providing such a secure base is one of the prime functions of the therapist. With his insistence on the role in psychopathology of early environmental failure, Bowlby also anticipated the rediscovery of the importance of sexual abuse in childhood as a formative factor in neurosis, and the mourning of loss as a central feature of psychotherapy.

In the US, interpersonal psychotherapists, such as Sullivan (1953), have likewise emphasized the importance of the patient's social environment as a cause and potential cure of neurosis, and interpersonal therapy (IPT) is a systematized form of psychotherapy designed to address such difficulties (Klerman *et al.* 1984).

Ferenczi (1955) was troubled by the tendency of analyses to become 'interminable' (as was Freud 1937), and proposed 'active techniques' in which the therapist was overtly supportive and confirming of the patient's value as a human being, coining the famous (but dangerously simple) thesis that 'it is the analyst's love that cures the patient'. His model of brief therapy was taken up by Alexander (1957). Through the work of Malan (1963, 1976), Sifneos, Mann and others, brief dynamic therapy (see Chapter 3) has become a psychotherapeutic mode in its own right, overlapping with psychoanalytic psychotherapy. Malan (1979) emphasized the importance of motivation and the therapeutic alliance, the development of a therapeutic dialogue, similar to Hobson's (1985) 'conversational' model of therapy, the centrality of transference interpretations as vehicles of change, and the need for the therapist to maintain a 'focus' rather than adopting a meandering and passive style.

Contributions from psychotherapy

Several non-psychoanalytic influences have, often unobtrusively, affected the evolution of psychoanalytic psychotherapy. Jerome Frank and J. B. Frank (see Chapter 1) (1974, 1991) believed that different therapies have more in common than their quarrelsome proponents would like to believe, a view later confirmed by research evidence that, on the whole, no one therapy is more effective than any other, a finding summarized by Luborsky *et al.*'s (1975) famous 'dodo-bird verdict': 'All have won and everyone shall have prizes.' His anthropological studies of healing suggested the 'common factors' to be found in all effective methods of psychological treatment. He summarized these as: (a) 'remoralization'—instilling hope in the sufferer; (b) providing a relationship with the therapist; (c) offering an explanatory theory of the illness or problem; and (d) suggesting practical steps to be taken to overcome the difficulty. In psychoanalytic therapy, the last would include learning to focus on one's dreams, to attend for therapy regularly, and to associate freely.

Carl Rogers (1951) introduced the idea of 'client-centred therapy', and the research findings based on his ideas that effective therapists possess (and can be trained to develop) a combination of empathy, genuineness, and 'non-possessive warmth' (Truax and Carkhuff 1967) suggest the prerequisites of successful psychoanalytic psychotherapists, whatever their level of theoretical sophistication. Finally the work of Aaron Beck (Beck *et al*. 1979), which has had a huge impact, must be mentioned. Cognitive therapy, while originally developed as an antidote to psychoanalysis, has much in common with it, especially as it moves into longer-term treatments for patients with personality disorders (Beck 1993). Psychoanalytic psychotherapists regularly issue cognitive challenges to their patients, for example when they question the dichotomized or catastrophizing assumptions that underlie the transference. Thus, it might be suggested to a patient who had been physically abused by his father and whose attitude towards the therapist is one of sulky compliance: 'It looks as though you assume I can only be either a depressed mother or a violent father.'

The efficacy of long-term individual psychotherapy

Several outcome studies of psychoanalysis have shown that about two-thirds of patients improve, and that these improvements are maintained at long-term follow-up (Rosser *et al*. 1987; Kantrowitz *et al*. 1990). Controlled studies of long-term therapy, however, are logistically virtually impossible, but several controlled studies of brief dynamic therapy suggest that it can produce effect sizes of around 0.6–0.8 (Dimascio *et al*. 1979; Woody *et al*. 1990; see Crits-Cristoph, 1992, for a meta-analysis of brief dynamic therapy and a critical review). It is clear, as the Wallerstein (1986) study already mentioned showed, that the strictly psychoanalytic elements in long-term therapy contribute only partially to overall outcome, and that supportive or 'non-specific' factors are also of great importance. Process-outcome studies of long-term therapy remains a field ripe for research (Fonagy 1993).

ASSESSMENT AND FORMULATION: INDICATIONS AND CONTRAINDICATIONS FOR LONG-TERM THERAPY

The word 'assessment' derives from the Latin *assidere*, 'to sit beside', but also has connotations of taxation and reckoning of assets (Holmes 1991). Assessment for long-term therapy contains both these elements:

a warm empathic attempt to enter into and understand the patient's inner world, and a cool analysis of strengths and weaknesses.

Before embarking on a course of psychoanalytic psychotherapy, the therapist will want to consider the patient's psychiatric and developmental diagnosis, to establish inclusion and exclusion criteria, to evaluate his behaviour at interview, and to arrive at a psychodynamic formulation.

Diagnostic considerations

The scope of psychoanalytic therapy has, since its inception, both narrowed and widened. Psychoanalysis was originally devised by Freud and Breuer as a treatment for neurosis, especially hysteria. Freud soon came to see the Oedipus complex as the 'kernel of the neuroses' and conceptualized anxiety disorders including obsessional neurosis, sexual dysfunction and psychosomatic difficulties in Oedipal terms. The Oedipal situation was seen as a 'three-person problem' (Balint *et al.* 1972): an unequal struggle comprising the child and his two parents, each vying for exclusive possession of one another, with attendant feelings in the sexually immature child of guilt, exclusion, anger, rivalry, and inadequacy, dealt with by defence mechanisms especially repression, the breakdown of which leads to the emergence of psychological symptoms.

In the early days, psychoanalysis was more or less the only form of therapy available and these Oedipal ideas were applied, with varying success, to a wide range of diagnoses and emotional difficulties. Today, many effective non-psychoanalytic treatments are available for specific disorders including behaviour therapy and drugs in obsessional neuroses, couple therapy and behaviour therapy in sexual dysfunction, and anxiety management techniques in anxiety. As a result, the focus of psychoanalytic psychotherapy has shifted increasingly towards the personality disorders. This has been paralleled by the development of object relations theory and self-psychology mentioned above which have opened up understanding of 'pre-Oedipal' or 'two-person' psychology, that is, the first year or two of life in which the developing infant's world is mainly concerned with himself and that of his principal caregiver, usually the mother.

Thus, candidates for long-term individual therapy will usually be those with enduring personality difficulties (see Stevenson and Meares 1992, for a study showing the efficacy of long-term therapy in borderline personality disorder), and those whose symptoms are pervasive and long-lasting rather than discreet and circumscribed. Patients with recurrent depressive disorders or prolonged grief reactions, long-standing and intractable anxiety, repeated relationship difficulties, and especially borderline and narcissistic personality disorder, form the bulk of the work of psychoanalytic psychotherapists. Many will have experienced severe childhood trauma including neglect, and/or sexual and physical abuse.

As well as reaching a psychiatric diagnosis the assessor will want to decide on a psychodynamic formulation, focusing particularly on the level of disturbance. A patient who shows mainly 'paranoid-schizoid' features, splitting his world absolutely into good and bad, treating people as part-objects, or narcissistically defending himself against depression by a grandiose view of himself, will be seen as suffering from early disruption of two-person relatedness and will be a correspondingly difficult propositon for therapy. The evidence suggests there is an optimum level of disturbance for psychoanalytic psychotherapy (Wallerstein 1986; Horowitz *et al.* 1984). Very disturbed patients need a large measure of support, while the less disturbed can be managed with cognitive and other techniques. Those in between—'sick enough to need it, healthy enough to stand it' (Thoma and Kachele 1987) or 'ill enough to merit it, well enough to benefit from it' (Bateman and Holmes 1995)—are potential psychoanalytic psychotherapy patients.

Inclusion and exclusion criteria

The principle of 'to whom it hath it shall be given . . .' applies, however unfairly, to psychoanalytic psychotherapy. Several decades of psychotherapy research have shown that patients with positive attributes are more likely to benefit from therapy (this applies to all types of therapy, however) than those who lack them. Young, attractive, verbal, intelligent, and successful (YAVIS) people tend to do well in therapy (Luborsky *et al.* 1971)—it should be remembered that these qualities are not in themselves proof against developing an emotional illness. Malan (1976, 1979) found that a history of at least one good relationship, or evidence of positive achievement in life through work, sport, artistic talent, or even a good sense of humour, were associated with good outcome in brief dynamic therapy.

Malan also proposed his 'law of increased disturbance', which suggests that a person's previous history of disturbed behaviour—addiction, promiscuity, violence, or self-harm—is likely to manifest itself at some time in the course of therapy. This implies that patients with a history of substance abuse, recurrent self-injury, psychosis, entrenched somatization, and obsessional neurosis should not be taken on for long-term therapy without careful thought. Often treatment is possible (and what is psychoanalytic psychotherapy for if not to help such disturbed patients?), but requires close collaboration between the therapist and other professionals such as the general practitioner, psychiatrist, or community psychiatric nurse, with the option of brief admission to hospital at times of crisis.

Behaviour at interview

The assessment interview is a microcosm of future psychodynamic therapy. A number of different but probably overlapping constructs have been found to predict good outcome in dynamic therapy (Malan 1973; Sifneos 1969). These include motivation for change, the capacity to show emotion at interview, the development of a positive working alliance (Bergin and Lambert 1986), and 'psychological-mindedness'. The latter captures such features as the ability to see oneself from the outside, to tolerate psychic pain, and fluidity of thought. Malan (1979) writes of 'leapfrogging'—a psychotherapeutic dialogue in which the patient describes some aspect of their feelings, the therapist responds with a comment or interpretation, and the patient then further opens up in response to that, and so on. For example (simplified):

Patient: (depressive illness precipitated by divorce): 'Whenever I begin to get close to someone I seem to back off and start trying to escape . . .'
Therapist: 'Do you think that could have something to do with your mother's death when you were young, and a feeling that it just isn't safe to trust anyone, including me . . .' [transference interpretation]
Patient (silence, cries): 'I remember at the funeral how my granny tried to put her arms around me and I just pushed her away. My dad really had a go at me about that, it was embarrassing in front of everyone, I just hated him for it . . .'

As with YAVIS, there is an inherent paradox in viewing those patients who are most able to participate in the psychotherapeutic process, and are therefore perhaps the least ill, as most suitable for treatment. As one patient put it when asked to 'free associate' at the start of therapy: 'If I could do that I wouldn't need to be here in the first place.' Nemiah *et al.* (1976) coined the term 'alexithymia' to describe those with difficulty in putting their feelings into words, who he claims are particularly prone to develop somatization disorders. While absolute alexithymia might be a contra-indication to therapy, some degree of it might be seen as the reason a person needs treatment, the skill of the therapist residing in his or her ability to help the patient to overcome their difficulty in finding a language for emotions. Similarly 'motivation', which is not a fixed category (Entwistle and Wilson 1977), may increase dramatically if therapy is felt to be helpful. In general, research findings and clinical experience indicate that a strong working alliance early in treatment is the best predictor of good outcome.

The psychodynamic formulation

The formulation is an attempt to find a core theme which underlies the patient's presenting problems (Hinshelwood 1991). Patient and therapist collaboratively act here like the interpreters of a literary text or musical score trying to grasp the deep structure of the work (Holmes 1992). The formulation brings together the presenting problem, past difficulty, or trauma, and the reactions of the patient at interview, into what Malan (1979), following Menninger and Holzman (1958), called the 'triangle of insight'.

Thus, in the example above the therapist had noticed within himself a sense of rejection and of being brushed off whenever he had tried to make emotional contact with the patient in the early part of the interview, and had felt some counter-transferential feelings of failure and annoyance about this. The formulation suggested that the patient responded to loss by withdrawal and angry rejection, and that this had been triggered by his divorce which activated the earlier loss of his mother, and which manifested itself subtly in his response to the approaches of the therapist. Malan also proposed a 'triangle of defence', which in this case would include a deep longing for closeness, anxiety that this would be followed by loss, and a resultant defensive avoidance of intimacy (see below for further discussion of Malan's triangles).

Luborsky (Luborsky and Crits-Cristoph 1988) and others have systematized the process of formulation, both to sharpen therapeutic thinking and for the purposes of research. For Luborsky the formulation consists in identifying a wish within the patient, the responses of others to that wish, and the response of the self to those responses (i.e. in the case above, wishing to be close, anxiety about loss, and avoidance of closeness, respectively). Ryle (1990) emphasizes the self-fulfilling nature of neurotic difficulty, in which a person's core state—here an inner loneliness—is reinforced and maintained by his reactions and behaviour: the more the patient rejects and pushes away, the more that feeling of isolation is maintained.

STARTING PSYCHOTHERAPY

Preparation

Patients need to be encouraged into therapy, coaxed sometimes; certainly they require appropriate information to decide about it, why the therapist considers therapy necessary, and what it involves in time and expense. Attitudes reflected in such phrases as unconditional positive regard, warmth and empathy should be expressed by the therapist and hope instilled into the patient; the therapist should feel he wants to help and that he can. That careful attention needs to be paid to this preparatory phase is now widely accepted. A therapist must conduct this preparation in his own way. While the ground rules are clear, he must be himself, not act the part of 'the therapist' or of someone else being a therapist. Styles of therapy and of therapist obviously vary. Therapy induction procedures must therefore be developed and adopted by therapists to suit their own style and to the different patients they treat. For example, some patients need a challenge, others persuasion when starting therapy.

The therapeutic contract

The arrangements—both general and specific, partly fixed and partly negotiable—made between therapist and client constitute the therapeutic contract. Flexibility is the key word. The only fixed, or relatively fixed, components to the contract are the initial logistics: times, lengths, and frequency of sessions. Even these may be modified later but they should be agreed on at least for a specified period; therapists' and patients' lives need some framework. Throughout therapy, any alterations should, as far as possible, not be made on impulse but should be thoroughly discussed and worked through. This allows the time to understand the full implications of change in terms of the patient's personality, his problems, his life-situation, his relation with the therapist (transference), or whatever else is relevant, and may contribute to the patient's insight.

Goals of therapy: finding a focus

Setting goals is a controversial subject. One advantage of long-term
therapy is that a relatively leisurely attitude can be taken to the task
compared, for example, with crisis intervention. Broad objectives
should be discussed like resolution of symptoms or increased work
satisfaction, but where basic personality change is an aim it can often
not be seen clearly either by patients or therapist during the early stage
of treatment. Establishment of a 'dynamic focus', which takes account
of the patient's goals in therapy is part of a continuously negotiable
implicit therapeutic contract. Malan (1976) and Sifneos (1969) writing
of brief psychotherapy suggest that a clear focus on specified goals is
mandatory. Thoma and Kachele (1987) see psychoanalysis as a focal
form of therapy, in that at any one time there will be a dynamic focus
around which the work is organized, but allowing for a gradual shift.

Trials of psychotherapy

Most patients can be allocated fairly easily into two groups: those
unlikely to benefit from long-term psychotherapy (although they may
benefit from another approach and should be guided toward it); and
those that probably will. In a third group, assessment leads only to a
tentative decision: here a trial of treatment may be agreed on between
patient and therapist. This usually involves 3–6 sessions, after which
the question of suitability becomes clearer.

Significant others

Psychoanalysis has traditionally treated the patient alone with the
argument that the changes he achieves will lead to appropriate changes
in those around him. In recent years, however, as more interest has
focused on marital and family therapy it has become clear that one
ignores significant other persons in the patient's life at great peril to
the future both of the therapy itself and of the patient's relationships,
particularly with his spouse, and children. There are, therefore, ethical,
as well as clinical, issues involved (Crown 1977).

Should we alter a patient's intimate relationships without at least
being aware of what we are doing and taking appropriate caution?
Thus, it is often appropriate for significant others, usually the spouse
or other partner, to participate in important therapeutic decisions.
This may involve an interview and discussion at the stage of

assessment so that everyone knows what is entailed—although the impact of such a meeting on the subsequent transference will have to be borne in mind. Full participation of relevant people in this way is a helpful adjunct to treatment by discouraging any possible sabotage by them and promoting their co-operation. The therapist's responsibility may extend to helping the spouse or significant other to obtain treatment in his or her own right if this should prove necessary; if, for example, changes in the designated patient prove too difficult for the partner to tolerate reasonably.

BASIC THERAPEUTIC TECHNIQUES

Free association; active listening

Long-term psychotherapy, although it now tends to take place in a more informal atmosphere, the patient usually sitting in a chair rather than lying on a couch, still uses, as far as possible, Freud's fundamental rule that the patient should try and say everything that comes into his mind without self-control or censure. This is, of course, an ideal not truly possible. Some patients do, however, have a facility for working this way; others soon learn to do so; while others continue to have great difficulty. This in itself can be informative: there is evidence that 'autobiographical competence' (Holmes 1992)—the capacity to describe facts and feelings about oneself in a fluent and coherent way—is linked to secure attachment in childhood, while insecure patterns of attachment are associated either with alexithymia or an emotional enmeshment in past trauma (Holmes 1993). Note too that fluent free association can be used defensively—to placate or ingratiate oneself with the therapist as a 'good' patient, thereby avoiding feelings of helplessness or hatred. In any event, the basic principle remains: once therapy actually starts it is the patient who initiates the sessions and sets the agenda—as he sees it. The therapist accepts the material presented as primary data which say something significant about the patient and his problems.

One of Freud's early patients dubbed psychoanalysis the 'talking cure': a more apt term is the 'listening cure'. The therapist's counterpart to the 'fundamental rule' is the technique of active listening. While silent the therapist aims for a state of active receptiveness, 'beyond memory and desire' (Bion 1978, quoting

Eliot), based on what Freud called 'evenly suspended attention', empathically attuned both to the emotional import of the patient's material, and his own counter-transferential reactions to it. Winnicott (1971), Kohut (Stolorow *et al.* 1987) and others (see Stern 1985; Holmes 1994) have linked this aspect of therapy with the sensitivity of effective parents to their children's needs, the provision of a 'holding environment', and the picture of a secure and self-absorbed child happily playing 'alone' in the presence of a watchful but non-intrusive parent.

Transference and counter-transference

The hallmark of psychoanalytic psychotherapy is the understanding and use of transference and counter-transference, which at their most general can be defined as the unconscious aspects of the therapeutic relationship as they affect patient and therapist. Freud originally conceived of both as impediments to progress but—by bringing the patient's interpersonal difficulties directly into the consulting room in a way that can be worked on—both are now seen as the keys to unlock the patient's psychological entrapment.

Two vital contemporary distinctions need to be made. Sandler and Sandler (1984) differentiate the 'past transference', which corresponds with the classical Freudian view of a repetition in therapy of feelings, attitudes, and assumptions derived from early parental relationships, with the 'present transference', which is more akin to the classical notion of the 'pre-conscious', referring to the immediate impact of the therapeutic relationship on the patient. Understanding and interpreting current transference should always precede that of past transference which otherwise may seem stereotyped and unconvincing. Transference is not some sophisticated phenomenon only available to the cogniscenti but is present in any therapeutic encounter. For example, on collecting a patient—a young man with paranoid feelings—from the waiting area the therapist noticed that he looked a little startled. When asked about this later in the session the patient reported that he had expected his therapist to be short, fat, bald, bearded and with a middle-European accent, and had assumed therefore that he was facing an imposter! This misperception in the 'present transference', and his suspiciousness generally, could subsequently be linked with a disrupted childhood in which his mother had frequently been hospitalized with depression, and, at times of her illness, had seemed to him alien and changed in a frightening way.

The classical notion of counter-transference as comprising the therapist's blind spots due to his misperceptions of the patient, based on his own childhood experience, remains valid. The 'compulsive caring syndrome' for instance, so often seen in health workers, may represent an attempt to assuage the guilt associated with childhood aggression towards siblings, or be a continuation of a childhood role reversal in which the therapist-to-be was expected emotionally, or even physically, to look after his or her parent. However, Heimann (1950), Winnicott (1971), and others emphasize the positive aspect of counter-transference by showing how emotions and fantasies aroused in the therapist may be a vital guide to the inner world of the patient (see Casement 1985). This links with the idea of projective identification mentioned earlier, in which primitive communication takes place by inducing feelings in a nurturing other. The therapist's task becomes one of observing his counter-transference, sifting that which relates to his own life from what has been projected by the patient, containing rather than acting on it, and translating these feelings into interpretations which can be useful for the patient. Here, too, the process need not be complicated: the patient who makes one angry is probably furious himself; a patient in tears may arouse in the therapist a variety of responsive feelings such as overwhelming sadness, irritation, anguish, or indifference, each of which can be linked to the particular patient's situation and problem.

In general, the concepts of transference and counter-transference reflect a growing recognition that the classical picture of the therapeutic relationship as a one-way street with therapist as neutral observer of the 'seething cauldron' of the patient's emotions is no longer appropriate. More relevant to a post-modernist world is a model in which patient and therapist each contribute to a 'bipersonal field' (Langs 1976), asymmetical in that each is assigned a different role, but to which each contributes with the conscious and unconscious parts of their mind. Thus, for example, after a difficult session, the therapist may 'forget' to write up his notes, while the patient for his part may 'forget' to turn up next time. If these unconsciously driven muddles can be identified and taken up, much progress can emerge from disentangling them; if they are ignored, the therapy may founder.

THERAPEUTIC STRATEGIES

The first psychotherapy session

In a sense this is the second stage of the preparation process, with the patient looking more deeply into therapy. It is important that the therapist be both careful and helpful. The first session should not be an agony for a patient who is too tense to say anything that 'comes into his mind'. If a patient is so tense it is reasonable to adopt a simple stratagem like taking an obvious part of his history and suggesting that he may like to talk about this. Most people will respond with relief and gratitude whether or not they actually go ahead and talk about what has been suggested. Later, they will need this help less and less often.

Some articulate patients need no help to begin; the less sophisticated, perhaps less educated, may need considerable help and it should be given willingly. In particular, attention should be paid to any communication difficulties by, for example, using concrete rather than abstract terms ('stress' rather than 'anxiety') and assisting the naïve patient to learn how to function effectively in the psychotherapy situation. The 'analytic honeymoon' should be a reasonable period for the patient, one for him and his therapist to learn how to work together and a little about each other's personalities.

After this phase, progress inevitably becomes more difficult; in terms of psychoanalytic theory resistances or unconscious blocks to clinical progress emerge and, in order to overcome these, therapeutic strategies have been formulated. The first and most important consideration is that of transference and counter-transference, as already mentioned. There are in addition five main types of intervention: clarification, linking, reflecting, interpretation, and confrontation.

Clarification

Clarification is a common therapist activity: if unclear about what a patient is saying, ask. Patients' lives are complex; the history obtained during assessment covers only a tiny fragment. As facts emerge it will be necessary from time to time to seek further elaboration or clarification. This applies particularly to patients from other cultures: if the therapist does not for example know about marital or family customs in Trinidad or Bombay he simply asks; similarly where patients have some technical expertise with which the therapist is unfamiliar, for example, instrumental technique in a professional musician where this is relevant to his problem. Another use of clarification, described by Kernberg (1977), is to detect a patient who may be more seriously disturbed than the therapist has suspected: unclear speech may reflect unclear thought. Unclear thought may in turn reflect neurotic anxiety or represent schizophrenic thought disorder and thus point to an unsuspected psychosis. As a generalization, when asked or challenged to clarify, a neurotic patient does so, whereas a schizophrenic patient's thinking may be thrown further into disarray.

Linking

A therapist often helps the patient by explicating links that as an observer he has noted but the patient has missed (between, for example, the extreme jealousy of a young man for his girlfriend, and his feelings of abandonment when at the age of seven, he was put into care when his mother became depressed after the sudden death of his sister). Indeed, the overall aim of therapy can be seen as an attempt to link and therefore make more coherent a life that feels fragmented and inchoate. One of the most emotionally powerful forms of linking is the use of metaphor (Holmes 1992). Much of the language of therapeutic conversation is, quite unselfconsciously, metaphorical ('I feel as though I don't really have a safe haven to go to'—a young woman having enormous rows with her adoptive parents; 'I always feel I'm on the fringe of things'—a young man with sexual difficulties especially with penetration). Metaphor and transference are etymologically identical: both mean a 'carrying across'.

As mentioned above, Malan (1979) has systematically described his 'two triangles' of psychoanalytic psychotherapy: the 'triangle of person' (or triangle of transference) which links together the relationship with the therapist, the patient's current relationship patterns with significant others, and parental relationships in childhood. At each 'point' of the triangle—therapist, other, parent—there is a 'triangle of defence', comprising anxiety, defence, and hidden fear. Thus, for the man described above who was jealous of his girlfriend the anxiety was manifest in his symptom of jealousy, his defence was his possessiveness and aggression towards her, his hidden fear was of abandonment (Holmes 1994). The work of psychoanalytic psychotherapy can be understood as, through interpretation, the gradual exploration and making conscious of the links between the different aspects of these two triangles.

Reflecting

Reflecting is a basic technique derived from Rogerian client-centred therapy. Its essence is that a problem or situation presented by the patient is sifted through the therapist's mind, drawing on his experience, and reflected back in a way that makes the problem or situation clearer. Even simple reflective techniques can be immensely helpful. For example, in a patient faced with a career decision the therapist comments: 'It seems to me that this conflict is between what you want to do and what you feel you should do.' The chief feature of reflecting is that nothing is added to, or taken from, what is produced by the patient.

Interpretation

Interpretation, the fundamental technique of psychoanalysis, is an attempt to make unconscious motives, attitudes, and feelings conscious in order that the patient can learn more about himself. Insight is a fundamental way in which psychotherapy leads to personal change (Crown 1973), and interpretations, if successful, should increase this insight. Interpreting applies to any facet of apparently unconscious behaviour that the therapist observes and thinks may be important. Any manoeuvre that the patient uses in order apparently to avoid the discussion of problem areas, for example, claiming that he is too busy to attend sessions, or of intra-psychic conflicts, (e.g. a family conflict of earlier life), should be interpreted.

Malan's ideas, described above, can be traced to Strachey's (1934) seminal paper on the 'mutative interpretation', bringing together the patient's current difficulty, his relationship with the therapist, and the past into a single theme; this has led to the prevalent view that transference interpretations are particularily powerful in effecting change. This was certainly not Freud's original view, who believed that non-transference interpretations were equally important. Indeed, an empirical study by Piper *et al.* (1991) suggests that in some circumstances a high frequency of transference interpretations can even be associated with deterioration, as the therapist desperately tries to salvage an ineffective therapeutic alliance.

Offenkrantz and Tobin (1974) have spelt out four conditions under which transference should be interpreted: when the patient shows undue emotion with no obvious cause within the therapeutic situation and particularly if this occurs repeatedly; when the patient's flow of associations becomes blocked; when the therapist considers it likely that a transference interpretation will increase a patient's understanding; and when the link between infantile attitudes to important figures in the past and attitudes to the therapist are close to the patient's awareness.

Conscience (super-ego) manifestations like excessive guilt need interpretation in an effort to discover their source and to modify their harmful effects: like cognitive therapists, analytic psychotherapists often try to help free patients from the 'oughts' and 'shoulds' which unconsciously and sometimes masochistically dominate their lives.

Dream interpretation remains a central part of psychoanalytic psychotherapy (Freud 1900; Flanders 1993). Dreams reflect both present preoccupations and problems, and earlier conflicts, and represent a spontaneous and therefore unwilled or 'innocent' account of the patient's current state of mind (Rycroft 1979). The patient should, with appropriate interpretative help from the therapist, learn to decode a dream as experienced (manifest content) so as to understand its underlying meaning (latent content).

Steiner (1993) has usefully distinguished between 'patient-centred' and 'therapist-centred' interpretations. In the early stages of therapy the therapist may have to contain and 'metabolize' (Bion 1978) projections without translating them into interpretations, which, to the uninitiated, can seem intrusive and confusing. Therapist-centred interpretations are usually reserved for later and deeper phases of therapy.

An interpretation is an hypothesis to account for a certain attitude, emotion, or aspect of behaviour: if accurate there should be a change in the patient towards increased insight, modified attitude, or more effective behaviour; if inaccurate there will be no effect. Sometimes the therapist may give a 'correct' interpretation early in treatment but which is rejected only for the same interpretation to 'click' later (Balint *et al.* 1972). This is not unlike the increasing insight that comes from repeated reading of a complex novel or listening to a piece of music. The main guideline is to interpret when it seems appropriate; the therapist should not be put off by the patient's negative response or, conversely, be too gratified by his overly ready acceptance. Too ready acceptance, compliance (Blackwell 1976), may itself be a defence and need further interpretation. The only way to judge the effectiveness of interpretations is via general progress towards deepening empathy in therapy.

Confrontation; acting-out

Periodically, patients need to be confronted with the consequences of their actions, although, in general, interpretation is always preferable and should always accompany it. Confrontation is basically a challenge: thus, for example, merely exploring the meaning of a patient's repeated lateness may not be enough: he may need to be faced with the fact that effectiveness of treatment is rendered null and void and may have to be abandoned.

Acting-out is a special problem that may need both interpretation and, later, confrontation. Acting-out reflects a patient's failure to acknowledge and to face up to his problems and anxieties; instead, a course of action, often self-destructive, is taken. Hence, the difficulty of dealing with impulsiveness in psychotherapy: an alcoholic patient, for example, at the first sign of increased anxiety may binge to alleviate this. Attempted suicide, self-mutilation, reckless driving, relationship-threatening behaviour such as promiscuity, and unnecessary challenges to supervisors risking dismissal, are common examples for which confrontation may be necessary.

Managing the unsuitable patient

Some patients reveal themselves as unsuitable for long-term psychotherapy, in a way that was not detectable at assessment—perhaps because they are impulsive, paranoid, histrionic with gross acting out, or hold unshakeable religious or political convictions impervious to therapeutic intervention. Management includes altering the basic approach from interpretive to supportive: this may include decreasing frequency of sessions; applying more direct support and less interpretation of unconscious motives; focusing less on reconstruction of the past; placing greater emphasis on the present reality (e.g. job and relationships); and the therapist becoming more 'transparent'.

FINISHING THERAPY

Positive and negative reasons for termination

There are both positive and negative reasons for finishing therapy. A positive reason is the feeling in both patient and therapist that as much has been achieved as is likely to be achieved—not necessarily of course all changes considered desirable initially—and that an agreed time for termination should be reached. Patients usually evaluate progress by using a subjective global rating of how they feel about themselves, but therapists should train themselves in the self-discipline of making a systematic assessment: symptom relief and personality change, the latter divided into work, social, and sexual areas. Psychotherapists are increasingly called upon to quantify the 'health gain' their treatments produce and many use standard questionnaires such as the Beck Depression Inventory, Social Adjustment Scale, and the Adult Attachment Interview (Main 1991) to evaluate progress (Bergin and Garfield 1994).

Termination is not difficult provided common sense and human kindness are applied. When it is clear to patient and therapist that termination is appropriate the patient's own pace should be considered: some like a few more sessions, most aim for a readily identifiable date such as the summer, Easter, or Christmas break. A 'negative therapeutic reaction' may occur, leading to apparent return of symptoms and loss of progress but analysis and discussion of the reasons for this are usually effective.

Negative reasons for breaking-off treatment may be situational (e.g. a patient's or therapist's job move) or as summed up in the term 'therapeutic failure'. In the case of the latter the therapist should try to ascertain where the problems lies: the patient's symptoms or personality, the therapist's actions, the patient–therapist relationship, or an incorrectly chosen modality of treatment. From this assessment it is desirable to help the patient to adopt the next course of action: no therapy, a different sort of treatment, or similar treatment with another therapist. Although these 'post-mortems' are painful for both protagonists they lead to further development in both.

Further treatment

Further treatment with the same therapist is always a possible option. The patient should be told in such a way that he knows it will be possible at a later stage if it proves necessary; that a new contract will then be negotiated; and that further treatment is neither expected nor forbidden by the therapist. Generally only a minority of patients return, but all feel grateful and relieved to know that they can do so if they wish. If a therapist knows he will not be available, a colleague's name can be provided or information about a suitable clinic.

THE THERAPIST AND HIS FRAMEWORK

Every therapist will, with increasing experience, develop his own particular style. Some are active, others more receptive; some more supportive, others managing to challenge without being destructive; some remain opaque, others reveal something about themselves without jeopardizing therapy. Humour is probably a vital, if little discussed, part of the successful therapist's repertoire (Bloch and McNab 1987). The more experienced a therapist, the more he learns to use his personal attributes to good effect. And just as the therapist provides a safe space with firm but flexible boundaries within which the patient can explore and mature, so, if he is to flourish as a therapist, he needs to function in a secure framework of ethics, supervision, and training.

Ethics

Psychotherapy should always be conducted within a clear ethical framework (Bloch and Chodoff 1991; Holmes and Lindley 1989). Ethical issues are mainly concerned with the boundaries of therapy which include the contract, fees if relevant, confidentiality, absolute prohibition of sexual contact, and discouragment of social as opposed to professional interaction between patient and therapist. The last does occasionally occur—for example, between trainees and their therapists in training organizations, or in small towns—and needs to be handled with sensitivity and circumspection. Reticence is the best policy (see Chapter 13 for a comprehensive account of these topics).

Supervision

It is a counsel of perfection that no therapist, however experienced, should work without supervision (Pedder 1986). Effective therapy requires a benign split within the therapist (and, as therapy progresses also to some extent within the patient) between an empathic experiencing part and an observing, rational part. Conceptualized developmentally, the father (but this might also be the grandmother) is a 'third term' who gradually balances the intense mutual interest of mother and infant, and provides the mother with objectivity, interest and nurturance (this could be seen as an aspect of the 'positive' Oedipal situation). Similarly, supervision can rescue the therapist when he becomes over-involved with his patient, help him if he is under-involved or bored, identify counter-transferential reactions, such as love, hatred, anger, frustration, stuckness, fear and detachment, and, by putting them into perspective, help put them to good use. Supervision has an almost mysterious capacity to keep therapy on track: simply talking over a session can, often without any apparent change of approach by the therapist, help resolve a problem. Supervision is the single most important safeguard against breaking of ethical boundaries. Supervision may be individual or in a group with an experienced therapist; if none is available, a mutual supervision model with a peer or group of peers is appropriate.

Training

A few therapists seem to have a natural knack of helping others, but even these may need their talents to be honed and extended. The vast majority require training, a slow process usually spread over several years. An explosion in the numbers of courses in psychotherapy has taken place since the 1970s. Most contain, in varying proportions, a combination of theoretical learning, supervised practice, and personal therapy. Training occurs in three main settings: as part of professional qualifications in, for example, psychology, nursing, social work, and psychiatry—psychotherapy training is now a mandatory requirement for psychiatric qualification in the United Kingdom (Grant *et al.* 1993)—finally bringing it in line with American and Australasian standards. In the private arena there is a dizzying array of courses of varying quality ranging through psychoanalytic, Jungian, eclectic, and humanistic trainings. University-based diplomas and postgraduate courses are also multiplying (Pedder 1989). Professional registers of psychotherapists have now been established in many countries; in Britain the organizing body is the UK Council for Psychotherapy which seeks to make registration a legal requirement for those who practise psychotherapy.

Most, if not all, therapists undertaking long-term individual psychotherapy will want, or be required, to aquire some personal experience of therapy. This may range from a work-based 'sensitivity' or Balint-type group (Balint *et al.* 1972), through brief therapy, to full psychoanalysis. The internalization of personal analytic experience is an invaluable template for the therapeutic relationship with patients, often freeing the therapist to make use of his counter-transference, as well as providing much-needed support and exploration for those—and they are not neccessarily a minority—who are drawn to therapeutic work partly in response to their own conflicts and doubts.

CONCLUSION

All psychotherapies, including psychoanalytically oriented psychotherapy, are limited in the degree to which they are capable of modifying behaviour. Every psychotherapy needs, through research, to explore its strengths and weaknesses. Paul's (1967) 'matrix paradigm' remains a guiding idea for research—'what treatment, by whom, is most effective for this individual, with what specific problem, and under which set of circumstances.' Psychoanalytic psychotherapy has been one of the last of the psychotherapies to come into the research fold, but increasingly sophisticated, often computerized, methods—such as the Adult Attachment Interview (Main 1991; Fonagy 1993), to take one example—mean that the subtle nuance of meaning and interpersonal communication can begin to be addressed. Long-term individual therapy remains central to psychotherapeutic training and treatment; its value and efficacy is likely to be both challenged and robustly defended well into the twenty-first century.

REFERENCES

Alexander, F. (1957). *Psychoanalysis and psychotherapy*. Allen and Unwin, London.

Balint, M., Ornstein, P., and Balint, E. (1972). *Focal psychotherapy*. Tavistock, London.

Bateman, A. and Holmes, J. (1995). *Introduction to psychoanalysis: contemporary theory and practice*. Routledge, London.

Beck, A. (1993). Cognitive therapy: past, present and future. *Journal of Consulting and Clinical Psychology*, **2**, 194–8.

Beck, A., Rush, A., Shaw, B., and Emery, G. (1979) *Cognitive therapy of depression*, (3rd edn), International Universities Press, New York.

Bergin, A. and Garfield, S. (1994). *Handbook of psychotherapy and behaviour change*, (4th edn). Wiley, Chichester.

Bergin, A. and Lambert, M. (1986). The evaluation of therapeutic outcomes. In (ed. S. Garfield and A. Bergin) (2nd edn.) *Handbook of psychotherapy and behaviour change*. Wiley, Chichester.

Bion, W. (1978). *Second thoughts*. Heinemann, London.

Blackwell, B. (1976). Treatment adherence. *British Journal of Psychiatry*, **129**, 513–31.

Bloch, S. and Chodoff P. (1991). *Psychiatric ethics*, (2nd edn). Oxford University Press, Oxford.

Bloch, S. and McNab, D. (1987). Humour in psychotherapy. *British Journal of Psychotherapy*, **3**, 216–25.

Bowlby, J. (1988). *A secure base: clinical applications of attachment theory*. Routledge, London.

Chodorow, N. (1978). *The reproduction of motherhood*. University of California Press, Berkeley.

Crits-Cristoph, P. (1992). The efficacy of Brief Dynamic Psychotherapy: a meta-analysis. *American Journal of Psychiatry*, **149**, 151–8.

Crown, S. (1973). Psychotherapy. *British Journal of Hospital Medicine*, **9**, 355–62.

Crown, S. (1977). Psychotherapy. In *Dictionary of medical ethics*, (ed. A. S. Duncan, G. R. Dunstan and R. B. Welbourn). Darton, Longman & Todd, London.

Crown, S. (1981). Psychotherapy research today. *British Journal of Hospital Medicine*, **25**, 492–501.

Dimascio, A. *et al*. (1979) Differential symptom reduction by drugs and psychotherapy in acute depression. *Archives of General Psychiatry*, **36**, 1450–6.

Entwistle, N. and Wilson, J. (1977) *Degrees of excellence: the academic achievement game*. Hodder & Stoughton, London.

Erikson, E. H. (1965). *Childhood and society*. Penguin, Harmondsworth.

Ferenczi, S. (1955). *Further contributions to the theory and technique of psychoanalysis*. Hogarth, London. (Originally published 1920.)

Flanders, S. (ed.) (1993) *The dream discourse today*. Routledge, London.

Fonagy, P. (1993). Psychoanalytic and empirical approaches to developmental psychopathology: can they be usefully integrated? *Journal of the Royal Society of Medicine*, **86**, 577–81.

Frank, J. D. (1974). Therapeutic components of psychotherapy. A 25-year progress report of research. *Journal of Nervous and Mental Disorder*, **159**, 325–42.

Frank, J. D. and Frank, J. B. (1991). *Persuasion and healing: a comparative study of psychotherapy*, (3rd edn). Johns Hopkins University Press, Baltimore.

Freud, A. (1937). The ego and the mechanisms of defence. Hogarth, London.

Freud, S. (1900). The interpretation of dreams. In *Standard edition*, (Vols 5–6, pp. 1–625). Hogarth, London.

Freud, S. (1922). *Two short accounts of psychoanalysis. Standard Edition*, Vol. 18, pp. 176–203. Hogarth, London.

Freud, S. (1923). The ego and the id. In *Standard edition*, Vol. 19, pp. 1–66. Hogarth, London.

Freud, S. (1937). Analysis terminable and interminable, In *Standard edition*, Vol. 23, pp. 209–53. Hogarth, London.

Grant, S., Holmes J., and Watson, J. (1993). Guidelines for training in psychotherapy as part of general professional training. *Psychiatric Bulletin*, **17**, 168–71.

Greenberg, J. and Mitchell, S. (1983). *Object relations in psychoanalytic theory*. Guilford, New York.

Heimann, P. (1950). On countertransference. *International Journal of Psychoanalysis*, **31**, 81–4.

Hinshelwood, R. (1989). *A dictionary of Kleinian thought*. Free Association, London.

Hinshelwood, R. (1991). Psychodynamic formulation in assessment for psychotherapy. *British Journal of Psychotherapy*, **8**, 166–74.

Hobson, R. (1985). *Forms of feeling*. Tavistock, London.

Holmes, J. (ed.) (1991). *A textbook of psychotherapy in psychiatric practice*. Churchill Livingstone, Edinburgh.

Holmes, J. (1992). *Between art and science: essays in psychotherapy and psychiatry*. Routledge, London.

Holmes, J. (1993). *John Bowlby and attachment theory*. Routledge, London.

Holmes, J. (1994). Clinical implications of attachment theory. *British Journal of Psychotherapy*, **11**, 62–76.

Holmes, J. and Lindley, R. (1989). *The values of psychotherapy*. Oxford University Press, Oxford.

Horowitz, M., *et al.* (1984). Brief psychotherapy of bereavement reactions: the relationship of process to outcome. *Archives of General Psychiatry*, **41**, 438–48.

Kantrowitz, J., Katz, A. and Paoletto, F. (1990). Follow-up of psychoanalysis five to ten years after termination. *Journal of the American Psychoanalytic Association*, **38**, 637–54.

Kernberg, O.F. (1977). The structural diagnosis of borderline personality organization. In *Borderline personality disorders*, (ed. P. Hartocollis). International Universities Press, New York.

Kernberg, O. (1984). *Severe personality disorders: psychotherapeutic strategies*. Yale University Press, New Haven, CT.

Klermann, G.L., Weissman, M., Rounsaville, B., and Chevron, E. (1984). *Interpersonal psychotherapy for depression*. Basic Books, New York.

Kohon, G. (1986). *The British school of psychoanalysis: the independent tradition*. Free Association, London.

Kohut, H. (1977). *The restoration of the self*. International Universities Press, New York.

Langs, R. (1976). *The bipersonal field*. Jason Aronson, New York.

Luborsky, L. and Crits-Cristoph, P. (1988). Measures of psychoanalytic concepts—the last decade of research from the 'Penn studies'. *International Journal of Psycho-Analysis*, **69**, 75–86.

Luborsky, L., Chandler, M., Auerbach, A. H., Cohen, J., and Bachrach, H. M. (1971). Factors influencing outcome of psychotherapy: a review of quantitative research. *Psychological Bulletin*, **75**, 145–85.

Luborsky, L., Singer, B., and Luborsky L. (1975). Comparative studies of psychotherapies: is it true that 'everyone has won and all must have prizes'? *Archives of General Psychiatry*, **37**, 471–81.

Main, M. (1991). Metacognitive knowledge, metacognitive monitoring, and singular (coherent) vs. multiple (incoherent) models of attachment. In *Attachment across the life cycle*, (ed. C. Parkes, J. Stevenson-Hinde, and P. Marris). Routledge, London.

Malan, D. (1963). *A study of brief psychotherapy*. Tavistock, London.

Malan, D. (1973). The outcome problem in psychotherapy research. A historical review. *Archives of General Psychiatry*, **29**, 719–29.

Malan, D. (1976). *The frontier of brief psychotherapy: an example of the convergence of research and clinical practice*. Plenum, New York.

Malan, D. (1979). *Individual psychotherapy and the science of psychodynamics*. Buttterworths, London.

Menninger, K. and Holzman, P. (1958). *Theory of psychoanalytic technique*. Basic Books, New York.

Mitchell, J. (ed.) (1985). *The selected Melanie Klein*. Penguin, London.

Nemiah, J. C., Freyberger, H., and Sifneos, P. E. (1976). Alexithymia: a view of the psychosomatic process. In *Modern trends in psychosomatic medicine*, Vol. 3, (ed. O. W. Hill). Butterworths, London.

Offenkrantz, W. and Tobin, A. (1974). Psychoanalytic psychotherapy. *Archives of General Psychiatry*, **30**, 593–606.

Paul, G. (1967). Strategy of outcome research in psychotherapy. *Journal of Consulting and Clinical Psychology*, **31**, 109–18.

Pedder, J. (1986). Reflections on the theory and practice of supervision. *Psychoanalytic Psychotherapy*, **2**, 1–12.

Pedder, J. (1989). Courses in psychotherapy: evolution and current trends. *British Journal of Psychotherapy*, **6**, 203–21.

Phillips, S. A. (1988). *Winnicott*. Fontana, London.

Piper, W., Hassan, F., Joyce A., and McCallum, M. (1991). Transference interpretations, therapeutic alliance, and outcome in short-term individual psychotherapy. *Archives of General Psychiatry*, **48**, 946–53.

Rogers, C. (1951). *Client-centred therapy*. Constable, London.

Rosser, R. *et al.* (1987). Five year follow up of patients treated with in-patient psychotherapy at the Cassel hospital. *Journal of the Royal Society of Medicine*, **80**, 549–55.

Rycroft, C. (1972). *A critical dictionary of psychoanalysis*. Penguin, Harmondsworth.

Rycroft, C. (1979). *The innocence of dreams*. Oxford University Press, Oxford.

Sandler, J. and Sandler A. (1984). The past unconscious, the present unconscious, and interpretation of the transference, *Psychoanalytic Inquiry*, **31**, 54–61.

Sayers, J. (1992). *Mothering psychoanalysis*. Penguin, London.

Segal, H. (1964). *Introduction to the work of Melanie Klein*. Heinemann, London.

Sifneos, P. (1969). Short-term anxiety-provoking psychotherapy. *Seminars in Psychiatry*, **1**, 389–98.

Staples, F. *et al.* (1975). Differences between behaviour therapists and psychotherapists. *Archives of General Psychiatry*, **32**, 1515–22.

Steiner, J. (1993). *Psychic retreats*. Routledge, London.

Stern, D. (1985). *The interpersonal world of the infant*. Basic Books, New York.

Stevens, A. (1991). *On Jung*. Penguin, London.

Stevenson, J. and Meares, R. (1992). An outcome study of psychotherapy in Borderline Personality Disorder. *American Journal of Psychiatry*, **149**, 358–62.

Stolorow, R., Brandchaft, B., and Atwood, G. (1987). *Psychoanalytic treatment: an intersubjective approach*. Analytic Press, Hillsdale.

Strachey, J. (1934). The nature of the therapeutic action of psycho-analysis. *International Journal of Psycho-Analysis*, **15**, 127–59.

Sullivan, H. (1953). *The interpersonal theory of psychiatry*. Norton, New York.

Thoma, H. and Kachele, H. (1987). *Psychoanalytic practice*. Springer, London.

Truax, C. and Carkhuff, R. (1967). *Towards effective counselling and psychotherapy: training and practice*. Aldine, Chicago.

Vaillant, G. (1977). *Adaptation to life*. Little, Brown, Boston.

Wallerstein, R. (1986). *Forty-two lives in treatment: a study of psychoanalysis and psychotherapy*. Guilford, New York.

Winnicott, D. (1971). *Playing and reality*. Penguin, Harmondsworth, Mddx.

Woody, G., Luborsky, L., McLellan A., and O'Brien, C. (1990). Corrections and revised analyses for psychotherapy in methadone maintenance. *Archives of General Psychiatry*, **47**, 788–9.

RECOMMENDED READING

Bateman, A. and Holmes, J. (1995). *Introduction to psychoanalysis: a contemporary synthesis*. Routledge, London. (An attempt to bring together the major psychoanalytic schools—Object relations, contemporary Freudian, Kleinian, self psychology—in a readable practical guide, illustrated with case examples.)

Casement, P. (1985). *On learning from the patient*. Tavistock, London (sensitive, jargon-free account of what goes on in the therapist's mind while with the patient, and, through self-supervision, how to make good therapeutic use of this.)

Freud, S. (1916–17). *Standard Edition, Introductory lectures on psychoanalysis*, Vol. 15/16. Hogarth, London. (Perhaps the most accessible of all Freud's texts.)

Malan, D. (1979). *Individual psychotherapy and the science of psychodynamics*. Butterworths, London. (Clear, logical account of the complexities of psychodynamic formulation and interpretation. Many fascinating case examples.)

Rycroft, C. (1972). *A critical dictionary of psychoanalysis*. Penguin, Harmondsworth. (Lucid exposition of psychoanalytic concepts by a master of psychological prose. Invaluable vade-mecum.)

Sandler, J., Dare, C., and Holder, A. (1992). *The patient and the analyst*, (2nd edn). Allen & Unwin, London (Scholarly but readable account of the concepts—the therapeutic alliance, transference, etc.—that underpin everyday therapeutic work.)

Symington, N. (1986). *The analytic experience*. Free Association, London. (Personal account, written with great *élan*, of the history and theory of psychoanalysis, with chapters on major figures like Klein and Fairbairn. Many illuminating case examples.)

3

Short-term dynamic psychotherapy

MICHAEL HOBBS

Short-term dynamic psychotherapy has flourished since the 1980s and brought into question the optimal duration of psychodynamically oriented treatment. In this chapter, Michael Hobbs draws our attention to the role of this time-limited approach. After providing a brief historical context he considers aims, assessment (including indications and contra-indications), and notable features—its brevity, the emphasis on a focus on which to work, and ending. The work of Sifneos, Davanloo, and Malan are highlighted. The application of the approach to adolescents, the elderly, grief, and post-traumatic disorders is examined. Typical problems that are encountered in treatment are discussed and the chapter concludes with brief sections on effectiveness and training.

The 1980s and 1990s have witnessed a substantial growth in interest in short-term psychological treatments. This renewed interest represents the conjunction of several powerful influences including the increasing demand for psychological treatments from groups resistant to the ready prescription of psychotropic medications, the progressive contemporary expectation of rapidly-effective treatments, and the economic imperatives of health care provision.

Short-term dynamic psychotherapy is characterized by its relative brevity, a focus on identified core problems, an active therapist style, and therapeutic exploitation of a time limit. Contemporary practice has emphasized flexibility of approach and modification of aims and techniques for specific patient groups.

Contrary to earlier misconceptions, short-term dynamic psychotherapies are *not* truncated versions of analytical psychotherapy, but planned treatments with their own inherent rationale. Fundamental to this rationale is the recognition that a focused short intervention can stimulate a powerful developmental process which, under the influence of ongoing life experience, continues and extends over time to generate substantial and lasting change.

Furthermore, short-term dynamic psychotherapy is not only effective in its own right but, although it may seem paradoxical, casts light on fundamental processes including the benefits of long-term analytical psychotherapies. Small (1971), in the foreword to his early account of the 'briefer psychotherapies', refers to the wisdom of those therapists who had 'penetrated the time barrier' in psychotherapy.

DEFINITION

This chapter describes a number of discrete but functionally interrelated short-term treatment approaches which, by virtue of their common psychodynamic basis, are here collectively called short-term dynamic psychotherapies (STDP). These include those treatments entitled by their authors 'focal psychotherapy' (Balint *et al.* 1972), 'brief psychotherapy' (Malan 1963, 1976), 'short-term anxiety-provoking psychotherapy' (Sifneos 1972, 1987), 'time-limited psychotherapy' (Mann 1973), 'time-limited dynamic psychotherapy' (Strupp and Binder 1984), 'short-term dynamic psychotherapy' (Davanloo 1980) and 'short-term psychotherapy' (Wolberg 1980).

STDPs are related to a number of other short-term psychological treatments such as the eclectic psychotherapies of Garfield (1989), cognitive analytic therapy (Ryle 1990), and interpersonal psychotherapy (Klerman *et al.* 1984). STDP also relates in application and technique to the psychodynamic aspects of crisis intervention (Sifneos 1972; Hobbs 1984), which is an integrative short-term therapy drawing also on behavioural, cognitive, systemic, and pragmatic principles (see Chapter 5).

Although differing significantly in practice, all STDPs are conducted within a conceptual framework which gives prominence to the influence of internal psychological processes, especially those of which the person is unconscious. In addition, they all emphasize the relationship between patient and therapist as both the medium for therapy and, through analysis of transference phenomena, its most important tool.

Despite their brevity, STDPs offer the patient an opportunity for reflective exploration and a search for meaning in experience. Self-awareness, understanding, and personal control is promoted rather than the resolution of symptoms; although, of course, symptomatology often recedes with the resolution of internal and interpersonal conflicts and the growth of insight. In these ways, STDPs share the basic features of psychoanalytic psychotherapies.

HISTORICAL DEVELOPMENT

STDP has its origins in psychoanalysis. Although some of its defining characteristics, particularly the brevity and focus, represent significant divergences from psychoanalysis, its theoretical basis and central methods are unequivocally psychoanalytic.

Nowadays, psychoanalytic psychotherapy is typically prolonged and intensive. As is stressed in most accounts of STDP, this was not initially the case. Freud's early treatments were aimed at the relief of neurotic symptoms, particularly those of conversion hysteria, and were surprisingly short. Derived from his earlier experimentation with hypnosis, his method was active and directive. Bruno Walter, the orchestral conductor, was treated by Freud in six sessions for a paralysis of his conducting arm. The composer Gustav Mahler's impotence was treated (although we cannot be sure about the outcome) by Freud in a single four-hour session.

As theory and practice evolved, treatment became progressively longer. Malan (1963) identified reasons for this, including the growing complexity of psychoanalytic theories of personality development and symptom formation, therapeutic perfectionism of practitioners, and expectation that exhaustive 'working through' would be accomplished during therapy, all of which conveyed a sense of timelessness to the patient. Eventually Freud (1937/1964) himself, in his succinctly entitled paper 'Analysis terminable and interminable', questioned the inexorable lengthening of psychoanalytic treatment.

Some of Freud's contemporaries opposed the tendency towards longer treatment. They challenged particularly the apparent passivity of therapist and therapy. Ferenczi (1920/1955), for example, adopted an active style to confront unconscious resistance. He used techniques like physical touch and embrace to remedy perceived deficiencies in the patient's formative emotional experience. Ferenczi's methods, however, eventually provoked Freud's displeasure (Marmor 1979), promoting hostile reaction in the psychoanalytic community to short, active therapies.

Rank (1936), best known for his identification of 'birth trauma' and separation anxiety, set and highlighted time limits in order to promote the patient's 'will' or motivation for the required work. In this, he pre-figured the central aspect of Mann's (1973) time-limited psychotherapy.

Alexander and French (1946) challenged the tendency of psychoanalysts to embark on treatment without taking a detailed history, arguing that the focus and effectiveness of therapy depended on an accurate psychogenetic formulation of the patient's problems. They also questioned the apparent emphasis on intellectual exploration, advocating instead the promotion of emotional experiencing in therapy. They argued that the recovery and expression of repressed feeling in an empathic atmosphere linked to increased self-awareness, offered the patient what they dubbed a 'corrective emotional experience'.

Despite clinical evidence for the effectiveness of planned short treatments and the fact that most psychotherapies were actually brief by design or default, most practitioners resisted development of short psychotherapies (Garfield 1989). Then, during the 1960s, several clinicians in the United Kingdom and United States began independently to devise short-term models which incorporated contemporary developments in psychoanalysis, particularly interpretation of defences and transference. Balint (Balint *et al.* 1972) and Malan (1963) at the Tavistock Clinic, Sifneos (1972) and Mann (1973) independently in Boston, and Davanloo (1980) in Montreal, developed short-term psychotherapies which differed substantially but shared a common psychodynamic identity. These models represent the basis for the contemporary practice of STDP and details of their respective concepts and techniques are outlined below.

Several notable clinical developments in STDP have taken place since the 1980s. First, selection and technique have been modified to permit extension of STDP to diverse patient groups. Secondly, integrative models, combining features of STDP and other approaches, have evolved. An example, widely practised in the United Kingdom, is cognitive analytic therapy (Ryle 1990). Time-limited dynamic group therapies have also been devised applicable both to broad diagnostic groups (MacKenzie 1990) and to specific problems such as pathological grief (Piper *et al.* 1992).

Over the same period, increasingly sophisticated scientific research has examined the process and outcome of short-term psychotherapies (Koss and Butcher 1986; MacKenzie 1988; Hobbs 1989). Confirmation for their power has been derived from a study of the dose–effect relationship which demonstrated that approximately 50 per cent of patients showed improvement by session 8 and 75 per cent by session 26 (Howard *et al.* 1986).

AIMS AND OBJECTIVES

Despite the brevity of STDP, its aims are radical. Small (1971) suggested that the primary goal of the briefer psychotherapies was to ameliorate or remove specific presenting symptoms; but, under favourable conditions, the dynamic intervention leads secondarily to progressive personality changes. The emphasis today is on the resolution of internal conflicts which have arrested, retarded, or distorted the development of personality and relationships.

STDP may entail exploration of historical origins of the patient's difficulties; but, more importantly for change, attention is focused on their current dynamic origins as evidenced by ways of feeling, thinking, communicating, and relating in therapy. This analytic work is the basis of the encounter in which problems are examined *in vivo* within the therapeutic relationship. It is also the basis for a 'corrective emotional experience', for the patient is enabled to examine uncomfortable personal aspects in a relatively safe, non-judgemental, and accepting atmosphere.

The high level of therapist activity, focus, and short duration of STDP are used by the therapist to combat development of a transference neurosis with all its attendant problems of regression and acting-out. Short-term therapies always involve a challenge to the universal illusion of timelessness, which is seen by Mann (1973) as a fundamental feature of neurosis. From the existential perspective then, STDP requires that the patient (and therapist) confronts and comes to terms with the finiteness of time. This is uncomfortable, even disturbing, but offers an important step towards redefining personal reality in a way which promotes responsibility and autonomy, and so ultimately reduces alienation from self and others.

In contrast to the wide-ranging remit of conventional analytic therapy, STDP involves the establishment of specific, personalized aims for treatment. These are defined in relation to the focus chosen in operational terms. Progress and outcome can be measured in relation to these defined aims as well as more generally.

In summary, the therapist's objective in STDP is to engage the patient in active exploration of his difficulties, especially as these impinge on the therapeutic relationship, and thereby to liberate his adaptive capacities and developmental potential. This objective is addressed through use of highly specific techniques.

ASSESSMENT, SELECTION, AND PREPARATION

The related processes of assessment and selection are fundamental to the competent practice and effective outcome of STDP. As with any powerful treatment, STDP should be prescribed with care to those who can be predicted to benefit.

Indications

In terms of diagnostic categories, the indications for STDP are:

(1) neurosis, especially when internal or interpersonal conflicts predominate;

(2) unresolved developmental crises, (e.g. a separation conflict, morbid grief); and

(3) uncomplicated post-traumatic disorders.

Sifneos (1987) suggested that patients who benefited most were those manifesting Oedipal conflicts, particularly those who 'lingered too long' in patterns of relating typical of a child's relationships with each parent. Other interpersonal dynamics amenable to STDP include those associated with rivalry, separation, and loss. Malan (1976) and Mann (1973) advocate STDP for a wider range of neurotic disorders. Davanloo (1980) has even treated patients with entrenched obsessive-compulsive disorder and moderately severe personality disorder, asserting that they are amenable to his own particularly confronting style providing that the core dynamics can be identified and addressed.

Other contemporary practitioners argue for broad applicability. Ashurst (1991) suggests that a broad spectrum of neuroses and personality disorders may be treatable by STDP if the patient has the capacity for adaptation; but she cautions that the therapist must be realistic about the aims of therapy and, while maintaining optimism, avoid over-ambition.

Contra-indications

A number of contra-indications have been demonstrated by clinical experience, including patients unable to use an active psychological method of treatment and to tolerate the unavoidable levels of anxiety generated by it.

Absolute contra-indications

The assessment procedure begins at the point of referral, for STDP is contra-indicated when a patient has a history of: psychotic illness; severe depression; gross destructive or self-destructive behaviour; severe somatizing disorder; marked personality disorder, especially when characterized by negativism or poor impulse control; serious substance misuse; and excessive dependency in relationships.

Relative contra-indications

For those patients not excluded by the above, the initial interview still includes a comprehensive psychiatric history and examination because STDP can prove destructive for psychologically fragile people. For example, a patient preoccupied with self-destructive thoughts could be precipitated into suicidal action by the challenge of STDP.

Patients should not be selected for STDP if, at assessment, evidence is found of: failure to make positive emotional contact with the therapist; rigid or primitive defences; a propensity for regression manifest by seeking reassurance or advice; low tolerance of frustration or anxiety; lack of motivation for the work of therapy; absence of a feasible focus for short-term therapy; a negative response to a 'trial' intervention designed to test defences and capacity to use a focused approach.

Prognostic criteria

A number of criteria have been shown clinically to have prognostic significance (Sifneos 1987): a capacity to identify a 'circumscribed chief complaint' and to prioritize difficulties; a history of at least one 'meaningful' relationship; flexible interaction with the assessor; capacity to express feelings, both directly and in words; psychological-mindedness, including reflectiveness, an ability to make mental links, and the capacity to construe experience in terms of internal psychological processes rather than attributing difficulties to bodily dysfunction or external events; motivation for change, as evidenced by open and honest participation in the work of therapy, introspective curiosity, realistic expectations of therapy, and a desire for significant internal change rather than symptom relief alone.

Malan (1976) emphasizes also the importance of a capacity for insight, or self-scrutiny and self-understanding, tested by trial interpretations.

Clinical experience points to other useful attributes in selecting patients: humour, an inclination to play with ideas, concern for others, sense of responsibility, and capacity to feel appropriate guilt. These qualities, in conjunction with evidence of some achievement in study, work and relationships, can be regarded as evidence of *ego strength*, a feature fundamental to change in STDP.

Availability of social support is important in sustaining the patient's commitment to an anxiety-provoking therapy. Further support for the prognostic significance of a history of mutual relationship, and capacity to interact flexibly with the therapist, derives from research which demonstrates a correlation between pre-therapy patterns of relating and the rapid establishment of an effective therapeutic alliance (Moras and Strupp 1982). The strength of this alliance at sessions 3–4 has been shown independently to correlate positively with outcome (Morgan *et al.* 1982).

Preparation for therapy

The assessment and selection procedure may extend over more than one interview, and ideally leads immediately into therapy. Selection is concluded, and therapy begins, with agreement on the focus and negotiation of a contract. The latter includes a clear statement that therapy will be short term, even if its exact duration is not determined at the outset, and sets administrative boundaries. Experience and empirical research show that patients engage in therapy more readily and successfully if adequately prepared.

The initial consultation can be therapeutic in itself since the exploratory assessment and trial interpretation generate greater awareness and self-understanding. Some practitioners, most notably Davanloo and Mann, undertake a preliminary screening but then proceed to an encounter with the patient designed to be both diagnostic and therapeutic. In this sense, assessment embodies a trial of therapy.

Dynamic focus

The focus is central to STDP. It is not the same as the patient's presenting complaint but a psychodynamic hypothesis which links the patient's current experience (including the presenting complaint) with formative past experiences, both recent and remote. The focus is identified during the psychodynamic assessment, both from historical information elicited and the interaction. By definition, the focus must be circumscribed. Patients whose difficulties require an extended and complex dynamic formulation are unlikely to benefit substantially from STDP. The focus must also be feasible for short-term therapy. For example, a patient's self-defeating guilt may be formulated succinctly in terms of repressed vengeful hostility towards his sadistically violent father; but this focus could not be explored safely and productively in a brief period.

Dynamic focus: clinical illustration

A feasible focus for STDP was identified in a young man who presented with a generalized anxiety state. Mr A's academic achievements at school and university were substantial, and he was expected to accomplish rapid promotion in his chosen profession. Instead, he became progressively more anxious and was passed over for prestigious assignments. Furthermore, after a brief sexual relationship in his teens with an older married woman, his fear of sexual impotence had caused him to avoid close relationships. He returned each weekend to his parents' home, where his doting mother laundered his clothes and prepared his meals for the week. The warm tones with which he spoke of his mother contrasted with his anxious, negative account of his father whom he described as formidably high-powered, critical and intimidating.

At interview, the patient was conspicuously anxious and related deferentially to the male therapist. Eventually the therapist began to feel irritated by the deference and passivity, but construed his own irritation as another (unconsciously projected) facet of the patient's transference. He used the information derived from the patient's account of his father and the transference/counter-transference development to construct a trial interpretation, suggesting to the patient that his deference to his father masked his deep, unacknowledged resentment. The young man appeared momentarily angry; but, after reflection, he agreed that he felt very angry towards his father for belittling him repeatedly.

This simple dynamic intervention proved therapeutic through enabling the patient to face his repressed anger. It also provided the therapist with the material with which to formulate the dynamic focus for the STDP he then recommended. The patient's anxious deference, which prevented him from asserting himself confidently in front of his (male) employers, was a product of his fear of standing up to his intimidating father; or, more accurately, was a product of his fear of the potential destructiveness of his own anger. This unconscious process was associated inextricably with the patient's continued, exclusive intimacy with his mother. With unconscious but disabling guilt, he identified his mother in each potential girl-friend. His impotence with men and women in adulthood was the result of an enduring internal dynamic process, one characterized in psychoanalytic terms as an Oedipal conflict, which offered a coherent focus for STDP.

The dynamic foci which are most readily amenable to STDP are those associated with such internal conflict.

For STDP to be most effective, the focus must be adhered to throughout treatment. Although other issues may emerge these should not be pursued unless they can be analysed in terms of the focus. Of course, the focus can be refined, and may be modified if shown to be inaccurate; but divergence on to other dynamic issues will diminish the power of therapy. The maintenance of high motivation and high 'focality' (Malan 1976) are associated with maximal effect.

THE PROCESS AND TECHNIQUE OF STDP

STDP makes substantial demands on both patient and therapist. The required level of activity and sustained tolerance of powerful emotions tests commitment and adaptive strength to the full.

For the patient, STDP is inevitably, and necessarily, anxiety-provoking. Well-established defences are challenged putting him in touch with powerful feelings and memories which were hidden hitherto. Intense negative feelings, perhaps including anger and fear, are re-kindled and focused on the therapist. The patient's trust in the therapist, and his security in the relationship, are tested.

As the core dynamic conflict is exposed and examined, the patient must alternate between experience and reflection on that experience. He may be gripped by discomfort in his relationship with the therapist which gives expression to unresolved childhood experience, and then be required by the therapist's observation or interpretation of this development to stand back in order to examine the origins and impact of the recapitulated experience. The oscillation between experience and reflection is taxing, particularly when pressed by the time limits of therapy. Furthermore, the patient cannot slip back into old defensive patterns between sessions. He is likely to remain unsettled, and is expected to maintain the introspective process in his personal and interpersonal experience outside of therapy.

For the therapist, the repeated challenge to the patient's defences, and exploration of de-repressed material within defined time limits require sustained vigilance, activity, and enthusiasm. At the same time, he must maintain empathic contact with the patient and an analytic stance, for otherwise there is a real danger that the confronting therapeutic activity will feel persecutory to the patient and repeat, rather than resolve, old conflicts. Clearly, the nature of STDP contrasts markedly with the relative leisurely exploration of longer-term analytic psychotherapy. Just as some patients are not able to tolerate or benefit from STDP, some therapists are not suited temperamentally or technically to practise it.

Although STDP is characterized by specific principles and technical ingredients, which will be outlined below, the way therapist and patient work together depends on the needs of the patient. The process with a patient suffering uncomplicated neurotic conflict, as in the example of Mr A above, will differ significantly from that of a moody adolescent, or of someone traumatized psychologically by bereavement. However, there is a common structure and technical repertoire for the spectrum of STDPs, and these features are enumerated below.

(1) Contract for therapy

The therapeutic contract between patient and therapist may be established during the initial assessment but, if another clinician undertook the assessment, the therapist needs to renew the contract at the start of treatment. Although neither legalistic nor necessarily written, the contract emphasizes key features including focus and time limit.

Focus

The dynamic focus derived from the assessment is reviewed and, if necessary, revised. Most practitioners see it as important to state their understanding of the dynamic underlying the presenting problems, and to obtain the patient's agreement to both its validity and the adopted focus. The focus may be revised in the light of emerging material, but adherence to the agreed focus is essential.

Time limit

The other central component is the short duration of therapy, and arrangements for it. Sessions are usually held weekly at a regular time, but flexibility is possible. Practitioners vary in their management of the time limit. Mann adopts a universal policy of 12 hours, usually involving one-hour sessions at weekly intervals but, where considered necessary, beginning twice weekly or concluding with shorter (perhaps

30-minute) sessions at increased intervals. In this way of working, the time limit is explicit and the date of the last session identified from the outset. Mann uses the limit as a subsidiary focus to combat the patient's illusion of timelessness and to promote a sense of reality and responsibility.

Other therapists do not establish duration firmly but clarify from the start that this will be short and within specific limits, for example, a maximum of 20 weekly sessions.

(2) Setting

Face to face

Whereas in long-term analytic psychotherapy the patient may be encouraged to lie down on a couch in order to promote free association and therapeutic regression, the patient in STDP sits up, facing the therapist. This setting promotes the tension, transference development, and direct confronting atmosphere required for active work. This is maximized, where necessary, by the therapist sitting directly in front of and relatively near to the patient rather than at the conventional angle.

Privacy

As in any psychotherapy, the consulting room must afford the quiet, neutral environment, and privacy essential for the patient to feel secure enough to express innermost thoughts and feelings. Although patients can often tolerate routine audio- and video-recordings if valid reasons for this are presented, few can work successfully if exposed to unexpected intrusions.

(3) Therapeutic alliance

The process is necessarily challenging and unsettling to the patient. The early creation and ongoing maintenance of an alliance between patient and therapist is a prerequisite for effective work and a successful outcome.

The strength of the alliance will be tested, sometimes to its limits, when the therapist confronts defences and when transference embodies anger, fear, and other negative feelings. The therapist will need to interpret such negative transference actively in order to preserve the alliance. It is from a secure base (Mackie 1981) that the patient can explore his anxiety and inner conflicts, as they become evident in de-repressed memories, feelings, and transferences.

(4) Therapist style

Within appropriate technical limits and professional boundaries, the therapist adopts an active, interactive, and flexible style. Touch is rarely appropriate. Within treatment there is not enough time for long monologues by the patient (or the therapist) or for prolonged reflective silences. The emphasis is on *active* reflection and dialogue, reinforcing the value of the patient's ability to express feelings and thoughts openly.

The therapist should communicate in everyday language, free from jargon. A competent therapist does not need the illusion of superiority which comes with mystifying the patient. On the other hand, there is no place for a collusive familiarity between therapist and patient.

The face-to-face setting and interactive style enables the therapist to use positive aspects of his personality to maximum effect in relating and communicating. Nothing is gained in adopting an inscrutable 'blank screen' facade, the caricature of the psychoanalyst: the patient will develop transferences regardless of the therapist's relative transparency and openness. However, he will need to monitor the significance of his emotional and other reactions to the patient rather than giving direct expression to them. His counter-transferences will be used by him as sources of information with which to generate or confirm hypotheses and to guide interventions.

(5) Therapist technique

The therapist's activity should have purpose and direction. His interventions are designed to facilitate patient disclosure, exploration of salient feelings, thoughts, and perceptions within the framework of the focus. To this end, interventions tend to be comments, statements, or (sparingly) questions which aim to facilitate, clarify, challenge, or interpret the patient's verbal and non-verbal expressions. The purpose of challenges and interpretation will be examined further below.

(6) Adherence to focus

The elucidation and agreement of a focus is central and adherence to it correlates positively with successful outcome (Malan 1976; Keller

1984). This need not be rigid or restrict the content of the dialogue. Since the focus is a dynamic formulation of the patient's problems rather than the presenting complaint or symptom itself, it is possible for the therapist to link a wide range of material to the focus. The patient is allowed to associate freely and to express thoughts openly, the therapist maintaining focality through 'selective attention' to relevant material and 'selective neglect' of extraneous matters (Balint *et al.* 1972).

(7) Challenge to defences

STDP necessitates active challenge of the patient's defences. This is not the same as confronting him as a person, although inevitably it may feel like this initially. The therapist utilizes the alliance with the patient to foster a collaborative analysis of the nature and neurotic functions of his defences.

Assessment is designed to ensure that patients selected for STDP can withstand the challenge to their defences as a basis for therapeutic work. Evidence during treatment that they cannot tolerate the levels of anxiety generated, such that they decompensate or disintegrate in the face of such challenges, leads the therapist to adopt a more supportive approach and, if necessary, to abort the STDP.

The degree of confrontation should be titrated to the patient's capacity to use such challenge. It also varies according to the intentions and skills of the therapist. Among the founders of STDP, emphasis on challenge has varied. Both Sifneos (1987) and Davanloo (1980) espouse particularly confrontative models while Malan (1980) came to regard Davanloo's systematic challenges of defences as 'the most important development in psychotherapy since the discovery of the unconscious'.

Sifneos

Sifneos's technique consists of repeated confrontations but without any systematic attempt to explain or interpret unconscious factors. A successful challenge releases feelings and memories which leads to further exploration, eventually permitting reconstructive analysis of the core conflict. The method works if the patient can tolerate the anxiety generated and if the core conflict is not overly complex.

Davanloo

Davanloo's method goes further, starting with the identification and 'relentless' challenge of defences, but proceeding to an active exploration and explanation of their dynamic purpose. Although relentless in this pursuit, and thereby appearing persecutory or even sadistic to sceptical observers, Davanloo works empathically. He seeks to break through defences to repressed feelings permitting de-repression and active analysis of the core conflict. He attaches importance to addressing the development of negative feelings towards the therapist, encouraging the release of anger and the patient's discovery that the expression of anger can be healing rather than destructive (Molnos 1986). Davanloo aims to achieve this breakthrough and demonstration of the healing potential of therapy in the first or second session. Like Malan, Davanloo's reconstructive work draws on his analytic understanding of the dynamic relationship between defences, anxiety and the unconscious feelings and motives central to the core conflict.

(8) Reconstructive analysis

In psychodynamic terms, the task is to enable the patient to understand and resolve his internal conflict and its relationship to the other people in his life, past and present. This is achieved through analysis of the patient's current patterns of relating, especially as they manifest through transference, and through linking these patterns to formative past experiences in relationships.

The two triangles

Malan (1979) introduced a diagrammatic representation of the unconscious processes which underpin and maintain conflict through the years. This map, combining the triangles of conflict and of person offers a guide in the navigation of the patient's unconscious.

The triangle of conflict (Fig. 3.1) represents the dynamic conflict associated with a hidden feeling (F) or impulse (e.g. Mr A's anger towards his controlling and belittling father), the potential expression of which generates such anxiety (A) of the fantasized consequences (e.g. Mr A's destruction of his father, or his father's retaliatory destruction of him) that defences (D) operate to render the forbidden feeling unconscious (e.g. Mr A represses all awareness of his anger, and manifests instead a compliant deference to older male figures).

The triangle of person (Fig. 3.2) represents the interaction between the patient's perception of, and feelings or attitudes towards, significant figures in his past (P) and current (C) life, including the therapist as a transference (T) figure. For Malan (1979) the aim of

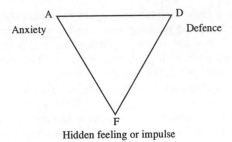

Figure 3.1   Triangle of conflict

most dynamic psychotherapy is 'to reach, beneath the defence and the anxiety, to the hidden feeling, and then to trace this feeling back from the present to its origins in the past,' usually to the relationships with one or both parents. This certainly applies for STDP, although it should be remembered here that the formative experience (P) may have occurred in the more recent past, and the hidden feeling (F) may be intense sadness, grief, or fear rather than anger.

Utilization of the two triangles can be illustrated by the following development of the case of Mr A.

In STDP with the male psychotherapist who originally assessed him, Mr A remained deferential and passively compliant, again masking unconsciously the anger which had been exposed during assessment by the trial interpretation.

Although appearing to work in therapy, Mr A showed little emotion and talked about his problems in an intellectualized manner. The therapist, in the second session, challenged defences: 'You're talking now about your father in a very detached way, as if you have no feelings for him.' The patient, visibly irritated and anxious, started to disagree but then fell silent.

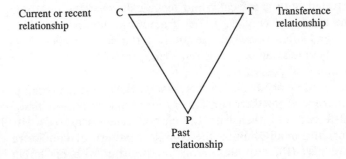

Figure 3.2   Triangle of person

Later in the same session the therapist again challenged the defence, but this time the patient concurred passively and without evident feeling: 'I suppose you're right.' This time the therapist pursued his challenge: 'Now hold on, you're avoiding my point by just agreeing with me.' The patient became very anxious, again evidently irritated, but said nothing.

Drawing on his understanding of the triangle of conflict, the therapist made an interpretation of the manifest conflict: 'I think you're cutting off [D, defence] from your irritation with me because you're afraid [A, anxiety] that you'll hurt me with your anger [F, hidden feeling]—or that I will retaliate and hurt you.'

The patient responded, atypically, with an angry outburst: 'Oh, you think you're so bloody clever. You psychotherapists are all the same.' Without rising to the bait of the transference, the therapist asked what the patient meant. Initially the latter remained angry, but then became deflated and apologetic.

Pursuing the defence, now manifest by apology, the therapist pointed out that the patient was hiding his anger again and asked whether this pattern was usual in his relationships. The patient mulled this over sullenly, then burst out angrily: 'I'd tell my boss to get lost except that he would fire me.'

At this point the therapist made a full transference interpretation, drawing on the triangle of person: 'Your problem in expressing your anger towards me [T] is the same problem that you experience with your male seniors at work [C]. This is just how you've always been with your father [P], isn't it, because you're terrified that, if you showed your anger, he'd "fire" you—whatever that would mean.'

The patient became tearful but calmer. He thought for a bit before responding: 'Yes, that's right. I was always afraid that, if I showed I was hurt or angry, he would blow up and reject me altogether.' The patient's need for his father's love prevented him from giving any expression to the pain and anger caused by his father's insensitive commands and criticism.

This model was extended usefully by Molnos (1984) who demonstrated both graphically and technically that the two triangles could be combined (Fig. 3.3). Her framework reminds us that it is possible, and often necessary, to analyse the core conflict (D–A–F) successively in relation to people representative of two or more corners of the triangle of person.

In the example of Mr A, the therapist worked with the (triangle of) conflict in each of the three corners of the triangle of person, first, with the transference (T), then with the current relationship (C) with his employer, and finally linking the common pattern of conflict to the formative past (P), but continuing, relationship with his father. In analytic therapy, long or short, the TCP interpretation is considered to be most powerful and mutative.

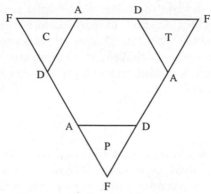

Figure 3.3   Combined triangles

Work with emotions

The clinical example demonstrates the importance of galvanizing feelings. The impact of exploratory and interpretive work is significantly less if the patient operates exclusively in a cognitive or intellectual mode. The power of the experience is heightened when the patient is emotionally charged, getting in touch with and expressing hitherto repressed feelings.

Sometimes, of course, the emotional experience is therapeutic in itself. To be able to release feelings without receiving from the therapist the anticipated and feared reaction, as in Mr A's case, offers a 'corrective emotional experience' which can accelerate change.

(9) Adherence to time limit

Active treatment which draws on the above principles and techniques can bring about a dramatic breakthrough to a core conflict and the beginning of powerful reconstructive changes in early sessions. Davanloo would expect, with suitable patients, to achieve this point within the first session or two. Thereafter, therapy involves a systematic re-working of the dynamic focus from successive perspectives, and in progressively greater depth. This process is akin to the working through of long-term psychotherapy.

However tempting it may be for patient and therapist to extend treatment, the power of STDP requires adherence to the time limit. Each session is used to maximum effect. For Mann, the middle phase revolves around the confrontation of the finite reality of time. The patient's unconscious fixation in past patterns of perceiving and relating, his longing for the illusory timelessness of dependent childhood relationships, is challenged by emphasis of the time limit. His disappointment and disillusionment is addressed, paving the way for the end phase.

(10) Ending

For many patients, the time limit and emphatic ending activate issues to do with unresolved experiences of loss. If not included in the primary focus, these become a subsidiary or secondary focus.

Whether or not the number of sessions was identified at the beginning, the therapist's initial statement of the finite duration of therapy and his progressive emphasis of the limited time available ensures that the ending is well anticipated. Practitioners who decide the ending date once the focal work has been largely completed nevertheless ensure that adequate time remains for dealing with ending.

The focus of the end phase is on the patient's anticipation of loss, and all that this stirs up. Of course, the focus on loss is central to the therapy for patients suffering unresolved grief, as will be addressed below. For them, the end phase may be particularly powerful, even painful. Other patients too may recover buried feelings associated with frustration, separation and perceived rejection in previous relationships, including those in early life. Many are ambivalent about the ending, relishing its conclusion and the prospect of independence on one hand, but fearing loss of security and increased responsibility on the other. This ambivalence, which may reflect ambivalence in other relationships, can be elucidated in the end phase. The therapist works with the framework of the triangles of conflict and person to illuminate how earlier experiences have influenced expectations and reactions in later relationships.

The aim of the end phase then is to enable the patient to learn from his emotional experience of separation and loss, and thereby to promote autonomy and individuation. The opportunity to examine his emotional reactions, in the relative security afforded even by the ending relationship, ensures that the patient does not experience the loss alone. Of itself, this may constitute a corrective experience.

Sifneos (1987) encourages the patient to initiate the ending but takes responsibility for doing so if the patient avoids the issue. He also introduces an educative dimension encouraging the patient to anticipate what could happen after therapy is concluded, thereby pre-empting avoidable crises. A problem-solving approach is promoted for any anticipated difficulties. The patient is encouraged to experiment with his new-found awareness outside of therapy, so generating increasing confidence, adaptive coping, and independence. New ways of coping and relating are rehearsed.

Although active work is continued until the very end, the dynamic process initiated by therapy can continue under its own momentum. This will be so particularly for young people and others whose natural development has been freed from neurotic or other obstacles. The patient becomes the agent of further change, having internalized the therapist's function. In this way, the end result may reach far beyond the point achieved at the final session.

MODIFICATIONS OF TECHNIQUE FOR SPECIFIC GROUPS

STDP has been advocated particularly for adult patients presenting with neurotic problems which have a clear psychodynamic basis, and the prognostic framework outlined above reflects this. In addition, practitioners have used this model successfully with patients presenting with more complex problems, including those complicated by a degree of personality disturbance. Nobody would suggest, however, that STDP is appropriate for patients manifesting more severe personality disorder. For these, successive short, structured, anxiety-reducing therapies during times of crisis may be beneficial in restoring limited adaptive capacities; but substantial change and maturational development, if any is viable, can be achieved only through more prolonged treatment.

In recent years, however, modifications of STDP have been applied with good effect in treating other patient groups.

Adolescent patients

Many adolescent patients who present with emotional or conduct disorders are struggling with dynamic conflicts which, with appropriate modifications of technique, respond well. Indeed, in view of the adolescent's age, temperamental characteristics, and developmental potential, STDP may be the treatment of choice. Yet, if conventional selection criteria were applied rigidly, few adolescents would be offered STDP.

The developmental tasks of adolescence, the phase of transition from childhood dependence to adult independence, revolve around the impact of bodily changes and issues of separation and individuation. The adolescent who, for internal or external reasons, experiences difficulty in negotiating these tasks may be volatile emotionally, oppositional in attitude, particularly with parents and other authority figures, and preoccupied with body image and identity (Wilson 1991).

Consequently, the adolescent patient, especially if referred unwillingly for treatment, may react negatively to the therapist at first. He may be passive, uncommunicative, and hostile, keeping his thoughts and feelings to himself. He is unlikely to relate flexibly and may display little capacity to express his difficulties or to co-operate in identifying a focus. He appears to have little psychological-mindedness and no motivation for therapy.

Nevertheless, the therapist who appreciates the phase-dependent dynamics underlying the adolescent's truculence will not be deceived. Despite initial resistance, the adolescent may respond more readily to STDP than other treatment because it is short, active, oriented to present issues outside and within therapy, and directed primarily towards emotions rather than cognitions. The therapist is experienced as authentic exactly because he addresses the adolescent's powerful and stormy transferences in the relationship without fear or rejection.

At first, however, the patient may be unco-operative and dismissive of the therapist's efforts. He needs to work flexibly in order to minimize the intensity of resistances; and, in particular, to avoid being provoked into an authoritarian stance. With tact, consistency, and a willingness to confront the patient's mistrust and hostility, the therapist is able gradually to overcome his initial resistances and engage him in the alliance (Uribe 1988). The adolescent develops a degree of trust and may then disclose his troubles with disarming openness. Fired by his youthful energy, the therapy may progress rapidly.

Some significant modifications of structure and technique are necessary. Initially, the frequency of sessions may need to be greater than weekly in order to overcome resistance and engage the patient, particularly for the adolescent with limited adaptive capacity; but should be reduced progressively in order to promote independence. Reflective silences should be avoided since they are experienced as persecutory; a conversational style is therefore maintained. The therapist needs to work actively with aggressive and sexual transferences, where necessary setting limits gently but firmly on behaviours which threaten progress. In the same way, the therapist needs to monitor his own counter-transferences, for adolescents can provoke powerful aggressive or sexual feelings.

Uribe (1988) suggests that it may be necessary, with the patient's consent, for the therapist to meet with the parents in order to explore their contribution to the adolescent's emotional or behavioural problems. Where indicated, parents may be referred for couple therapy; or the whole family may be engaged in parallel family therapy.

Elderly patients

Many elderly people benefit from psychotherapy, including STDP. Advancing age does not necessarily diminish psychological-mindedness, the ability to mobilize feelings, or motivation for change. Although the elderly patient may have time for a long-term approach, goals must be realistic and increasing awareness of the finite duration of life lends itself to STDP.

The demands and developmental tasks of advancing age are concerned primarily with loss. In particular, the elderly person is having to come to terms with diminishing physical and mental powers, changing sexuality, the upsurge of primitive and regressive emotions, the perceived discontinuity between past and present lives, and the accelerating succession of external losses—of spouse, other relatives, and friends. Perhaps the most painful loss is the loss of independence. Ultimately, there is the prospect of loss of life itself (Porter 1991).

There may be difficulty in establishing an alliance if the patient is wary or envious of the therapist's relative youth, or if the therapist is threatened by the patient's apparent helplessness, dependence, or fear of death. The patient may perceive the therapist, transferentially, as a child or grandchild at one time but as a parent or authority figure at another. Such transferences may be unfamiliar to the younger therapist, as may the powerful counter-transferences evoked.

Therapy with an elderly patient may be less confrontative than with a younger and more robust patient, but it is still possible to challenge defences and to release repressed feelings. Interpretations addressing links between present and past may be central, encouraging recollection and reminiscence, and promoting re-establishment of the continuity of life. In addition, particularly in the end phase, the patient is encouraged realistically to anticipate the future—with all it means, including further loss and eventual death. Many elderly people welcome the opportunity to talk honestly of their hopes and fears.

In this way, the patient is offered an opportunity to bring together past, present, and future. The ending, addressed openly, offers a new beginning even to the elderly person.

Pathological grief

STDP has an important place in the treatment of abnormal grief reactions, particularly when grief is prolonged, exaggerated, or masked by somatic or behavioural symptoms (Worden 1991). It is an effective treatment for unresolved grief following loss of a spouse (Marmar *et al.* 1988) and perinatal loss (Leon 1987).

Grief therapy must not be confused with grief counselling, the goal of which is to facilitate grieving in the recently bereaved. Its goal is to identify and resolve obstacles to mourning. Worden identifies factors which can complicate mourning:

(1) the nature of the relationship with the deceased, particularly ambivalence and unacknowledged hostility, intense dependency, or a history of sexual or physical abuse;

(2) the circumstances of the loss, such as sudden and unexpected death, the absence of a body, multiple losses, or violent and mutilating death;

(3) a history of previous unresolved loss, including loss of a parent in early life;

(4) personality factors, such as particular vulnerability or its converse, the 'strong' type who does not grieve but cares for others; and

(5) social factors that discourage active grieving, such as the absence of a supportive family, social network, or cultural rituals which sanction mourning.

Time-limited therapy is appropriate for the treatment of all but the most complicated grief reactions, because the time limit and emphasis of the ending serves to highlight the focus on loss without promoting an unhealthy dependency on the therapist. A psychodynamic approach is appropriate when significant degrees of repression, ambivalence or other unconscious processes are encountered in pathological grief. Gentle challenge to defences, recovery of epressed memories and feelings, and interpretive linking of present with past experience are important techniques. The therapist may become a transference representation of the deceased, a target perhaps for the ambivalence which characterized the lost relationship; its analysis can facilitate the recognition of the feelings and dynamic processes obstructing mourning, such as anger or guilt. This unblocks grieving, as a result of which the patient comes to accept the finality of the loss and lets go of the deceased. Sensitive handling of the ending is essential, for the conclusion of treatment acts as a symbolic opportunity to say goodbye and move on to a new phase.

Post-traumatic disorders

As with pathological grief, which itself may be the result of traumatic loss, post-traumatic disorders may be amenable to treatment by STDP. Traumatic events are those which, by virtue of being sudden, unexpected, and violent or violating, penetrate the person's defences to injure the very core of the self. Traumatic events usually involve death, the threat of death, or serious threat to the person's physical and psychological integrity. Psychological reactions to trauma are immediate or delayed; but, like grief, are construed as abnormal only if prolonged, disabling, or masked by somatic or behavioural symptoms. Evidence suggests that early pro-active interventions, which discourage denial and promote emotional and cognitive processing of the traumatic experience, may reduce later post-traumatic disorder.

Post-traumatic symptoms are categorized into three clusters: (1) re-experiencing (e.g. intrusive recollections, flashbacks, nightmares); (2) avoidance (e.g. emotional numbing or denial, avoidance of the scene of the incident or any reminder of it, social withdrawal); and (3) arousal (e.g. persistent tension, irritability, hypervigilance). Only if features of all three clusters persist is a diagnosis of post-traumatic stress disorder (PTSD) made, but other permutations can be as severe and disabling. Apart from a symptomatic presentation, severe trauma can damage personality development and structure, giving rise to post-traumatic personality disorder (PTPD).

Terr (1991) differentiates two types of trauma. Short, intense, and unanticipated traumatic experiences (Type 1), for example involvement in a road accident, give rise to reactions characterized by vivid, detailed, and intrusive recollections of the event, associated with intense arousal and provoking avoidant behaviour, the pattern typical of uncomplicated PTSD. Prolonged, repeated, and anticipated traumatic experiences (Type 2), such as repeated sexual abuse in childhood, torture, or exposure to prolonged danger or depravity in warfare, result in reactions typified by psychic numbing, denial, and dissociation, extremes of passivity, rage and guilt, and distortion of personality. This is the pattern of PTPD.

STDP can be an effective treatment for Type I reactions, that is relatively uncomplicated PTSD, even years after the traumatic experience (Marmar 1991). Complicated PTSD and PTPD however require prolonged treatment.

STDP addresses the dynamic experience of the trauma as the focus and gives subsidiary prominence to issues of loss, particularly of the ubiquitous illusions of safety and immortality. An exposure strategy is central, the patient encouraged in the secure therapeutic context to recollect and narrate the traumatic experience with its associated emotions, repeatedly if necessary. Thereby he becomes desensitized and integrates the traumatic experience into a revised view of his life and identity.

Again, it may be necessary to challenge maladaptive defences against the fear, anger, sadness, and guilt generated by the trauma, and to explore unconscious links to previous unresolved traumatic experiences or losses if these obstruct emotional and cognitive processing of the more recent trauma. However, there is a danger of re-traumatizing the patient if the therapist cuts through defences prematurely or forcibly; or he allows de-repression to proceed unchecked without active processing of recovered memories and affects. Particular dangers are evident when the therapist makes incisive challenges to the defences of a patient who suffered penetrative sexual abuse or rape, and especially if the therapist is of the same sex as the perpetrator. For these reasons, the pace and style should be managed sensitively.

The end phase represents a chance to render the trauma past, and to incorporate the experience into the continuity of life. In this way the victim becomes a survivor, wiser, more compassionate, and more appreciative of life.

THERAPEUTIC FACTORS AND THE PROCESS OF CHANGE IN STDP

Ashurst (1991) has identified a number of therapeutic ingredients common to all psychodynamic therapies:

(1) *Therapeutic alliance*. Fundamental to all therapies, this represents more than just the vehicle for treatment. In STDP the relationship with the therapist, although short, offers a vibrant encounter in which honesty and openness are prized, the patient can feel accepted despite his perceived faults and failures, and psychological change is tangible and valued.

(2) *Emotional catharsis*. Expression of feelings, including those previously hidden, provides relief from tension and contributes to the resolution of neurotic conflict, grief, or traumatization.

(3) *Corrective emotional experience*. Therapy may constitute a corrective experience for the patient exactly because the therapist responds in an accepting and enabling manner. This constructive response may contrast significantly with attitudes and reactions of previous formative figures, including parents.

(4) *Cognitive learning*. The analytic work, confronting defences and examining transference developments, promotes greater self-understanding as a result of which new ways of thinking are generated.

(5) *Modelling*. Consciously or unconsciously, the patient may adopt the qualities of active curiosity, confidence in addressing negative feelings, and capacity to think about difficult issues which are exhibited by the therapist.

(6) *'Working through'*. Although short, STDP actively encourages the patient to experiment with his growing insight both within therapy and in relationships and activities outside. This contrasts with the working through of long-term analytic psychotherapy, which is primarily a prolonged internal process, but may achieve similar ends.

A number of researchers have added to our understanding of the change process in STDP.

Llewelyn *et al.* (1988), through study of the patient's perception of significant events in therapy, found that those which enhanced awareness (particularly getting in touch with previously hidden feelings), a sense of relief and hope, the relationship with the therapist as a person, and the opportunity to identify and rehearse new ways of problem-solving were particularly valued in short exploratory therapy. The experience found to hinder progress most was for the therapist to focus on unwanted feelings and thoughts in an 'unhelpful' way. This suggests that it may be counter-productive to expose uncomfortable thoughts and feelings without addressing and resolving them, a danger identified particularly in work with people who have been abused sexually or otherwise traumatized.

A collaborative alliance is fundamental and interpretations are framed in a way which promotes it at the same time as extending insight and conscious control over patterns of thought, feeling and behaviour (Piper *et al.* 1991; Westen 1986). This process of 'making the unconscious conscious' is tolerable and productive only if managed sensitively in patients carefully selected and prepared for it.

PROBLEMS IN THE PRACTICE OF STDP

Problems encountered in STDP can be categorized as the products of faults in selection or technique.

Faults in selection

Attention has been drawn repeatedly to the problems which can result from inadequate assessment. Particular dangers may arise in the attempted treatment of borderline patients, who may become psychotic or act-out destructively, of patients with a propensity to become suicidal, and of those with strong regressive potential who may decompensate at the conclusion of therapy (Malan and Osimo 1992).

Difficulties can emerge in STDP, even when assessment was apparently thorough, if aspects of the patient or his history remained hidden. This occurs particularly if the patient is aware that he is being assessed for short-term therapy, for he may present only the 'short-term' part of himself (Coren, personal communication). During the course of STDP, a history of severe childhood abuse or other Type 2 trauma may emerge which cannot be ignored, but which is not a feasible focus. In this situation, discretion is the better part of valour. The therapist needs to acknowledge that another form of therapy is required and either prolong the treatment, or end it carefully while arranging to transfer the patient to another therapist.

Faults in technique

The therapist's failure to adhere to the defined focus and to the time limit are obvious sources of failure. This may be particularly difficult for therapists trained in long-term psychotherapies, used to a different pace and an expansive framework in treatment.

Other technical faults are associated with over-zealousness in confrontation of defences and premature uncovering of unconscious material. Provision of a supportive alliance and opportunities for exploration and resolution of uncovered material are essential, particularly when memories and feelings associated with traumatic experience are de-repressed.

Particular problems are presented by the generation of powerful transferences. If the patient develops a pervasive negative transference, which may be the result of the therapist's faulty technique, the alliance may be destroyed, the patient is likely to drop out. As dangerous is the emergence of an idealizing or even eroticized transference both of which are likely to be the product of undiagnosed personality disorder.

The therapist's counter-transference may be problematic because the brevity and high activity level both diminish the therapist's ability to monitor his own transferences and create an atmosphere in which the predisposed therapist can become sadistic. The repeated challenge to defences in particular requires that the therapist maintains empathic contact, and effective control of his own aggressive impulses, if an unwarranted and anti-therapeutic attack on the patient is to be avoided. For this reason continuing supervision is essential for good practice, even for experienced therapists.

TRAINING

Malan and Osimo (1992) confidently state that supervised practice of STDP is an excellent training experience. Working with patients selected for their capacity to interact dynamically with the therapist and for the clarity of their psychopathology, trainees obtain ready opportunity to learn principles of active dynamic psychotherapy, to appreciate the dynamic structure of psychopathology, and to experience the satisfaction of early, tangible results.

Many psychotherapists believe, however, that is is not possible to learn the skills of STDP before acquiring competence in long-term analytic psychotherapy, particularly because it takes time to recognize and work effectively with resistance and transference. The therapists in Malan and Osimo's retrospective study were senior trainees obtaining specialized training experience in dynamic psychotherapy.

Nevertheless, more junior trainees can develop skills and confidence in STDP, particularly if working with carefully selected cases and supervised closely (Ashurst 1991). In parallel with training in other short psychological treatments, such as cognitive therapy, exposure of trainees to basic training in STDP is highly relevant. It is also important they learn to recognize indications for STDP, and to value its effect.

CONCLUSION

STDP is an economical and effective treatment for patients with a wide spectrum of presenting problems, ranging from entrenched neuroses to developmental disorders to unresolved grief. The technical ingredients and style of therapy are modified according to the patient's personal characteristics and psychopathology. The attention to preliminary assessment, dynamic focus, analysis of defences, and adherence to time limit are defining features common to all versions.

STDP is not a panacea. Only a minority of patients presenting to a psychiatric service could benefit; many patients referred to specialized psychological treatment services are too vulnerable or disturbed for this anxiety-provoking therapy.

Psychiatric treatments rarely produce 'cures', and STDP is no exception. Clinical and research evidence suggests that STDP, in common perhaps with other psychological treatments, unlocks and promotes adaptive psychological processes. The effects may generalize and extend over time, but further episodes of treatment may be required. The patient with more complex problems may benefit from successive episodes of focal psychotherapy, perhaps including family, couple, and group therapies at different points.

It has been shown that STDP is an effective treatment (Crits-Christoph 1992), although other studies suggest that it is marginally less so than cognitive-behavioural therapy (Shapiro and Firth 1987). Further research is required to establish whether or not this difference is a methodological artefact, and to identify patient characteristics and components of outcome which are responsive to STDP.

In the end, however, the demonstration that one therapy is superior to another can be misleading. Psychotherapists are more concerned to resolve the old but unanswered question: Which therapy is indicated for which patient at which point in time? The further application and study of STDP may well assist in the elucidation of an answer.

REFERENCES

Alexander, F. and French, T. (1946). *Psychoanalytic therapy: principles and application*. Ronald Press, New York.

Ashurst, P. M. (1991). Brief psychotherapy. In *Textbook of psychotherapy in psychiatric practice*, (ed. J. Holmes), pp. 187–212. Churchill Livingstone, Edinburgh.

Balint, M., Ornstein, P. H., and Balint, E. (1972). *Focal psychotherapy: An example of applied psychoanalysis*. Tavistock, London.

Crits-Christoph, P. (1992). The efficacy of brief dynamic psychotherapy: a meta-analysis. *American Journal of Psychiatry*, **149**, 151–8.

Davanloo, H. (ed.) (1980). *Short-term dynamic psychotherapy*. Aronson, Northvale, NJ.

Ferenczi, S. (1950). *Further contributions to the theory and technique of psychoanalysis*. Hogarth, London. (Originally published 1926.)

Freud, S. (1964). Analysis terminable and interminable. In *Standard edition*, Vol. 23. Hogarth, London. (Originally published 1937.)

Garfield, S. L. (1989). *The practice of brief psychotherapy*. Pergamon, New York.

Hobbs, M. (1984). Crisis intervention in theory and practice: a selective review. *British Journal of Medical Psychology*, **57**, 23–34.

Hobbs, M. (1989). Short-term dynamic psychotherapy. *Current Opinion in Psychiatry*, **2**, 389–92.

Howard, K. I., Kopta, S. M., Krause, M. S., and Orlinsky, D. E. (1986). The dose–effect relationship in psychotherapy. *American Psychologist*, **41**, 159–64.

Keller, A. (1984). Planned brief psychotherapy in clinical practice. *British Journal of Medical Psychology*, **57**, 347–61.

Klerman, G. L., Weissman, M. M., Rounsaville, B. J., and Chevron, E. S. (1984). *Interpersonal psychotherapy for depression*. Basic Books, New York.

Koss, M. P. and Butcher, J. N. (1986). Research on brief psychotherapy. In *Handbook of psychotherapy and behaviour change*, (2nd edn), (ed. S. L. Garfield and A. E. Bergin). Wiley, New York.

Leon, I. G. (1987). Short-term psychotherapy for perinatal loss. *Psychotherapy*, **24**, 186–95.

Llewelyn, S. P., Elliott, R., Shapiro, D. A., Hardy, G., and Firth-Cozens, J. (1988). Client perceptions of significant events in prescriptive and exploratory periods of individual therapy. *British Journal of Clinical Psychology*, **27**, 105–14.

MacKenzie, K. R. (1988). Recent developments in brief psychotherapy. *Hospital and Community Psychiatry*, **39**, 742–52.

MacKenzie, K. R. (1990). *Introduction to time-limited group psychotherapy*. American Psychiatric Press, Washington, DC.

Mackie, A. (1981). Attachment theory: its relevance to the therapeutic alliance. *British Journal of Medical Psychology*. **54**, 203–12.

Malan, D. H. (1963). *A study of brief psychotherapy*. Tavistock, London.

Malan, D. H. (1976). *The frontier of brief psychotherapy*. Plenum, New York.

Malan, D. H. (1979). *Individual psychotherapy and the science of psychodynamics*. Butterworths, London.

Malan, D. H. (1980). The most important development in psychotherapy since the discovery of the unconscious. In *Short-term dynamic psychotherapy* (ed. H. Davanloo), pp. 13–23. Aronson, Northvale, NJ.

Malan, D. H. and Osimo, F. (1992). *Psychodynamics, training, and outcome in brief psychotherapy*. Butterworths-Heinemann, Oxford.

Mann, J. (1973). *Time-limited psychotherapy*. Harvard University Press, Boston.

Marmar, C. R., Horrowitz, M. J., Weiss, D. S., Wilner, N. R., and Kaltreider, N. B. (1988). A controlled trial of brief psychotherapy and mutual-help group treatment of conjugual bereavement. *American Journal of Psychiatry* **145**, 203–9.

Marmar, C. R. (1991). Brief dynamic psychotherapy of post-traumatic stress disorder. *Psychiatric Annals*, **21**, 405–14.

Marmor, J. M. (1979). Short-term dynamic psychotherapy. *American Journal of Psychiatry*, **136**, 149–55.

Molnos, A. (1984). The two triangles are four: a diagram to teach the process of dynamic brief psychotherapy. *British Journal of Psychotherapy*, **1**, 112–25.

Molnos, A. (1986). Anger that destroys and anger that heals: handling hostility in group analysis and in dynamic brief psychotherapy. *Group Analysis*, **19**, 207–21.

Moras, K. and Strupp, H. H. (1982). Pretherapy interpersonal relations, patients' alliance, and outcome in brief therapy. *Archives of General Psychiatry*, **39**, 405–9.

Morgan, R., Luborsky, L., Crits-Christoph, P., Curtis, H., and Solomon, J. (1982). Predicting the outcomes of psychotherapy by the Penn Helping Alliance Rating Method. *Archives of General Psychiatry*, **39**, 397–402.

Piper, W. E., Azim, H. F. A., Joyce, A. S., and McCallum, M. (1991). Transference interpretations, therapeutic alliance, and outcome in short-term individual psychotherapy. *Archives of General Psychiatry*, **48**, 946–53.

Piper, W. E., McCallum, M., and Azim, H. F. A. (1992). *Adaptation to loss through short-term group psychotherapy*. Guilford, New York.

Porter, R. (1991). Psychotherapy with the elderly. In *Textbook of psychotherapy in psychiatric practice*, (ed. J. Holmes), pp. 469–87. Churchill Livingstone, Edinburgh.

Rank, O. (1936). *Will therapy: an analysis of the therapeutic process in terms of relationship*. Knopf, New York.

Ryle, A. (1990). *Cognitive-analytic therapy: active participation in change*. Wiley, Chichester.

Shapiro, D. A. and Firth, J. (1987). Prescriptive v. exploratory psychotherapy: outcomes of the Sheffield psychotherapy project. *British Journal of Psychiatry*, **151**, 790–9.

Sifneos, P. E. (1972). *Short-term psychotherapy and emotional crisis*. Harvard University Press, Boston.

Sifneos, P. E. (1987). *Short-term dynamic psychotherapy: evaluation and technique*, (2nd edn). Plenum, New York.

Small, L. (1971). *The briefer psychotherapies*. Brunner/Mazel, New York.

Strupp, H. H. and Binder, J. L. (1984). *Psychotherapy in a new key*. Basic Books, New York.

Terr, L. C. (1991). Childhood traumas: an outline and overview. *American Journal of Psychiatry*, **148**, 10–20.

Uribe, V. M. (1988). Short-term psychotherapy for adolescents: management of initial resistances. *Journal of the American Academy of Psychoanalysis*, **16**, 107–16.

Westen, D. (1986). What changes in short-term psychodynamic psychotherapy? *Psychotherapy*, **23**, 501–12.

Wilson, P. (1991). Psychotherapy with adolescents. In *Textbook of psychotherapy in psychiatric practice*, (ed. J. Holmes), pp. 443–67. Churchill Livingstone, Edinburgh.

Wolberg, L. R. (1980). *Handbook of short-term psychotherapy*. Grune & Stratton, New York.

Worden, J. W. (1991). *Grief counselling and grief therapy* (2nd edn). Routledge, London.

RECOMMENDED READING

Bauer, G. P. and Kobos, J. C. (1987). *Brief therapy: short-term psychodynamic intervention*. Aronson, Northvale, NJ. (A comprehensive summary of the historical development, principles, and practice of STDP. Valuable practical guidance for therapists.)

Davanloo, H. (ed.) (1980). *Short-term dynamic psychotherapy*. Aronson, Northvale, NJ. (Davanloo's chapters include verbatim transcripts which give a clear picture of his challenging method of STDP.)

Flegenheimer, W. V. (1982). *Techniques of brief psychotherapy*. Aronson, New York. (A comparative account of the techniques employed by leading practitioners of STDP.)

MacKenzie, K. R. (1988). Recent developments in brief psychotherapy. *Hospital and Community Psychiatry*, **39**, 742–52. (Useful summary of research and developments in STDP.)

Malan, D. H. (1979). *Individual psychotherapy and the science of psychodynamics*. Butterworths, London. (In this readable book, which is peppered with clinical illustrations, there is a valuable account of the application of the 'two triangles' in therapy.)

Malan, D. H. and Osimo, F. (1992). *Psychodynamics, training, and outcome in brief psychotherapy*. Butterworths–Heinemann, Oxford. (A detailed evaluation of the long-term results of brief psychotherapies undertaken by trainees at the Tavistock Clinic, demonstrating method and outcome.)

Mann, J. (1973). *Time-limited psychotherapy*. Harvard University Press, Boston. (Mann's influential text includes a lucid rationale for his emphasis of a time limit and an annotated transcript of a 12-session treatment.)

Sifneos, P.E. (1987). *Short-term dynamic psychotherapy: evaluation and technique*, (2nd edn). Plenum, New York. (A clear presentation of Sifneos's short-term anxiety-provoking psychotherapy, including illustrated accounts of his selection process and method.)

4

Group psychotherapy

SIDNEY BLOCH and MARK AVELINE

The goals of long-term individual therapy discussed by Jeremy Holmes and Sidney Crown in Chapter 2 can also be tackled in group therapy. In this chapter an interpersonal model of small group therapy is described with special emphasis placed on therapeutic factors. Sidney Bloch and Mark Aveline cover selection, group composition, preparation of members, group development and the mature group. The final section deals briefly with other applications of the group approach and with training.

Human beings live, work, and play in diverse groups, and find and express their identity through social interaction. Not surprisingly many of the emotional problems they may experience stem from disturbed relationships within the groups in which they have learned to be the people they are. With increasing recognition of the interpersonal factor in psychiatric theory and practice has come the development of psychotherapies which have as their target problems between people rather than within the individual. Chapters in this volume on family, marital, and sex therapy partly reflect this focus. In addition to these naturally occurring groups, 'stranger' group therapy, both small and large, has been widely used in a variety of settings: wards of psychiatric hospitals, the therapeutic community, the human potential movement, the out-patient clinic, the private therapist's office, and many more. Today, group therapy of many types is a commonly used psychological treatment.

In this chapter we consider the long-term group composed of patients who appreciate they have recurrent difficulties in relating and wish to change them. The model we describe is based on the interpersonal theory of psychiatry of Harry Stack Sullivan (1953). For comprehensive accounts of this model see Yalom (1985) and Whitaker (1985), and for a summary, Aveline and Dryden (1988). A long-term group is the optimal training ground for the novice and much of what

ıe learns there can be transferred to other group therapy settings. Brief
mention is made of other uses of the group at the end of the chapter,
ınd reading recommended on them.

3ACKGROUND

The systematic use of groups in psychotherapy practice is a twentieth-
century development (Scheidlinger 1994). But the healing properties of
groups have long been recognized particularly in religious practice; the
shrine at Lourdes is an excellent example.

Joseph Pratt (1974), a Boston physician, is usually designated the
father of group therapy. At the turn of the century he assembled together
patients with tuberculosis in order to instruct them on medical aspects of
their illness. Apart from this didactic dimension he also promoted a
group climate through which patients provided mutual support. Several
years later a number of American psychiatrists incorporated Pratt's ideas
forming structured groups of patients who were viewed as 'students' and
tutored on mental ill-health. This educational approach soon waned, to
be replaced by the pioneering efforts of psychoanalysts treating patients
in groups. Freud (1955) himself never practised group therapy but
recognized the significance of group phenomena, as reflected in his
Group psychology and the analysis of the ego. Jung (1974) was distinctly
biased against the therapy group; since psychological illness was an
individual experience, it required individual analysis. Alfred Adler, in
contrast, considered social factors in treatment using the group format in
child guidance centres and with alcoholic patients.

Several American psychoanalysts attempted to transfer their methods
to a group format. Trigant Burrow (1974), for example, regarded
phenomena like resistance and transference as pertinent in group as in
individual therapy. A group had particular advantages—the patient
could see that he was not unique, and derive support from his peers; as
a result his resistance would diminish and he would take greater risks.

The Second World War was a watershed in the development of
group therapy. It proved an economical method to cope with the large
patient numbers among the military; some analysts in the British army
had a marked impact on clinical practice with their application of
groups. The Northfield Military Hospital was a centre of innovation
and there Wilfred Bion (1961) and Michael Foulkes (1946) tried out
new approaches. Bion's work later influenced therapists at the
Tavistock Clinic in London while Foulkes was the force behind the
founding of the influential Institute of Group Analysis in London.

Another key contribution was that of a group of social psychologists led by Kurt Lewin in the United States (1951). His field theory—that a person's dynamics are intimately associated with the nature of the social forces around him—was the basis for extensive research into group process. In 1946 the State of Connecticut invited Lewin to help train community leaders in an effort to reduce interracial tensions. In this way the sensitivity-training group (or T-group) was born. Four years later the National Training Laboratory (NTL) was formed as a training centre for human relations and group dynamics. Participants from a range of backgrounds, such as teachers and managers in industry, could both experience and study group functioning and interpersonal dynamics in a group workshop, and as a result act more effectively in their home settings.

A decade later the NTL emphasis changed, from group to personal dynamics, paralleling the swell of interest in the human potential movement. The goals of the T-group became greater self-awareness and personal growth. Before long it had spawned the encounter-group movement, and with it, the development of the 'growth centre'. Although many centres sprang up in the United States during the 1960s and 1970s, the encounter movement subsequently declined both in terms of membership and originality of its concepts.

ASSESSMENT

Indications for group therapy depend to a great extent on the kind of treatment offered. Obviously, a self-help group like Alcoholics Anonymous (AA) suits a specific range of people only. For the group therapy considered in this chapter, that is, long-term treatment whose aim is personality change, indications are not as clear-cut. We have limited research findings to assist in selection, and yet a group's success hinges on the patients chosen (Bond and Lieberman 1978; Aveline 1994; Piper 1994) and on the group's culture. None the less, guidelines can be set: a range of clinical problems can be dealt with effectively in a group; desirable patient features are specifiable; and, within certain diagnostic groups, particular attitudes, perceptions, and behaviours mitigate against effective participation.

Problems that can be and are commonly tackled in group therapy include:

Interpersonal—pervasive difficulty in initiating and sustaining relationships is a pre-eminent indication. The patient may identify an inability to achieve intimacy, either in friendship or sexual, discomfort in social situations, and maladaptive interpersonal style (e.g. lacking trust, overly dependent, abrasively assertive).

Emotional—unawareness of feelings in oneself or in others, inability to express feelings like love or anger, poor emotional control (i.e. explosive and volatile), obsessive (i.e. controlled and rigid).

Self-concept—blurred identity, poor self-esteem, lack of purpose and direction.

Symptomatic—anxiety, depression, somatization, poor work or study performance, ineffective coping with stress. These symptoms need to be regarded by the patient as closely linked to problems in the first three categories rather than as independent.

More suited to group than individual therapy—some patients pose major difficulty when treated individually (e.g. the person who settles into such an intense, regressed relationship that satisfaction derived outweighs motivation to become more independent; or the sadistic patient who may 'damage' the therapist in individual therapy). These sorts of patients may benefit from a group experience, without the group itself being dominated by the particular pressures they tend to bring to bear.

Desirable patient characteristics include the following (see Bloch 1979, for a review of the topic of assessment for psychotherapy generally, and Aveline 1994, on that for focal therapy):

(1) He is motivated to change and prepared to work for it; his wish for therapy is his choice, not the result of pressure by others. In the selection process, as we shall see, setting up hurdles for the candidate to surmount is a means to demonstrate motivation.

(2) He has sufficient trust to share his life, and a capacity for mature relationships so that, when interpersonal conflicts are enacted in the group, he can allow them to be examined constructively.

(3) He expects the group will prove beneficial and, ideally, has a high opinion of group therapy.

(4) He is psychologically minded, able to use verbal and conceptual skills, in order to engage in challenging self-exploration and to

reflect on the group's process. Psychological-mindedness however, is not synonymous with intelligence, professiona occupation or high socio-economic status. Indeed, patients from diverse backgrounds can participate in the same group to everyone's benefit.

Diagnostic categories in ICD 10 or DSM–IV are a relatively poor guide to assessment of suitability for group therapy and prediction of outcome. Much depends on the group's cohesiveness, its stage of evolution (see the section on group development), and the scope of change sought. Conventional diagnosis is best viewed as an indication of particular difficulties a person brings to the group and has to wrestle with in order to benefit. Should the difficulties prove severe, the likelihood of productive engagement diminishes. Some of these patients, however, may be helped by more structured group approaches; we refer to these in the list that follows.

Diagnoses presenting particular problems for interpersonal group therapy include:

(1) *The severely depressed*—mild or moderate depression is a common feature of patients entering groups. Signifying a human reaction to problems, it often lifts or at least improves after the first few months of therapy. The severely depressed patient, in contrast, feels too hopeless even to enter a group. Efforts by both therapists and fellow members to reach out fail and result in frustration and guilt. Unable to influence the patient, the group itself becomes dispirited. The patient may need antidepressants or other psychiatric intervention, either as a prelude or concurrently, in order to raise his level of functioning to the point where psychological issues can be explored.

We should note carefully that affective disorders are becoming a significant focus of attention in various ways, for example, post-partum depression (Gruen 1993); bipolar affective disorder (Kanas 1993; Graves 1993); and grief (McCallum *et al.* 1993; Yalom and Vinogradov 1988; Lieberman and Yalom 1992).

(2) *The acute schizophrenic patient*—a patient in the midst of an acute episode is an inappropriate candidate. Out of contact with reality and disturbed in thinking, he has little chance of engaging. In contrast, a patient who has emerged from such an episode and is now stable is a potential candidate. Kanas (1986) has conducted a useful review of group therapy's application in schizophrenia as

well as reporting on his own systematic research (Kanas and Barr 1982).

(3) *Severe personality disorders*

(a) *The paranoid personality*—in theory this category points to interpersonal difficulties that could benefit from a group experience. Crucial questions are the degree of suspiciousness and the capacity to be flexible. Marked paranoid attitudes preclude the establishment of trusting relationships, an essential component for participation.

(b) *The severe schizoid personality*—group therapy challenges members to do interpersonally what they find most difficult. Patients with marked traits of detachment, coldness, and hypersensitivity manifest a style which is the antithesis of the group's striving to achieve open communication and intimacy. Often, such patients feel that what is asked of them is beyond their experience. The less severely schizoid person is a good candidate since the group establishes a cohesive, trusting environment in which he is encouraged to risk involvement. With both this and the previous category, having more than two such members imposes a severe burden on a group's adequate functioning (see later section on composition).

(c) *The antisocial personality*—again the problem of long-term commitment is pertinent. A low frustration threshold and a lack of a sense of responsibility make both for poor candidacy and a potentially disruptive influence. The patient is likely to profit more from a homogeneous group in which limits are set and a solid structure provided. Being an 'expert' in antisocial behaviour enables him to recognize it in others and, given the right setting, challenge it.

(d) *The narcissistic personality*—insensitive to others, he alienates himself from the group. He claims attention exclusively and has great difficulty in learning how to interact.

(4) *The patient with substance abuse*—tends not to make a long-term commitment. Easily frustrated, and intolerant of the anxieties inherent in group work, he seeks relief from the drug on which he is dependent, often with disastrous effects for the group. He tends to benefit more from a highly structured group composed entirely of patients with the same problem (Yalom *et al.* 1978). Flores and Mahon (1993) have advocated and implemented an approach blending Yalom's (1985) interpersonal model and concepts from

object relations theory and self-psychology. For a comprehensive review of the whole field, see Stinchfield *et al.* (1994).

(5) *The somatizing patient*—patients in group therapy commonly present with somatic complaints as part of their clinical picture but the intense somatizer who cannot be deflected from bodily concerns or translate them into psychological terms does not gain. Moreover, his relentless focus on the body frustrates other members.

SELECTION

Since a group's fate is bound so closely to the patients who constitute it, selection should be done methodically. Therapists are often eager to launch their group and in their haste may generate avoidable difficulties for themselves. Long before any patient is seen, the leaders, preferably in conjunction with a supervisor, should have worked out a format and aims and addressed their personal preferences which may affect collaboration. Selection is both for group therapy *and* for a particular group. Furthermore, the process is closely linked to preparation (see later section).

Each referred patient should be interviewed in depth on two occasions. A useful procedure is to conduct an interview in which information is gathered, the capacity to construe problems in interpersonal terms tested and developed, and willingness to have them examined and modified in the group explored. To help the patient make an informed choice, goals and process are elaborated; in written form, they constitute the basis of an informal agreement (see the Appendix). As well as describing the process, guidelines spell out the importance of confidentiality, regular attendance, and punctuality. One of us (MA) has shown potential patients a film which opens with an account of how groups work, is followed by a discussion among members of a well-established group about their experience and what they needed to do to get the most out of it, and ends with a member reviewing his progress after 'graduating'.

Before the second interview, a homework assignment is given involving preparation of a list of problems the patient wishes to tackle, their associated goals, and a brief biography. Attention paid to these tasks also serves the purpose of assessing motivation. The second session is used to review the material after which therapists and patient can jointly reach their decision. We emphasize *jointly*, as patient and therapists must sense they can work well together. Once the patient is selected, the therapists prepare him for the experience as outlined later in the chapter. Occasionally, a third assessment session is required.

Having accepted a patient, the therapists then pose the question based on observed and inferred interpersonal style: how will he manifest interpersonal difficulties in the group? What, if any, are the potential hazards of his participation? Will he monopolize, withdraw, moralize, and the like? Is there a way to avert these hazards?

COMPOSITION

That a patient may be suitable for treatment but not necessarily for the group being formed raises the question of composition. Should a group be balanced in a specific way or admit all patients assessed as likely to benefit? There is no definite answer but a few principles help in selection.

Homogeneous groups, comprising patients with similar problems (e.g. abusing alcohol), are relatively easy to form as they entail common goals for all members. Heterogeneous groups require more careful thought. Patients, presenting with a variety of problems, need a multifaceted 'social world' (or 'social microcosm' in Yalom's apt phrase; 1985) to learn about themselves and others and to try out new adaptive behaviours. This implies diversity in composition. For instance, a group consisting only of passive-dependent or schizoid members permits minimal scope for learning alternative ways of relating. Similarly, a unisex group is limited in helping a patient with heterosexual difficulties.

A typical group has eight members (a minimum of five is necessary for any learning to occur while more than eight prevents members obtaining sufficient time for themselves) and is characterized by an equal balance of men and women, an age range of about 20 to 60, mixed social, economic, and occupational backgrounds, and a wide assortment of clinical problems and personality types. The therapist avoids including a patient who obviously stands out, for example, one woman only or a patient markedly older than the rest; such members tend to drop out.

Whitaker (1985) advocates formation of a group in which patients have a variety of problems and coping styles but are similar in their tolerance of anxiety. This principle is an excellent basis for selection. In practice, groups almost always contain patients with a range of problem severity. Too great a span is to be avoided lest the more disabled impede the development of the more fortunate members, thereby generating frustration and a sense of failure.

Groups may be open or closed. The closed group begins and ends with the same membership. For pragmatic reasons this arrangement is uncommon in long-term therapy as some patients graduate earlier than others and some drop out prematurely. The closed system is appropriate for a relatively short-term group and for training groups. The open group permits members to terminate at different points and their substitution by new patients. The disadvantages are obvious: cohesiveness is threatened with each departure and arrival and a new patient must integrate into an established social group. These difficulties, however, are transient since the solid working group can afford both to lose members and absorb newcomers. Moreover, advantages of the open model include a successful graduate inspiring the rest of the group, both patients and therapists, and the newcomer invigorating and offering new opportunities for interpersonal learning.

PREPARATION

Both clinical and research evidence confirm the value of preparing patients for their experience (Kaul and Bednar 1984). Most novices harbour diverse concerns: Is group therapy not inferior to individual treatment? Will I be forced to make a confession? Can I be assured that confidentiality will be respected? Will I be affected adversely by other members? How can others with problems help me? The concept and the initial experience of group therapy are often baffling and unsettling; indeed, most drop-outs take place in the first three months. The guidelines in the Appendix ask new members to commit themselves for six months, a period necessary to note how the group can confer benefits.

Anxiety and confusion can be reduced considerably through preparation. It is our practice to explore concerns and fantasies and to hand out the document mentioned above (see the Appendix). Any misconceptions are discussed in a second meeting. The patient may fail to assimilate all this information because of anxiety thus requiring the therapist to cover the ground repeatedly.

Confirming the expectation that the patient's problems will be addressed, albeit at a pace that he and the group can handle, is a vital aspect of preparation. We find it helpful to identify explicitly problematic aspects of interaction that will inevitably manifest in the group, and need to be 'owned' and worked on by the patient. It is these problems that often lead to premature termination. As an example, Jonas had never experienced an intimate relationship. He expected others to attack him even while holding out a hand of friendship. His remedy was to attack and to annihilate others pre-emptively. Once they got too close few were given a second chance. Having agreed on the nature of this pattern, preparatory work was directed towards how this problem would be tackled. Jonas agreed to disclose the pattern, to invite the group to intervene when it happened, and to try to let people get closer than was his wont. The benefit would be in learning to do precisely what he found so daunting.

On a lesser level, Jim was overly cautious; he was apt to make carefully considered comments but by the time he spoke the conversation had moved on. If he could talk in generalities rather than more personally, he would. His caution had resulted in an isolated life. He was able to see that he ran the risk of becoming an outsider in the group—passed over through his passivity. The task was agreed upon; he would try to act more spontaneously and to take risks.

This procedure of anticipating problematic interactions and making them a focus can be formalized in a system of reviews. Prior to joining the group, the patient documents his problems and their impact on his relationships, and prepares a 'wish list' of changes that, realistically, he intends to grapple with in the succeeding four months. Every four months, all members review work done by each other, taking as their baseline what has been documented. A new wish list is then formulated and the original statement of problems revised as necessary. The procedure helps to maintain momentum and focus and makes it more likely that members will continue to examine their interpersonal difficulties.

THERAPEUTIC FACTORS

The novice is apt to become bewildered by the diversity of the many extant theoretical schools, each claiming merit for its own approach (see Recommended Reading). Fortunately, the methodical study of therapeutic factors helps to deal with this. We can conclude that certain components of group therapy are of value. For a full account of the relevant research see Bloch and Crouch (1985). We should also note that therapeutic factors depend on the group's goals and that different factors are relevant at particular times in the group's life.

Corsini and Rosenberg (1955) were the first to review the group therapy literature on these factors, delineating nine categories. Later workers refined these categories (see, for example, Yalom 1985, and Bloch and Crouch 1985). What follows is a brief account of these factors. It should be borne in mind that the list is to an extent arbitrary and that the factors are not entirely discrete. An updated review is to be found in Crouch *et al.* (1994).

Group cohesiveness (acceptance)

This factor is a *sine qua non* for effective group therapy and a foundation for all other factors. A group is cohesive when members have a sense of belonging and mutually support one another. The patient feels secure, enjoys close contact with his peers and the therapists, takes risks without disastrous repercussions, and is not judged. Lest this sounds like a haven, we should note that cohesiveness also entails negative feedback, anger, and conflict but all expressed constructively and as a feature of caring. As William Blake once said: 'Opposition is true friendship.'

Research repeatedly confirms the pre-eminent role of cohesiveness (Bloch and Crouch 1985; Crouch *et al.* 1994). Cohesive groups have better attendance, punctuality, member activity, and stability.

Learning from interpersonal action

A patient's intra-group behaviour typically resembles the way he acts in general. Thus, for example, clinging, explosive, or self-centred members enter the group with these patterns which have proved troublesome in their lives, and before long they emerge and became obvious to the membership. This continuity is fundamental to all explorative psychotherapy making it possible to address directly in treatment what is problematic beyond it.

In group therapy, the pattern is addressed by feedback from others about its impact, and disclosure of trigger feelings, and past, formative interactions by the initiator. The interpersonal problem is then 'publicly' identified, reasons for its genesis and continuation explored, and the stage set for trials of new ways of relating (Ratigan and Aveline 1988). In practice, the sequence moves fitfully.

There are various views in the group, some objecting to the pattern, others, perhaps those who share in the dynamic, making light of it. Insight is resisted. Patterns gradually become clearer to members. Insight deepens as the question of 'why' is tackled—at the level of triggers and in the form of remembered, formative experiences. It is not clear if linking present behaviour to such influences is necessary for change. Certainly, it helps some patients to place their behaviour in context. What is important—and uniquely beneficial in group therapy—is interpersonal learning through taking novel action in the here and now (see the section on the mature working group).

As an example, Bill had a record of several failed relationships and had never achieved intimacy with either men or women. Within the first few meetings, he alienated himself when he monopolized the group and incessantly grabbed attention. He sulked when deprived of the centre stage.

Schematically, learning from interpersonal action follows the above sequence but in practice, is more complex. First, Bill perceives that a problem exists; he relates poorly to members and is not accepted. They react to his style and inform him that they feel anger at his insensitivity. They have avoided him, since engagement only leads to further monopolizing. Bill recognizes the feedback (this is not so simple, as resistance may render him defensive and disgruntled; weeks or months usually pass before he is willing to see himself as the group sees him). He begins to evaluate the awkward ties he has with his fellows and comes to understand that his domineering style is responsible.

Bill now has to commit himself to change by becoming less egocentric, a major step. It is one thing to be aware of an undesirable trait, quite another to eradicate it. Yet there is no change without interpersonal action. The group plays a pivotal role by encouraging and reinforcing Bill's efforts. It applauds risks he takes to relate anew. On discovering that he not only survives but is also rewarded, Bill experiments beyond the group.

In this example, Bill benefited from his willingness to relate constructively and adaptively within the group. He did not need to learn why, at a deeper level of insight, he had related domineeringly in the past. Some therapists would pursue this issue to unravel sources usually located in early family relationships. Thus, unresolved sibling rivalry might emerge which he could then explore. In our view, this is fine as long as the exploration does not supplant the here and now focus (Yalom 1985).

Insight (self-understanding)

Insight, or some form of cognitive processing, is a central common feature of most psychotherapies. A strict behaviourist might view cognitive change as a secondary phenomenon, or an epiphenomenon of behavioural change. However, most contemporary therapists would unite in regarding change in self-concept and behaviour as intimately related and agree that causality is bidirectional. In other words, behaviour can lead to shifts in self-concept, and vice versa. Several types of self-understanding may occur: *inter alia*, recognizing defences, understanding the origin of symptoms, appreciating the meaning of dreams, and becoming aware of how behaviour affects others.

In their early attempt to classify therapeutic factors, Corsini and Rosenberg (1955) used the term 'intellectualization' to identify a process of learning that leads to insight. This distinction between intellectualization and insight is problematic since the former has been used to reflect a defence mechanism. Yalom (1985) argues that interpersonal insight is the form of learning most relevant to group therapy, psychogenetic insight (understanding the origin of symptoms) subsidiary.

As a therapeutic factor, insight occurs following feedback from and interpretation by other members, both patients and therapists. It operates when patients: (1) learn something important about themselves (understanding overt behaviour, assumptions they hold about themselves, underlying motivations of their behaviour, uncovered fantasies); (2) learn how they come across to the group; (3) learn more clearly and comprehensively about the nature of their problems; and (4) learn why they behave as they do and how such behaviour developed (psychogenetic insight).

Universality

Before entering the group the patient commonly perceives himself as uniquely burdened with problems. Universality operates within the first few sessions in that a 'we're all in the same boat' feeling soon replaces the 'I am unique' one. In one early group, Peter's disclosure of shame about masturbation was followed by the male members sharing problems about sexuality. Peter experienced relief that he was not special in this regard. The therapist reinforces this factor with comments like 'It seems as if everyone shares this problem in one way or another.'

Instillation of hope

Hope is inherent in all therapies. The patient begins treatment with the expectation of gaining relief from problems (Frank and Frank 1991). The factor operates when a patient perceives that his peers improve and the group can be beneficial and thus becomes optimistic about the prospect of change.

Altruism

A unique benefit of group therapy is its potential to facilitate mutual help. The occasion frequently arises for a patient to support a co-member, to enjoy the sense of giving of himself: 'I can be useful to others and I am therefore of value'. This is particularly useful in patients who suffer from poor self-esteem. Altruism also enhances sensitivity to others, reducing morbid self-preoccupation.

Guidance

We saw earlier that pioneering group therapy was didactic. Advice still plays a role but much less so. In early meetings, the therapist shapes the culture by promoting interaction, self-reflection, and reducing distress and confusion through openness to personal experience and making sense of it through exploration. As the group matures, these functions are increasingly held by members themselves. Less helpfully, they easily slip into offering advice on how to solve problems 'Why don't you simply discuss it with your wife?' or 'You should change jobs'. Although this reflects caring and should not be undermined, it usually has a negligible effect. The group comes to see that no short-cut remedies exist. Occasionally, advice signifies retreat from facing unsettling experiences and then needs to be highlighted.

Vicarious learning

A member has, in his peers, potential models from whom to learn. Herein lies a distinct advantage of group treatment. Every patient does not need to go through the work to tackle a shared problem but benefits in noting how a peer deals with it. Furthermore, each patient may have a quality which another wishes to emulate. For example, a passive member may attempt to model herself on an appropriately assertive peer.

Identification is also a mechanism to lay down desirable group norms. Noting that a patient takes risks, reveals aspects of himself, expresses feelings and survives, encourages others to act similarly. The therapist also acts as a model although this may work both ways. A passive, reticent therapist, for example, is unlikely to promote an interactive, risk-taking group.

Catharsis and self-disclosure

This pair of factors embraces ventilation of feelings like anger, anxiety, depression, guilt, and shame, and the disclosure of previously concealed information, often embarrassing and painful. Although the factors often occur together, they are distinctive because of their specific effects. Emotional release has had a hallowed tradition in individual psychotherapy (see Chapter 1). The same is true for group therapy. But catharsis itself is of limited value unless the patient makes sense of the experience. What happened when I cried so bitterly? What was the significance of the tears? What should I do now that I have a greater understanding?

Through self-disclosure the patient divulges hidden aspects of himself about the past, current life, fantasies, or held-back feelings about members. Its value lies in sharing, which reduces isolation, demonstrates trust, and is often the first step of a process in which patient and group explore the ramifications of 'secrets' in their lives.

GROUP THERAPY IN PRACTICE

What happens in a group depends on the leaders, members, ambitions that both have, time available, and the negotiation of inherent developmental phases. It is history written by many hands, an evolution of nature shaped by nurture.

The role of the leaders

Essentially, leaders assist members to realize the group's potential. The effective group has the capacity to develop from a position of apprehension and relative ignorance to a maturity typified by solidarity, trust, and confidence. The more the group's culture approximates to the latter, the better able it will be in achieving results. The leader acts an expert guide in this progression (Aveline 1993). (See also the classic account of the 'work group' by Bion 1961.)

Two therapists are generally better than one since they share the rigours of leadership and place multiple perspectives at the service of the group: their first task is to create and maintain the group, the second to promote a facilitative culture. The leaders determine the givens of the group—size, frequency and time of meeting, duration, and whether open or closed. They arrange for a comfortable, quiet room free from interruption. They select and prepare members as previously described.

Once the group is launched the leaders have many means at their disposal to help members to realize the group's potential especially by promoting a climate of spontaneity and authenticity. The leaders encourage members to address each other directly; create a space for reticent members; are respectful and even-handed; address important neglected issues; adjust the group's pace to minimize harm; foster the group's sense of responsibility for its actions and direction; seek to release therapeutic forces in members and in the group as a whole; encourage members to act determinedly at opportune moments; model openness, spontaneity, and honesty in a responsible way; and cultivate a reflective, analytic attitude. Exercising these means effectively requires a keen appreciation of the continuing experience of each member and the group generally, its history and developmental phase.

Developmental phases

A group in which therapeutic factors operate optimally does not arise automatically; chaos and demoralization can occur. Although each group is unique and therefore somewhat unpredictable in its development, clinical observation and systematic research suggest that groups pass through a series of stages before achieving maturity. The pattern is not necessarily orderly; there may be movement to and fro between stages and not every patient may be in the same stage at the same time. Schutz's (1958) illuminating account, although dating back to the 1950s, is still a most useful model.

In–out is the stage of dependency. The leaders have created the group and members rely heavily on them, awaiting guidance from experts who are seen as knowledgeable. Dependency is heightened by the group's apparent uncertainty. There is no explicit agenda; each patient is more aware of his personal goals than of the group's to evolve into a mature system. Because of his need to survive, the patient is on his best behaviour, participating but superficially and diligently to avoid risks.

Top–bottom is the stage of conflict in which counter-dependence replaces dependence. The leaders inevitably disappoint the group since they are not ideal and cannot be relied on. The trainee therapist may be seduced into this role and collude with the patients' infantile wishes by attempting to be all-loving and wise. The experienced therapist, however, provides cues that he expects the group to assume responsibility for itself.

Counter-dependence manifests itself as conflict and competitiveness. The patient has to secure his place other than through dependency and he has rivals. This is a time of disappointment, frustration, and anger, the last directed at both therapists and fellow patients. Commonly, the former will be criticized for 'not telling us what to do'. Differences between them will be accentuated through splitting. Unpunctuality and absenteeism also reflect patient frustration. Peer criticism manifests as sniping, scapegoating and impatience. Carl Rogers (1973), in discussing the comparable stage of an encounter group, suggests that expression of negative feelings is the patient's best way to test the group's trustworthiness: 'Can I really express myself, even negatively?' The expression of positive feelings is more hazardous because of possible rejection.

Top–bottom is stressful but confers some benefits. Patients learn that they can express anger without disastrous repercussions, this leading to confidence in risk-taking.

Near–far is the stage of intimacy. With a more realistic view of the leaders and disappointment in their lack of omnipotence worked through, conflict between patients wanes. Successful passage through the top–bottom phase brings relief. Patients 'pulling one another apart' is replaced by 'pulling together'. Now the quest is for intimacy. Can I get closer (nearer) to others? In an effort to achieve this, the group shows greater trust. Negative feelings may still be expressed but they now occur in a more secure framework, based on mutual understanding.

Problems arising during group development

The passage between creation and transformation into a mature group has taken many weeks, even some months, and called for skilful leadership. Threats to its welfare are encountered even by experienced therapists. Dropping out is the most serious. Loss of membership is inevitable no matter how rigorous the selection. The group's morale is undermined when a patient departs and others may become ambivalent about continuing. Eight patients can stand the loss of one or two peers but greater attrition calls for replacement. Two useful caveats are pertinent. Addition of a pair of members simultaneously is less anxiety-provoking for the newcomers. A new patient should not be introduced into a group which is in a state of crisis as there is a danger that he will be scapegoated. All newcomers require the same preparation as foundation members, plus focused help to examine their expectations of entering an established group.

Absenteeism and lateness also undermine a group's welfare. Regular, punctual attendance is crucial and the leaders need to reinforce its importance repeatedly, both by comment and behaviour. A member unable to attend or knowing he will arrive late should inform the therapist. Absenteeism or unpunctuality invariably represent important communications: resistance, anger, defiance, testing (does it care about me?), and the like. For example, Jenny repeatedly arrived late and demanded a résumé of events she had missed. The group soon resented her but she seemed to thrive on this insisting that punctuality was not essential. Later it became clear that only by acting provocatively could Jenny feel part of the group.

Drop-outs, missed meetings, and tardiness are matters of concern and always need to be dealt with head-on.

The mature working group

Following this developmental sequence, the group becomes a mature working system (Bion 1961). Hitherto, a principal goal has been cohesiveness. With this achieved—although always threatened through, *inter alia*, regression, stagnation, and conflict—patients tackle their problems and those of their peers. Now the therapeutic factors discussed earlier are fully operative, the most central being insight and learning from interpersonal action. Therapy is facilitated by a here and now focus, that is, what transpires in the group, between patients, between patients and leaders, and between each patient and the group. Change is a consequence of patients recognizing and evaluating ways they relate and then taking action to change. The pre-therapy list of goals compiled by the patient helps to emphasize a future orientation, reinforced by periodic review. As the patient learns more about himself he is encouraged to be future-minded: What options do I have? How will I choose between them? How will I translate my choice into action?

A there and then focus is discouraged. 'There' refers to events outside the group, most commonly crises. The danger prevails that the group may become crisis-bound, the patient with the most pressing crisis dominating the session and the group bouncing from one crisis to another. Crises are indeed inevitable and may be significant either in terms of individual or group dynamics but an exclusive focus on them jeopardizes the core purpose, that of individual change catalysed by group interaction. When such events arise the leaders bring them into a here-and-now context.

'Then' implies an historical inquiry, a search for causes of current behaviour. The danger here lies in preoccupation with the sources. A patient's disclosure of his family and personal history is helpful both in allowing members to know him better and for greater self-understanding but the group can get bogged down in unlimited archaeological exploration.

During the group's early life the leaders had the task of steering the patients into the here and now and explaining its relevance. In the mature group the pattern is more automatic although the leaders may be required to cut into there and then activity. There are infinite ways to maintain a here and now approach, the choice depending on clinical circumstances. Some illustrations follow:

'Who do you feel closest to/most intimidated by/most dominated by/etc. in the group?' (The patient has referred to intimacy, fear of others, or submissiveness.)

'Who in the group is most like you with respect to indecisiveness/passivity/ aggressiveness, etc.?' (Patient has indicated that he has one of these traits.)

'What has been the most difficult thing to share with the group today?' (The patient has mentioned his difficulty in acting spontaneously.)

Here and now comments may also focus on the group as a whole:

'Each of you seems buried in private thoughts.' (Following an extended silence.)

'How does each person see the meeting today?' (Half-way through a tense session.)

'How do you feel about Peter's absence?' (Peter has not arrived after 15 minutes and has not left any message.)

Another feature of the mature group is its ability to examine and understand its own process or dynamics (i.e. the how and why of the group's events, communications, interactions, and moods). Beyond what occurs overtly, the group operates at several levels. Content is obviously necessary and things must happen but this is not sufficient. The group needs to examine carefully events in the context of how and why—the level of process.

Commenting on process is mainly the leaders' task. Patients are too mired in the actual happenings in the group to view clearly what lies behind them; they may also resist immediate, emotionally charged interaction. This task is undoubtedly demanding for leaders who need to keep the group process moving forward. Even Whitaker's (1985) excellent account on group dynamics does not suffice to cover the myriad complexities involved. Group analysis has produced many useful concepts including group matrix, mirroring, resonance, polarization, and scapegoating (Aveline 1990; Roberts and Pines 1992). The therapist, however, gains much of this knowledge through clinical training (to which we turn later in this chapter).

Commonly made comments on group dynamics follow. These may be addressed to the group as a whole, to a subgroup or to a particular patient.

Group-directed

'There is a tension in the room today as if we were all on tenterhooks awaiting Jim's arrival.' (An absent member has not informed the group that he would not attend.)

'The group is split, those supporting Claire and those critical of her.'

'The group is being protective of Ann. Perhaps there is part of them in Ann they would like to be protected too.' (Projection and mirroring.)

'It feels like we are unable to identify with Jack and his problem.' (Silence following his disclosure about his homosexuality.)

'The group is finding fault with Jim for not being entirely open. Surely this is something that everyone in the group is struggling with.' (Scapegoating.)

'The group has moved completely away from Jane as if her distress is too painful to bear.' (The group is in flight, as described by Bion 1961.)

Patient-directed

'You come across as extremely angry in talking about Paul's lateness.'

'You tell us things are O.K. but your body tells another story; you look shaky and tense.'

'I have the feeling that you're saying to the group "I want the group's attention on my terms or not at all".'

Since the group roams boundlessly, an infinite number of comments is possible. Some general points apply to the process that serve as useful guidelines. The main objective is to facilitate learning, not to display the therapist's observational skills, his wit (although there is a distinct place for humour; see Bloch *et al.* 1983), or his cleverness. A patient only benefits from the therapist's comments if he understands, integrates, and can make use of them. The clearer the link between here and now content and the comment the better. Putting it another way, the more inferential and obscure the contribution the more difficult for the patient and the less effective its impact. A direct statement is preferable to a question. In the face of uncertainty it is reasonable to preface a comment with: 'I have the feeling that . . .' or 'I could be off the mark but . . .' 'Why' questions are unhelpful and again should be replaced by a statement (e.g. 'James seems critical of you today' rather than 'why do you think James is critical of you today?') Comments on non-verbal behaviour like seating arrangements, lateness, change in appearance, or silences are as important as those on verbal content and need to be made regularly.

Timing must be appropriate and generally is best related to here and now material while this is fresh. Sometimes, it is better deferred to a point when the patient is less distressed, the level of inference less ambiguous, or the therapist better able to highlight a consistent pattern. For instance, it may be more effective to wait a couple of meetings before commenting: 'Chris has been relatively quiet for the last few meetings and participates only when invited. His mind seems to be elsewhere.' There is also a risk of flooding the patient with comments to the extent that he becomes perplexed.

The written summary

This technique has been described fully elsewhere (Yalom *et al.* 1975). In brief, the therapist prepares a brief account of each meeting (one to two pages) and mails it to members. The summary contains a narrative of the main events interleaved with commentary. Although the technique has not been objectively tested, therapists who have prepared many such summaries are impressed by their utility. They serve several functions: help to bridge sessions; offer a second chance to the therapist to press home a point made in the meeting; enable him to reinforce group norms; and facilitate new observations not conceived of during the meeting. Further, the summary allows an absent member to keep up with the group. The therapist also profits from its preparation; since it is a 'public' document, he must ensure accuracy and clarity. Written reports also have a role in training (Aveline 1986).

Ending therapy

When a patient should end treatment is as much of an issue in group as in individual therapy. The concept of cure is raised. Should a patient stop treatment when he has achieved goals originally set? Should he 'graduate' with a certain fund of knowledge and experience on the premise his 'education' will continue thereafter?

The termination process differs in group therapy compared to individual treatment. The reason is obvious; the group can resort to a jury system to decide the questions of when and how. Ideally, a patient raises the issue and asks members for their reactions. If there is consensus, it is likely that termination is reasonable. Disagreement suggests it is premature. The process of leaving should last some weeks enabling the graduate to share what he has achieved, his hopes, and why he feels ready to depart. Both he and the group also need time to say farewell and to work through separation.

Termination based on consensus is also a time to celebrate. The patient feels confident to manage independently. The remaining members should be urged to note the change and to take encouragement from it; they are thus reminded that they are also potential graduates and the group is beneficial (the therapeutic factor of instillation of hope).

The above applies to an open group. In a closed one termination is often predetermined, all members ending at the same time. An open group may also agree to terminate as a group on a set date because of circumstantial factors such as therapists moving to other jobs. As the group mourns the loss of a member who leaves so it must work through its own termination. Approaching the group's end is akin to dying; it is a sad period and needs to be faced fully.

It must also be accepted that the leaders in conjunction with the group have to discharge a member in rare cases. Reasons for this drastic step include repeated breaches of rules, coming drunk to meetings, and forming an intimate relationship with a peer which they refuse to discuss.

OTHER APPLICATIONS OF THE GROUP PROCESS

Space does not permit a consideration of alternative theoretical models that have been applied to out-patient groups. These include, for example, the psychoanalytic, existential, cognitive-behavioural, and one derived from the observations of Bion. The reader is referred to the Recommended Reading.

Although we have focused on the long-term, out-patient group, the group process has also been deployed in in- and day-patient settings, its mode of application dependent mainly on whether the unit is run on therapeutic community (Kennard 1983) or more conventional lines. In the latter, careful attention has to be paid to aims that can be realistically achieved. Thus, for example, in an acute ward where a patient's stay rarely exceeds two to three weeks it would be fanciful to expect that group membership could exert any radical changes. In this instance a model is needed which enables realistically set goals to be accomplished.

One such model, devised by Maxmen (1978), involves in-patients in a small, open group where they are guided to 'think clinically and respond effectively to the consequences of their illnesses'; that is, they learn to identify maladaptive behaviours and to avoid circumstances likely to precipitate recurrence of symptoms. Maxmen sets this objective on the premise that in a brief admission the primary goal is to modify efficiently a patient's disturbed behaviour so that he can return to the community without delay.

In similar vein, Yalom (1983) advocates considering each session on a psychiatric ward as complete in itself so recognizing temporal constraints and a rapidly changing membership. Differentiating two levels of psychotherapy he has devised two distinct approaches, one or high-functioning, the other for low-functioning patients. This advance gets away from the 'one-size fits all', an impediment to effective in-patient group therapy (Klein *et al.* 1994).

Therapeutic factors like instillation of hope, acceptance, universality, and altruism (see earlier) are especially promoted. In fact, these were found previously by Maxmen (1973) to be valued most highly by in-patients receiving brief group therapy. Leszcz *et al.* (1985) found similar perceptions in their patients. Other factors such as self-understanding do not feature as prominently on the premise that patients by virtue of their psychiatric state are not able to profit from their use.

In contrast, the small group conducted in a therapeutic community in which a patient's stay (or daily attendance) usually extends over several months and a specific selection policy operates, can function more similarly to a long-term out-patient group, that is, have as a primary goal not only symptomatic relief but also personality change. But even in these circumstances, the approach will not necessarily be identical (Kennard 1983, 1988). Clearly, detailed attention has to be paid to the continuous and varied contact experienced by the community's members in other group activities and in a host of informal ways.

A particular form of group meeting, the community group, may also be convened in either the conventional psychiatric ward or in the therapeutic community. Customarily, patients and staff assemble on one or more occasions during the week for periods ranging from 30 to 60 minutes. Despite their common application community meetings remain conceptually unsatisfactory (Kisch *et al.* 1981). Both patients and staff are frequently unclear about their purpose. Should they be regarded as therapeutic fora, say the equivalent of the small group? Or should they be confined to administrative matters (e.g. to sort out the legendary washing-up rota!). Or should they seek to identify and deal with tensions that exist between patients or between patients and staff that, if ignored, might jeopardize the unit's overall functioning.

The most appropriate way to tackle this sort of question is to identify the objectives of the ward's therapeutic programme as a whole and then to ascertain the specified methods whereby the community group can contribute to that programme. A great deal of informed conceptual thinking is still needed before the community group can confidently gain its proper place. A most useful achievement in this context is Kreeger's (1975) edited volume, *The large group* (see Recommended Reading).

The whole area of in-patient group therapy has deservedly gained more attention since the 1980s, both from the clinician and researcher. The interested reader is recommended to consult two illuminating reviews, those by Leszcz (1986), who helpfully stresses the differences between out-patient and inpatient groups, and by Klein *et al.* (1994), who concentrate on the empirical literature and, in addition, examine the in-patient group's application to a range of homogeneous clinical areas such as substance abuse, schizophrenia, social anxiety, and antisocial behaviour. Pam and Kemker (1993) offer eminently practical guidelines for the task of recruiting in-patients to the therapy group and promoting their active participation.

There is a place for structured exercises in group therapy; these stem mainly from the traditions of psychodrama. Various forms of creative expression can be incorporated into group practice many of which are ideally suited to the group format. Apart from psychodrama, dance, music, and art have been tried. The interested reader is referred to Davies (1988) and to Kaplan and Sadock (1993) for contributions on this aspect of group therapy.

A chapter on group therapy would be incomplete without mention of the self-help group. Although the purist may demur from designating this application of the group process as treatment, sufficient common ground is shared by self-help and therapeutic groups in terms of membership, underlying theoretical assumptions, and strategies applied. The self-help group, however, is distinctive in the sense that, classically, it is founded and run by its members without professional leaders (although some organizations do consult for advice). Alcoholics Anonymous, one of the most notable examples, has a membership composed exclusively of people dependent on alcohol who meet in order to provide mutual help and support. Such a group is perfectly compatible with professionally led group therapy. Indeed, there are good grounds to suggest that the two group forms are synergistic (Yalom *et al.* 1978).

In general, group therapists would do well to co-operate with the self-help movement since it is clear that the need for their expertise far exceeds the resources they can provide; the self-help group can contribute substantially to meeting some of that need. Research on self-help groups is one means to clarify their role in complementing conventional group therapy (and psychotherapy in general) (Goodman and Jacobs 1994). Rootes and Aanes (1982) have offered a useful conceptual framework for understanding the self-help group, while Lieberman (1986) has drawn an illuminating comparison between it and group therapy.

TRAINING

Training in group therapy comprises supervised practice, observation of skilled therapists, participation in a training group and knowledge of the relevant literature on theory and technique (Aveline 1988).

A supervised experience is the most important. Commonly, a pair of co-therapists meet with an experienced clinician at weekly intervals. Supervision should begin at the time of patient selection; as noted earlier the success of a group is heavily dependent on this and trainees require guidance. Supervisory sessions ideally take place soon after each meeting while its events are still fresh in mind.

Two difficulties in supervision are the time taken for the trainees to report what occurred and omission of material which may embarrass or threaten them (selective inattention obstructs supervision in all psychotherapy). A method to reduce both is the written summary described earlier (Bloch *et al.* 1975). The summary sent to patients is also given to the supervisor who reads the account before he meets the trainees. The leaders are less defensive as they have already 'exposed' themselves and can thus provide a more honest account of their participation. Supervision is best continued throughout the group's life.

Before and during their practical experience, leaders need to acquire knowledge of the salient aspects of theory and technique including pertinent research findings. Leading a group for the first time should not be like jumping into the deep end. Without basic knowledge, the therapist lacks a coherent framework in which to work and adopts poor techniques. Familiarity with various theories is also necessary. Inevitably, a trainee selects the approach prevalent in the institution in which he is being trained. As we have sparse knowledge on the relative effectiveness of different schools, a newcomer would probably be advantaged in applying the model described above which tends to the eclectic and non-doctrinaire. Later, attachment to a particular framework may arise which can be incorporated into her clinical work (see Recommended Reading for texts on theory).

Trainees often become members of a training group in order to become acquainted first-hand with what it is like to participate. They acquire valuable information about group dynamics as well as recognize how they come across to peers. The aim is twofold—the group conveys to the therapist an idea of what patients experience and uses the opportunity for self-exploration. Whether individual therapy is also a requisite for training is debatable; a thorough training group experience probably suffices.

Viewing skilled therapists through a one-way screen or on video tape has a place. The former is preferable as discussion with the therapists of their methods and of group events follows immediately.

SUMMARY

Group therapy has become an established mode of treatment in psychiatry. In this chapter we have concentrated on the long-term group, whose goal is personality change, as the optimal initial training experience. An interpersonal model has been offered; training in other schools may follow depending on personal preference and clinical need.

We should remember that a group approach is applicable to diverse clinical contexts, from the psychiatric ward to the self-help group. Space has permitted only brief mention of this range. Again, the recommended reading contains a guide to these applications.

APPENDIX 1: GUIDELINES FOR GROUP PSYCHOTHERAPY

Outlined below are features of group therapy you need to know about before making a commitment. They form the basis of a successful group and we believe members should be guided by them.

(1) The group works on the assumption that an important problem for all its members is difficulty in establishing and maintaining close and satisfying relationships. Members may experience their problems with other people in a variety of ways.

(2) The group is a special place where you can explore in an honest way your relationships with other members and with the therapists. If you have difficulty in the way you relate then a situation which encourages honest, open communication provides you with a good opportunity to learn valuable things about yourself.

(3) It is important that you are honest with your feelings especially towards other members and the therapists. In many ways this is an essential

element of group therapy and involves taking risks. This becomes progressively more possible as you develop trust in the group and feel comfortable in participating.

(4) Group therapy gives you the opportunity to try out new ways of behaving. It is important to recognize that this is probably the safest place in which you can experiment. The group tolerates experimentation and provides feedback about its effectiveness.

(5) Stumbling blocks occur along the way. As there is no agenda or formal structure to meetings, you may initially feel puzzled, even discouraged. We encourage you to weather the first few weeks. Working on personal problems and developing new ways of relating is not easy, indeed can be stressful. Group therapy may involve pain and distress but there are also many lighter moments.

(6) We shall ask you to identify the main difficulty you experience in your relationships with others and that you will be working on. Every four months, we will review progress by asking you to assess any change with the rest of the group, including the therapists; they will be invited to offer feedback. New goals will then be set to cover the next four months. We hope this will prove helpful and enable us to maintain focus.

(7) A basic aim is that each member accomplishes his set goals. Since problems requiring change have usually been many years in the making, members should commit themselves to at least six months' membership. Should there be unavoidable reasons for leaving, it is important to give notice as early as possible so that you and the others can come to terms with the departure.

(8) In the event of contact between members outside the group, we ask you to share this so that the work is kept within the group context.

(9) Regular attendance and punctuality are crucial. If you know you will be unable to attend a session or that you will be late, a telephone message spares members' and therapists' anxiety.

(10) What happens in the group is confidential. All members are duty-bound to respect that confidentiality. (The reader is directed to Appelbaum and Greer 1993, and Roback *et al.* 1993 for interesting commentaries on this important aspect of the group's culture.)

(11) Smoking and drinking are not permitted in the group.

REFERENCES

Appelbaum, P. and Greer, A. (1993). Confidentiality in group therapy. *Hospital and Community Psychiatry*, **44**, 311–12.

Aveline, M. (1990). The group therapies in perspective. *Free Associations*, **19** 77–101.

Aveline, M. (1986). The use of written reports in a brief group psychotherapy training. *International Journal of Group Psychotherapy*, **36**, 477–82.

Aveline, M. (1988). Issues in the training of group therapists. In *Group therapy in Britain*, (ed. M. Aveline and W. Dryden). Open University Press, Milton Keynes.

Aveline, M. (1993). Principles of leadership in brief training groups for mental health professionals. *International Journal of Group Psychotherapy*, **43**, 107–29.

Aveline, M. (1994) Assessment for focal therapy. In *The art and science of assessment* (ed. C. Mace). Routledge, London.

Bion, W. R. (1961). *Experiences in groups*. Tavistock, London.

Bloch, S. (1979). Assessment of patients for psychotherapy, *British Journal of Psychiatry*, **135**, 193–208.

Bloch, S. and Crouch, E. (1985). *Therapeutic factors in group psychotherapy*. Oxford University Press, Oxford.

Bloch, S., Brown, S., Davis, K., and Dishotsky, N. (1975). The use of a written summary in group psychotherapy supervision. *American Journal of Psychiatry*, **132**, 1055–7.

Bloch, S., Browning, S., and McGrath, G. (1983). Humour in group psychotherapy. *British Journal of Medical Psychology*, **56**, 89–97.

Bond, G. R. and Lieberman, M. A. (1978). Selection criteria for group therapy. In *Controversy in psychiatry*, (ed. J. Brady and H. K. Brodie). Saunders, Philadelphia.

Burrow, T. (1974). In *Group psychotherapy and group function*, (ed. M. Rosenbaum and M. Berger). Basic Books, New York.

Corsini, R. J. and Rosenberg, B. (1955). Mechanisms of group psychotherapy: processes and dynamics. *Journal of Abnormal and Social Psychology*, **51**, 406–11.

Crouch, E., Bloch, S. and Wanlass, J. (1994). Therapeutic factors: Interpersonal and intrapersonal mechanisms. In *Handbook of group psychotherapy*, (ed. A. Fuhriman and G. Burlingame). Wiley, New York.

Davies, M. (1988). Psychodrama group therapy. In *Group therapy in Britain*, (ed. M. Aveline and W. Dryden). Open University Press, Milton Keynes.

Flores, P. and Mahon, L. (1993). The treatment of addiction in group psychotherapy. *International Journal of Group Psychotherapy*, **43**, 143–56.

Foulkes, S. H. (1946). Group analysis in a military neurosis centre. *Lancet*, **i**, 303–10.

Frank, J. D. and Frank, J. B. (1991). *Persuasion and healing: a comparative study of psychotherapy*, (3rd edn). Johns Hopkins University Press, Baltimore.

Freud, S. (1955). *Group psychology and the analysis of the ego*. Hogarth, London.

Goodman, G. and Jacobs, M. (1994). The self-help, mutual-support group. In *Handbook of group psychotherapy*, (ed. A. Fuhriman and G. Burlingame). Wiley, New York.

Graves, J. (1993). Living with mania: A study of outpatient group psychotherapy for bipolar patients. *American Journal of Psychotherapy*, **47**, 113–26.

Gruen, D. (1993). A group psychotherapy approach to postpartum depression. *International Journal of Group Psychotherapy*, **43**, 191–203.

Jung, C. (1974). In *Group psychotherapy and group function*, (ed. M. Rosenbaum and M. Berger). Basic Books, New York.

Kanas, N. (1986). Group therapy with schizophrenics: A review of controlled studies. *International Journal of Group Psychotherapy*, **36**, 339–51.

Kanas, N. (1993). Group psychotherapy with bipolar patients: A review and synthesis. *International Journal of Group Psychotherapy*, **43**, 321–33.

Kanas, N. and Barr, M. A. (1982). Short-term homogenous group therapy for schizophrenic inpatients: A questionnaire evaluation. *Group*, **6**, 32–8.

Kaul, T. and Bednar, R. (1994). Pretraining and structure: Parallel lines yet to meet. In *Handbook of group psychotherapy*, (ed. A. Fuhriman and G. Burlingame). Wiley, New York.

Kennard, D. (1983). *An introduction to therapeutic communities*. Routledge & Kegan Paul, London.

Kennard, D. (1988). The therapeutic community. In *Group therapy in Britain*, (ed. M. Aveline and W. Dryden). Open University Press, Milton Keynes.

Kisch, I., Kroll, J., Gross, R., and Carey, K. (1981). In-patient community meetings: problems and purposes. *British Journal of Medical Psychology*, **54**, 35–40.

Klein, R., Brabender, V., and Fallon, A. (1994). Inpatient group therapy. In *Handbook of group psychotherapy*, (ed. A. Fuhriman and G. Burlingame). Wiley, New York.

Leszcz, M. (1986). Inpatient groups. In *Psychiatry update*, Vol. 5, (ed. A. Frances and R. Hales). American Psychiatric Press, Washington, DC.

Leszcz, M., Yalom, I.D., and Nordern, M. (1985). The value of inpatient group psychotherapy: Patients' perceptions. *International Journal of Group Psychotherapy*, **35**, 411–33.

Lewin, K. (1951). *Field theory in social science*. Harper, New York.

Lieberman, M. A. (1986). Self-help groups and psychiatry. In *Psychiatry update*, Vol. 5, (ed. A. Frances and R. Hales). American Psychiatric Press, Washington, DC.

Lieberman, M. A. and Yalom, I. D. (1992). Brief group psychotherapy for the spousally bereaved: A controlled study. *International Journal of Group Psychotherapy*, **42**, 117–32.

Maxmen, J. (1973). Group therapy as viewed by hospitalized patients. *Archives of General Psychiatry*, **28**, 404–8.

Maxmen, J. (1978). An educative model for in-patient group therapy. *International Journal of Group Psychotherapy*, **29**, 321–38.

McCallum, M., Piper, W. E., and Morin, H. (1993). Affect and outcome in short-term therapy for loss. *International Journal of Group Psychotherapy*, **43**, 303–19.

Pam, A. and Kemker, S. (1993). The captive group: Guidelines for group therapists in the inpatient setting. *International Journal of Group Psychotherapy*, **43**, 419-438.

Piper, W. (1994). Client variables. In *Handbook of group psychotherapy*, (ed. A. Fuhriman and G. Burlingame). Wiley, New York.

Pratt, J. H. (1974) In *Group psychotherapy and group function* (ed. M. Rosenbaum and M. Berger). Basic Books, New York.

Ratigan, B. and Aveline, M. (1988). Interpersonal group therapy. In *Group therapy in Britain*, (ed. M. Aveline and W. Dryden). Open University Press, Milton Keynes.

Roback, H., Purdon, S., Ochoa, E., and Bloch, F. (1993). Effects of professional affiliation in group therapists' confidentiality attitudes and behaviours. *Bulletin of the American Academy of Psychiatry and the Law*, **21**, 147-53.

Roberts, J. and Pines, M. (1992) Group-analytic psychotherapy. *International Journal of Group Psychotherapy*, **42**, 469-94.

Rogers, C. (1973). *On encounter groups*. Penguin, Harmondsworth.

Rootes, L. and Aanes, D. (1992). A conceptual framework for understanding self-help groups. *Hospital and Community Psychiatry*, **43**, 379-81.

Scheidlinger, S. (1994). An overview of nine decades of group psychotherapy. *Hospital and Community Psychiatry*, **45**, 217-25.

Schutz, W. C. (1958). *Firo: a three-dimensional theory of interpersonal behavior*. Rinehart, New York.

Stinchfield, R., Owen, P. and Winters, K. (1994). Group therapy for substance abuse: A review of the empirical research. In *Handbook of group psychotherapy*, (ed. A. Fuhriman and G. Burlingame). Wiley, New York.

Sullivan, H. S. (1953). *The interpersonal theory of psychiatry*. Norton, New York.

Whitaker, D. S. (1985). *Using groups to help people*. Routledge & Kegan Paul, London.

Yalom, I. D. (1983). *Inpatient group psychotherapy*. Basic Books, New York.

Yalom, I. D. (1985). *The theory and practice of group psychotherapy*, (3rd edn). Basic Books, New York.

Yalom, I. D. and Vinogradov, S. (1988). Bereavement groups: techniques and themes. *International Journal of Group Psychotherapy*, **38**, 419-46.

Yalom, I. D., Brown, S. and Bloch, S. (1975). The written summary as a group psychotherapy technique. *Archives of General Psychiatry*, **32**, 605-13.

Yalom, I. D., Bloch, S., Bond, G., Qualls, B., and Zimmerman, E. (1978). Alcoholics in interactional group therapy: an outcome study. *Archives of General Psychiatry*, **35**, 419-25.

RECOMMENDED READING

Aveline, M. and Dryden, W. (ed.) (1988). *Group therapy in Britain*. Open University Press, Milton Keynes. (Covers a range of theoretical models and applications as well as chapters on research and training.)

Bion, W. R. (1961). *Experiences in groups*. Tavistock, London. (The 'Tavistock' approach in which the theoretical ideas of Melanie Klein are central.)

Foulkes, S. H. and Anthony, E.J. (1973). *Group psychotherapy*. Penguin, Harmondsworth. (The approach of the London Institute of Group Analysis and influenced by psychoanalytic concepts and techniques.) *See also*: Foulkes, S. H. (1975). *Group analytic psychotherapy: methods and principles*. Gordon & Breach, London (Similar in content to *Group psychotherapy*.)

Fuhriman, A. and Burlingame, G. (ed.) (1994). *Handbook of group psychotherapy*. Wiley, New York. (A most comprehensive volume, which presents a synthesis of empirical and clinical research on every conceivable aspect of group therapy.)

Kaplan, H. I. and Sadock, B. J. (ed.) (1993). *Comprehensive group psychotherapy*, 3rd edn. Williams & Wilkins, Baltimore. (Contains chapters dealing with therapy of special groups such as married couples, adolescents, and the elderly, as well as chapters on different schools.)

Rosenbaum, M. and Berger, M. M. (ed.) (1975). *Group psychotherapy and group function*. Basic Books, New York. (A general text containing over 60 chapters on all aspects of group therapy including several interesting contributions on its history.)

Whitaker, D. (1985). *Using groups to help people*. Routledge & Kegan Paul, London. (A clear, comprehensive account of group work by a leading figure in the field; useful practical orientation.)

Yalom, I. D. (1985). *The theory and practice of group psychotherapy*, (3rd edn). Basic Books, New York. (An excellent account of the theory and practice of interactive group therapy, with an important section on therapeutic factors.)

5

Crisis intervention

JOHN BANCROFT AND CYNTHIA GRAHAM

Chapters 2 and 4 dealt with psychotherapies that are long term and have personality change as a main aim. In this chapter John Bancroft and Cynthia Graham focus on a completely different form of therapy, which is short term and designed to help a person who, overwhelmed by some stress, is in a state of crisis. In the first section they cover concepts basic to crisis intervention; then follows a description of two main forms of therapeutic help—intensive care and crisis counselling, each with its own series of strategies. The emphasis throughout is on practical application.

'Crisis intervention' as a concept has almost as many meanings as there are people writing about it. Moreover, the term has been applied to a diverse range of groups, for example, survivors of disasters (Joseph *et al.* 1992) and of sexual assault (Ellis 1983), and medical and surgical patients (Viney *et al.* 1985*a*); and settings, including telephone and walk-in counselling services, emergency psychiatric clinics (Winter *et al.* 1987) and residential crisis services (Stroul 1988).

The term 'crisis intervention' originated in relation to people with stable personalities and a history of adequate coping resources who are facing major but transitory difficulties (Caplan 1961). Although some of the groups listed above would fall into this category, it is clear that most patients presenting as psychiatric emergencies would not. Indeed, the applicability of crisis theory and intervention to psychiatric patients has been questioned (Szmukler 1987). However, in spite of the confusion surrounding crisis intervention, it has served a useful purpose in drawing attention to an aspect of health care where there is overlap among the roles of psychiatrist, casualty doctor, general practitioner, social worker, probation officer, and lay counsellor. While each of these can bring particular professional skill to the problem, there are also non-specialist skills that most people in crisis need. It is this non-specialist role that will be mainly considered below.

Our purpose is to provide a framework for carrying out crisis intervention and to put it in a medical treatment context. Literature on the subject is voluminous (for useful reviews, see Langsley 1981; Aguilera and Messick 1982; Hobbs 1984; Szmukler 1987), but unfortunately provides little in the way of practical guidance. Our focus will be on the use of the approach for those with a history of adaptive functioning but who currently face a major life crisis.

This chapter is written in an eclectic spirit but with a behavioural bias. While it cannot deal with all clinical contingencies, it does aim to provide a practical framework that can be built on and adapted. The approach was developed in a particular setting—a general hospital psychiatric service dealing predominantly with the patient who has attempted suicide; it evolved, however, within a multidisciplinary team and has wider relevance than to this setting alone. Much of it involves 'common sense' for which we make no apology. The field has been hampered by therapists' need to maintain special expertise for the sake of their professional identity.

Before describing the approach, we outline the main tenets of crisis theory. Crisis can be usefully regarded as a failure in or inadequacy of coping. What do we mean by coping and what happens when it fails? What problems commonly over-extend coping resources? When is it appropriate to consider someone in crisis as 'ill' or in need of treatment? How far should we go in taking over responsibility for other people's problems?

CRISIS THEORY

The evolution of crisis theory has been well outlined by Hobbs (1984), who noted contributions from social psychiatry, ego psychology, and learning theory. A most influential pioneering theorist, Gerald Caplan (1961), defined a crisis as occurring:

when a person faces an obstacle to important life-goals that is, for a time, insurmountable through the utilization of customary methods of problem solving. A period of disorganization ensues, a period of upset, during which many abortive attempts at solution are made.

The crisis is seen as a turning point or decisive moment: if the situation is resolved effectively the person may have learnt new skills which can be applied in future crises; on the other hand, if there is a poor outcome, maladaptive behaviour and possibly psychiatric disturbance may ensue. Caplan (1961) emphasized that crisis is self-limiting, lasting four to six weeks. It therefore calls for immediate but relatively short term help.

Most of the initial theorizing and practical developments in crisis intervention occurred in the United States; it is helpful to consider the social and political context in which this happened. The American pattern of health care, dependent for the most part on costly private practice or health insurance schemes, inevitably led to a social and political reaction in the 1960s. Free 'walk-in' clinics emerged in many cities, staffed by liberally minded, socially conscious professionals. This was followed by massive federal development of community mental health centres, run by staff keen to reject the health establishment on ideological grounds. As a consequence, this pattern of care developed determined as much by the need to discard traditional medical values and methods as by any clearly formulated set of principles. It is not surprising that conceptual confusion resulted, some order emerging years later. The need for alternatives to customary medically based care is difficult to refute, but because of our prevailing social structure, such care is commonly sought in medical settings as well as in non-medical agencies such as social work departments or Samaritan-type organizations. How to deal with a person in crisis is therefore an important matter for medical and for other helping professionals. For the doctor, there is the additional need to clarify the relationship between this type of help and conventional medical treatment. And for the non-medical counsellor, the question arises as to when to involve medical personnel.

BASIC CONCEPTS

Coping and failure to cope

'Coping behaviour' is how we respond to a problem or threatening situation. Traditional accounts of coping emphasized traits or 'styles', in other words, stable personality features. In contrast, theorists like Lazarus (1993), depicting coping as a process and acknowledging that stable coping styles do exist, stress that coping behaviour is mainly situation-specific. Moreover, the role of cognitive appraisal in mediating reactions to a stressful situation is crucial. Coping depends on an appraisal of whether anything can be done to alter the situation (Lazarus 1993). There are two types of coping processes:

1) *'Problem-focused' coping*

If appraisal suggests that something can be done to deal with a problem, problem-focused coping will most likely be used. This is considered further on p. 129.

2) *'Emotion-focused' coping*

If appraisal suggests that nothing can be done, a coping process that changes only the way we interpret or attend to a situation may be deployed. Denial and distancing are obvious examples. With denial, perception of reality is so distorted that the problem is no longer seen to exist. This may be effective if the problem resolves spontaneously but usually it only postpones and aggravates the problem. Regression, in which a person resorts to behaviour learned at an earlier stage of development, may be a helpful strategy, at least temporarily, with responsibility being transferred to others. Resort to alcohol or drug overdosage may be similarly used in this way. Another coping strategy is inertia, a state of inaction based on the judgement that there is nothing effective to be done; while inertia is appropriate at times, it usually reflects a feeling of hopelessness typical of depressive states.

Sex differences in coping styles have been found, with women more likely to show emotion-focused and men more problem-focused coping (e.g. Vingerhoets and Van Heck 1990). However, Lazarus (1993) concluded from his research that when the type of stress is held constant, women and men show similar coping patterns. Interestingly, evidence suggests that women may respond better to crisis intervention than men. In a group of medical and surgical patients, women receiving crisis intervention showed a better response than men (Viney *et al.* 1985*b*), in particular, demonstrating less anxiety and helplessness.

Another important facet of coping relevant to crisis intervention is *the expression of emotion*. Perception of a problem or threat usually generates such emotion. In some instances, for example, when anger leads to aggressive behaviour, its expression provides a direct and possibly adaptive way to cope with a problem or threat (e.g. the enemy retreats). This reaction, whether it be anger, fear, or any other emotion, is presumably a necessary and motivating force for coping behaviour. But frequently this becomes a problem in its own right, and has to be dealt with directly. Unless we can handle our feelings of anger, anxiety, grief, and the like appropriately, the ability to cope effectively becomes impaired. This is best regarded as 'second-order' coping (i.e. coping with emotional reactions to problems or threats) and underlies the method first formulated by Lindemann (1944).

We tend to use combinations of coping behaviours, but in certain circumstances they fail and problems remain unresolved. Various factors contribute: the problems may be too demanding, too numerous, or too unfamiliar; the person may use maladaptive coping methods; coping may be limited by physical or mental ill-health; support from friends or family that would have otherwise enabled a person to cope is unavailable.

When coping fails we recognize what Caplan (1961) described as the *four phases of crisis*:

Phase 1—arousal and efforts at problem-solving behaviour increase;

Phase 2—with increased arousal or 'tension', functional impairment ensues with associated disorganization and distress. Arousal reaches a level which hinders rather than promotes coping: the person becomes too anxious or too angry, is too perturbed to sleep properly and so becomes fatigued, and so on;

Phase 3—emergency resources both internal and external are mobilized and novel methods of coping tried; and

Phase 4—continuing failure to resolve the problem leads to progressive deterioration, exhaustion, and 'decompensation'.

Help can be offered in two quite different ways: at an early stage when the person attempts to mobilize help as part of adaptive coping, and later in the decompensation phase when intervention by others becomes a matter of necessity to prevent further disorganization. The relationship with the helping professional obviously differs in these two phases, a point of central relevance to intervention. Before developing that theme, let us consider briefly types of problems that commonly lead to the need for help.

Common problems tackled in crisis intervention

The diverse problems to which 'crisis intervention' has been applied have already been cited. Hobbs (1984) divided stressful situations which precipitate crisis into two: developmental and accidental. Developmental crises refer to the inevitable transitional periods from one stage of psychosocial development to another (e.g. childbirth, retirement). Accidental crises involve unexpected life-events and nclude natural disasters, physical illness and injury, bereavement, and redundancy. Hobbs suggested that situations where an accidental event occurs at the time of a developmental transition (e.g. the death of a partner at retirement) may, in particular, render a person vulnerable to a state of crisis.

The common problems these situations produce, and which are dealt with in therapy, include:

(1) *Loss*

This may involve loss of many forms—of a loved one by death or separation, of self-esteem, of body function (e.g. following amputation, when part of the body is also lost), and of resources such as financial. In the aftermath of trauma like sexual assault or disaster, a person may experience loss of trust, freedom, and a sense of identity. Loss leads to a response pattern typically experienced in bereavement and which was described classically by Lindemann (1944), and more recently by others (Parkes 1986). Initially, the person is in a degree of shock; then follows denial which gives way to the feeling of grief. When the grief is 'worked through', the person gradually restructures his or her life and fills the gap that has been created. Intervention, at everyday or clinical levels, focuses on helping the person to face, express, and 'work through' the grief.

(2) *Change*

Here, the problem is the development of a new situation that has to be contended with rather than the loss of a previous one. Principal types of change are: in role, such as work, marital status and parenthood; and in identity, accompanying changes of role (the transitional or maturational crises described by Erikson 1969, fall into this category). There is usually a positive aspect with such change—the element of challenge in expectation of new and potentially rewarding life experiences. But it can none the less prove threatening. A particular form of change which overlaps with effects of loss, is entry into a 'sick' role, with the threat of actual loss of health and bodily function.

(3) *Interpersonal*

An enormous degree of stress may stem from troubled interpersonal relationships, especially between spouses or other close family members. This is almost certainly the most common reason for non-fatal suicide attempts (Hawton and Catalan 1987). Interpersonal crises are also associated with the onset of depression, which Brown *et al.*

(1987) demonstrated in their studies of mothers. In these cases, the
helping professional needs to facilitate communication between the
protagonists in the disturbed relationship with the goal of achieving
satisfactory resolution of hostility or other problematic emotions.

(4) *Conflict*

Here, the person faces a difficult or seemingly impossible choice
between two or more alternatives. Principles of problem-solving,
described below, are highly pertinent in this context.

The patient–therapist relationship

Whatever type of problem, the therapist is faced with the
aforementioned distinction, between offering help to someone who is
mobilizing extra resources (i.e. is in phase 1 or 2 of a crisis), or taking
over responsibility for a person temporarily in a decompensated state
(i.e. in phase 3 or 4). The nature of the relationship between therapist
and the person in crisis is a fundamental aspect and yet usually the
least considered.

From time to time, health professionals debate the concept of
illness. Usually, the issue is the definition of illness for purposes such
as classification or epidemiological and aetiological research, and for
interprofessional communication (Lewis 1953; Kendell 1975). It is
much less often that they consider how their description of a patient as
ill affects not only their professional role and relationship with him,
but also the latter's self-concept. Paradoxically, it has been left to
people outside the health professions to comment. The concept of the
'sick role' was clearly formulated by the sociologist Talcott Parsons
(1951), who pointed out that, in general, the 'ill' person is not held
responsible for his or her incapacity and, even more important, is
exempt from responsibility for normal obligations on the premise that
appropriate medical help is being sought. These ideas stimulated
useful research (Mechanic 1977). They were provocatively discussed
by Illich (1975) who criticized the medical profession for fostering
dependency and weakening a patient's sense of self-efficacy. More
germane to crisis intervention is whether dependency is reasonable.

Clearly, there are instances when it is entirely appropriate to permit
a state of dependency and transfer of responsibility. The person who
breaks a leg needs the sick role to allow healing to occur, as well as
medical and nursing expertise. Responsibility is gradually handed
back to the patient who in the phase of recovery is expected to take on

the onus for his or her rehabilitation. This transfer is seldom made explicit and in most cases is not even recognized by patient or doctor. Consequently, it may well 'go wrong'; the sick role continues for too long or the patient has difficulty in relinquishing it.

We are faced with a further difficulty in the context of crisis intervention. It is important to bear in mind that a crisis is not in itself a pathological state, although its outcome might be (Hobbs 1984). Although, as already stated, transfer of responsibility from the person may be appropriate, do we, as a result, want to regard the person in crisis as ill? If so, we imply that the distressed state results from a morbid process, but in fact he or she may have been overcome by a 'natural disaster' (e.g. an old age pensioner whose house has burnt down) or simply lack adequate coping resources and hence become overwhelmed by circumstances that would be met by most people. Do we want to encourage the sick role in such cases? On occasion the answer is a clear 'yes' because the illness label protects the person's self-esteem or enables responsibility to be handed over. In other cases, the answer is 'no' since it may discourage a person from seeking and learning new coping skills that might improve his or her ability to handle similar stress in the future.

Two decisions, therefore, have to be made when helping someone in crisis. Is this person in or about to enter a decompensated state requiring urgent intervention and the therapist's assumption of responsibility? Is it therapeutically helpful to label the person as ill? These important matters are linked to clinical judgement. This is made more difficult in that people present in a decompensated state as a regressive method of coping; they have learnt to do this in the past and found that it worked, at least in the short term. The therapist may have difficulty recognizing that this is happening unless knowledge of the person's past history or evidence of similar behaviour on previous occasions is available. Obviously, in such a case it is in everyone's interest for the person to resume responsibility for his or her behaviour.

Generally, the role of the therapist should be flexible and active, working with patients to enable them to use their own internal resources.

One final issue concerns the importance of therapists judging what they are realistically able to offer, for example, with respect to contact between sessions and duration, and setting clear boundaries which are discussed with the patient. This is particularly important in dealing with people in crisis who are likely to be very distressed, and where the therapist may initially feel compelled to offer more than he or she is able to provide.

METHODS OF INTERVENTION

Given the wide range of problems to which it has been applied, it is not surprising that there is disagreement about what constitutes crisis intervention. However, Waldron (1984) has identified features common to most approaches:

(a) prompt assessment and provision of services for the person or family in crisis;

(b) intensive, focused, and time-limited intervention directed at here and now problems and at specific goals;

(c) active and flexible style.

Initial assessment

A basic tenet of early crisis theory involved a 'critical period' during which the person in crisis is most responsive to help. Obviously, the initial contact with someone presenting in crisis is pivotal. Aims are to establish trust and gain rapport, and to identify clearly relevant recent events, particularly those influential in leading the person to seek help. Much useful information is obtained through a detailed inquiry of what has taken place in the previous 48 hours or so. This usually points to the chief problems, though it may be some time before their precise nature or full extent become recognized. It is important to clarify what demands the person is facing, including practical obligations. When obtaining this account, attention should be paid to the mental state: suicidal ideas, degree of anxiety, agitation, or distress, and in particular whether his or her condition will enable practical steps immediately required to be implemented. The therapist also assesses the support the person can count on from family or friends and the nature of the home circumstances. The ultimate goal is to establish a picture not only about the background and development of the patient's problems, but also to determine how he or she has fared with them in the past and the quality of available coping resources. This clarification may have to wait until the disorganization and helplessness, often associated with a severe decompensated state, abates or until another informant can be interviewed.

By the end of the initial assessment, the first clinical decision has to be taken: does responsibility for the person's affairs need to be taken over temporarily? If yes, a form of intervention appropriately called 'intensive care' is organized; care because the patient has to be temporarily looked after and intensive because concentrated contact will be of the essence. If such care is not necessary, another form of help, 'crisis counselling' is offered. In many cases, the distinction between the two types is clear-cut, in others it is less so, as responsibility may be transferred only partially. What is important is the therapist's clear awareness of what is called for in this respect. In any event, as for the patient with a broken limb, intensive care is only a temporary phase following which responsibility is gradually handed back; the therapist–patient relationship shifts from doctor–sick patient to adult–adult, allowing for collaborative problem-solving or other forms of intervention.

Intensive care

The goal in intensive care is to reverse the state of decompensation, so enabling a return to adaptive coping as efficiently as possible. The following steps are taken:

(1) *Explicit transfer of responsibility*
The patient is informed that his or her usual responsibilities and obligations will be taken over by others for the time-being. Whether this is justified to the patient on grounds of illness is determined at this time, after carefully considering the implications.

(2) *Organization of the takeover of immediate tasks*
The therapist then ensures that the patient's obligations are assumed by others. Children may need to be looked after by relatives or taken into care; employers may have to be contacted. Homes have to be secured, pets fed, and so on. The help of family and friends is mobilized as far as is possible (although social services and community agencies may need to be recruited).

(3) *Removal of the patient from a stressful environment*
This is not always necessary or possible and depends on how pertinent the patient's home environment is in aggravating the problems and how supportive family and friends are. A move to friends or relatives may suffice. Admission to hospital or a crisis unit is another option which permits closer and continuing contact with professional aid and hence facilitates the objectives listed below.

(4) *Lowering arousal and distress*

Commonly the patient in need of intensive care is distressed, over-aroused, and emotionally or physically exhausted. Arousal should desirably be reduced by psychological means: by spending time with and talking to the patient in a reassuring and concerned manner. Instruction in anxiety management, such as deep breathing exercises or progressive relaxation, may help. Drugs may have a place, particularly if arousal is marked and unresponsive to these psychological methods, or sleep is severely impaired. But medication should be seen, and presented clearly to the patient, as a short-term measure only.

(5) *Reinforcing appropriate communication*

Decompensation may present as the exhausted, distressed state described above, or as a state of 'shock', perhaps of sudden onset, in which the patient becomes almost mute and immobile. In either case, an important goal is to re-establish communication: to reinforce normal and relevant conversation by paying attention to it, and to discourage agitated, perseverative, or non-communicative behaviour.

(6) *Showing concern and warmth and encouraging hope*

Underlying the two previous tactics is a need to convey to the patient that the therapist cares, is willing to listen, is empathic, and instils hope for a positive resolution. Raphael (1986), when discussing support in the aftermath of disaster, stresses the need for survivors to talk about their experience with those who do not make them feel worse. There are other ways whereby the therapist can help during intensive care particularly after the initial state of over-arousal has subsided, but these are also used in crisis counselling and are therefore described in the next section.

Crisis counselling

The key difference between crisis counselling and intensive care is that the counselled patient is not regarded as sick or dependent but rather as an adult with problems seeking help. Whether or not intensive care has been given previously, the nature of the relationship is made explicit. Objectives are agreed, frequency and duration spelt out, and the need for the patient to work actively emphasized. In other words, a verbal contract is negotiated. However, as counselling proceeds and circumstances change, this often needs to be modified, but always explicitly. For example, an initial objective may be to define the problems before a decision on further steps to be taken. Having achieved that goal, another contract might be made involving problem-solving.

Patients with difficulty in agreeing or conforming to contracts of this kind may seek a more dependent ('sick role') relationship. In these cases it is necessary to discuss with the patient the inevitable disadvantages of a passive and dependent position and the constraints this imposes on both therapist and patient. The patient's inability to modify expectations may reflect a need for long-term psychotherapy and precludes brief, goal-oriented crisis counselling.

Once an explicit contract has been implemented, the therapist may deploy one or more methods, discussed below, as appropriate; the choice is determined by the nature of the crisis and by the patient's resources.

(1) *Facilitating the expression of emotion*

As mentioned above, emotion generated in a crisis frequently becomes a problem in its own right, impeding resolution until dealt with. Good examples of this are grief, where cultural, family, or personality factors may inhibit its expression and hence prevent satisfactory resolution (Lindemann 1944), and anger, where early acquired attitudes to it (e.g. 'It is wrong to show anger or lose your temper') or fear of its consequences may inhibit its expression. Unexpressed anger, lingering in the patient and often manifested by sulking, withdrawn, or negative behaviour, can have a devastatingly destructive effect. Expression of anger, on the other hand, can, if expressed appropriately, improve the situation.

The therapist facilitates emotional expression by attending to cues, encouraging patients to share feelings, and making it clear their expression will be accepted non-judgementally. Where appropriate, expression of feelings between patients and their relatives is also encouraged. There are instances where emotions are a feature of a severely disturbed mental state, such as in agitated depression or morbid jealousy, and encouraging their expression is likely to aggravate the problem. But generally, if feelings are perceived as understandable reactions to the crisis and they have not been adequately ventilated, then their expression is bound to be beneficial.

(2) *Facilitating communication*

Problems arise not only in expression of feelings but also in communication of meaning. Once again this may be a reaction to crisis, but more often reflects communication difficulties which render the patient and his or her family more vulnerable at times of stress. The patient's customary methods of communication are observable in the context of the therapeutic relationship, or in a family or marital interview, or can be inferred from the patient's descriptions. Observational feedback helps demonstrate how communication fails and its effects on others. This leads to suggestions as to how it can be improved. The presence of a therapist in family sessions often makes this otherwise sensitive topic easier to discuss.

(3) *Facilitating patients' understanding of their problems and their responses*

Much distress results from patients' failure to comprehend why traumatic events have occurred to them and why they feel so upset. A good example is the tendency for women who have been raped to question, and often feel guilty about, their behaviour during the assault (e.g. 'Why didn't I fight back?'). A therapist can elucidate the nature of shock and also the sequence of emotions which women who have been raped commonly experience. Similarly, survivors of disasters can be informed that guilt or self-blame are common post-traumatic symptoms. Helping patients to appreciate these aspects is not only therapeutic in its own right but also serves to identify problems and possible solutions.

(4) *Showing concern and empathy and bolstering self-esteem*

Concern and empathy have been highlighted in relation to intensive care but are clearly pertinent to crisis intervention generally and there are occasions when it is the therapist's most useful task. Bolstering self-esteem, while frequently difficult when the patient is enveloped in failure, is nevertheless an important pursuit, all too often overlooked. Assessment of the patient's past life together with observation of current behaviour provide the therapist with material to identify available strengths and assets. The therapist also encourages the patient when progress is achieved.

(5) *Facilitating problem-solving behaviour*

Emotionally distressed people are not efficient at solving problems, tending to use impulsive or aggressive strategies (Rose 1986)—recall Caplan's (1961) definition that, during a crisis: 'many abortive attempts at solution are made.'

The term 'problem-solving' refers to a systematic process incorporating a step-by-step approach to help patients to grapple with difficulties. Problem-solving demands a collaborative approach in which the adult–adult nature of the relationship is paramount—problem-solving and associated decision-making are done by the patient, not the therapist. Haaga and Davison (1986) define five stages:

(1) *problem orientation*—the therapist instils in the patient a 'set' that will facilitate problem-solving, including the ability to identify problematic situations, feelings of self-efficacy, and the capacity to 'hold back' rather than acting impulsively to confront the problem;

(2) *problem definition and formulation*—obtaining information about the problem(s) in concrete, specific terms; deciding which to tackle first; setting realistic goals and specifying desired outcomes;

(3) *generation of alternative solutions*—this involves the patient suggesting an infinite range of potential solutions;

(4) *decision-making*—cognitively rehearsing each option, and becoming aware of its short- and long-term consequences;

(5) *solution implementation and verification*—the patient tries out the chosen option, and observes and evaluates the results.

The choice of an alternative in practice does not necessarily follow logically. Choice may still be intuitive. However, the ability to 'feel' what is right is enhanced by working through the stages.

The following techniques, many of them used in cognitive-behavioural treatment (Hawton and Kirk 1989), are helpful in promoting problem-solving skills:

(a) *explain principles of problem-solving*—that distress and maladaptive behaviour often result from inadequate problem-solving;

(b) *help the patient to define the problem* in terms that suggest realistic methods of dealing with it (e.g. by providing the patient with facts or feedback from informants which have a bearing on the problem).

Diaries that monitor fluctuations in mood or other symptoms can
assist in identifying the problem(s);

(c) *defining goals and recording them in writing*; one method is to ask
patients what they would like to see changed if they could wave a
magic wand;

(d) *problem-solving depends on creative thinking*, producing novel
ideas. In 'brainstorming', patients are asked to generate as many
possible solutions as possible, however unlikely they may seem.
Therapists also contribute their creative thinking in tandem with
specific skills in problem-solving;

(e) *assessing patients' previous coping resources* and so becoming aware
of strengths and weaknesses enables a clearer vision of alternatives
likely to succeed;

(f) ensuring that the patient has realistically considered practical
consequences and implications of each alternative (i.e. further *'reality
testing'*);

(g) *encouraging the patient to make a choice* after due consideration
and when the choice 'feels right';

(h) *helping the patient dissect the chosen method* into manageable steps
and to anticipate their likely implications and stumbling blocks;

(i) *negotiating a contract with the patient*. Once agreed, both short-
and long-term targets are recorded and the patient given a copy;

(j) *checking the effectiveness*, or otherwise, of the coping behaviour
selected.

In addition to these commonsense tactics, there is scope for the use
of customary therapeutic skills. By setting behavioural goals and
analysing the patient's difficulties in carrying them out, the therapist
effectively identifies key attitudes, resistances, and defences that
obstruct the behaviour. Various strategies are used to modify these
(see Chapter 9 on sex therapy for details).

Two further methods are part of crisis counselling: *offering expert
advice* and *prescribing psychotropic drugs*. These have been left till the
last because, in the case of the medically trained, they tend to be in the
forefront of their minds whereas they should be used sparingly. There
are obviously many clinical circumstances where these methods are
appropriate, but seldom so in crisis counselling. Nevertheless, special

advice is occasionally indicated either from the therapist or another helping agency. Medical, family planning, legal and financial advice come into this category. Agencies such as Citizens' Advice Bureaux are examples of community-based sources. The patient may be advised to withhold from a course of action, for example, to delay divorce proceedings because of the possibility of change in the marital relationship. The therapist is ideally aware of both the rationale for advising and satisfied that it is appropriate.

Psychotropic drugs may be indicated during intensive care (as has already been mentioned). There, it presents no problem as far as the therapeutic relationship is concerned. On the other hand, when used during crisis counselling the implication that 'prescription of drugs' equals 'illness' and hence the transfer of responsibility to the therapist must be counteracted. The therapist stresses that the drugs are only an adjunct, an aid to the patient's own problem-solving efforts.

Indications for medication are:

(a) to lower arousal where it seriously impairs ability to develop problem-solving behaviour or make decisions, and where psychological methods have failed. The aim is to reduce arousal so that effective coping can be resumed;

(b) to elevate mood in patients whose depression is of such severity that they are unable to carry out any problem-solving activity. Antidepressants are prescribed to improve mood sufficiently to enable the patient to participate actively in problem-solving but are not intended to solve those problems;

(c) to improve sleep disturbance—insomnia needs special attention because of its deleterious effect on patients' coping. Care is taken to avoid dependency by drugs being taken intermittently, for only a few successive nights.

CLINICAL ILLUSTRATION

Gerald, a 38-year-old accountant, and Elizabeth, a 35-year-old nurse, had been married for 12 years; they had two children aged 11 and 8. For the past three months, an old friend of theirs, Brian, whose marriage had broken up and who was having financial difficulties, had been staying with them. Twelve hours before Gerald was referred to a crisis unit, he had discovered Brian and Elizabeth having sexual intercourse. After an angry scene he had told them to get out, and they had both left in the middle of the night, driving off in Brian's car. A neighbour found Gerald the following morning in a distressed and agitated state. The children were also distressed having heard the angry ejection of their mother.

When seen in the unit, Gerald was still agitated, expressing intense anger at his wife and Brian and alarm at the prospect of being left to look after the children on his own. He was making suicidal threats if his wife was not prepared to care for them. After initial assessment it was decided that Gerald's reaction, involving anger, humiliation, and the threat of single parenthood rendered him unsuitable to care for his children or to be left on his own. Immediate intensive care was indicated and the following plan implemented:

(1) He was strongly advised to enter the unit for two to three days, and to pass over responsibility for his children temporarily to the unit staff.

(2) Arrangements were made for the children to be cared for by a family friend.

(3) He was given an opportunity to ventilate his intense feelings of distress and resentment with a staff member.

(4) He was given a hypnotic to help him sleep.

After 36 hours, he had largely regained his composure, and although still very angry was judged capable of returning home to look after his children. At this stage, intensive care came to an end. It was then made explicit that he would have to resume responsibility for himself and his children, but if at any time he felt incapable of doing so, he was to contact the unit immediately. He was also offered crisis counselling and an appointment was set to attend the next day. Over the next week, three sessions were held during which the following matters were covered:

(a) how to deal in the short term with his children—it was agreed that he would take time off work to be at home until the situation became clearer;

(b) what to do about his marriage—further ventilation of feelings occurred; it was agreed that the therapist should contact his wife with a view to a joint session later.

After further meetings during the next three weeks, it became evident that the marriage had ended and that Elizabeth had opted to stay with Brian. She revealed long-standing discontent with the marriage. Gerald arranged for a part-time housekeeper so that he could return to work. He later initiated divorce proceedings.

This case illustrates the use of brief intensive care, leading on to crisis counselling of about a month's duration—there were six sessions in all.

PRACTICAL ASPECTS

Provision of intensive care requires special resources. Although these can often be provided by family or friends, in many situations the professional needs to consider institutional settings. The use of traditional psychiatric facilities should be treated cautiously as these are often not designed to provide the type of support described here and may serve to prolong dependency. Special units have been developed to provide this type of intervention, utilizing a multidisciplinary approach.

Crisis counselling can be conducted in the patient's home or in a clinic setting. It may involve the patient's family or friends. Duration of therapy is most commonly between six and eight weeks, but decisions about the spacing of sessions should be based on particular needs. Group methods have been used, although interviews are generally on a one-to-one basis.

TRAINING AND CONCLUSION

There is much scope for skill and experience in carrying out crisis intervention. This involves empathy and sensitivity, attributes with which some therapists are well endowed, but which all can enhance by becoming aware and critical of their own performance. Clinical practice, ideally with a broad range of patients, under the supervision of an experienced therapist, is a vital aspect of training. Observation of the veteran practitioner on video-tape or through one-way screen is also helpful. Knowledge of the literature, although it is possibly confusing, is another facet of training, and to this end a recommended reading list is provided at the end of the chapter.

For much of what we do we need to recognize real alternatives open to us but also their limitations. Communicating a sense of competence combined with concern is a major therapeutic achievement, particularly in the stages of intensive care. Often, inexperienced therapists feel hesitant because they suspect there are forms of help with which they are unfamiliar. Although the details are few and the complexity not fully apparent in this chapter, the various forms of crisis intervention are more or less covered. This is the 'menu' from which to choose. For the most part, therapists will rely on skilful use of common sense rather than highly specialized techniques. Appreciation of these points increases the therapist's sense of competence as well as provides a framework within which to operate.

Given the range of approaches for which the term 'crisis intervention' has been applied, it is difficult to reach a conclusion about its effectiveness. Research has demonstrated that support provided during crisis situations is related to better outcome (Viney *et al.* 1985*a*; Joseph *et al.* 1992). However, few studies have incorporated random allocation of patients into treatment groups, or compared crisis intervention with a control group. The difficulties in executing outcome research with heterogenous types of crisis and considerable variability in competence at coping should not be underestimated. Nevertheless, limited systematic evidence of efficacy should not deter us from using an approach which is based on both caring and common sense.

REFERENCES

Aguilera, D. C. and Messick, J. M. (1982). *Crisis intervention: theory and methodology*, (4th edn). Mosby, St. Louis, MO.

Brown, G. W., Bifulco, A., and Harris, T. O. (1987). Life events, vulnerability and onset of depression. *British Journal of Psychiatry*, **150**, 30–42.

Caplan, G. (1961). *An approach to community mental health*. Tavistock, London.

Ellis, E. M. (1983). A review of empirical rape research: Victim reactions and response to treatment. *Clinical Psychology Review*, **3**, 473–490.

Erikson, E. H. (1969). *Childhood and society*. Penguin, Harmondsworth.

Haaga, D. A. and Davison, G. C. (1986). Cognitive change methods. In *Helping people change: A textbook of methods*. (ed. F. H. Kanfer and A. P. Goldstein), pp. 236–82. Pergamon, New York.

Hawton, K. and Catalan, J. (1987). *Attempted suicide. A practical guide to its nature and management*, (2nd edn). Oxford University Press.

Hawton, K. and Kirk, J. (1989). Problem-solving. In *Cognitive behaviour therapy for psychiatric problems. A practical guide*, (ed. K. Hawton, P. M. Salkovskis, J. Kirk, and D. M. Clark), pp. 406–26. Oxford University Press.

Hobbs, M. (1984). Crisis intervention in theory and practice: A selective review. *British Journal of Medical Psychology*, **57**, 23–34.

Illich, I. (1975). *Medical nemesis*. Calder & Boyars, London.

Joseph, S., Andrews, B., Williams, R., and Yule, W. (1992). Crisis support and psychiatric symptomatology in adult survivors of the *Jupiter* cruise ship disaster. *British Journal of Clinical Psychology*, **31**, 63–73.

Kendell, R. E. (1975). The concept of disease and its implication for psychiatry. *British Journal of Psychiatry*, **127**, 305–15.

Langsley, D. G. (1981). Crisis intervention: An update. In *Current psychiatric therapies*, Vol. 20, (ed. J. H. Masserman), Grune and Stratton, New York.

Lazarus, R. S. (1993). From psychological stress to the emotions: A history of changing outlooks. *Annual Review of Psychology*, **44**, 1–21.

Lewis, A. (1953). Health as a social concept. *British Journal of Sociology*, **4**, 109–24.

Lindemann, E. (1944). Symptomatology and management of acute grief. *American Journal of Psychiatry*, **101**, 101–48.

Mechanic, D. (1977). Illness behaviour, social adaptation and the management of illness. *Journal of Nervous and Mental Disease*, **165**, 79–87.

Parkes, C. M. (1986). *Bereavement: studies of grief in adult life.* (2nd edn). Penguin, Harmondsworth.

Parsons, T. (1951). *The social system.* Free Press, Glencoe.

Raphael, B. (1986). *When disaster strikes. A handbook for the caring professions.* Hutchinson, London.

Rose, S. D. (1986). Group methods. In *Helping people change: A textbook of methods*, (ed. F. H. Kanfer and A. P. Goldstein), pp. 437–69. Pergamon, New York.

Stroul B. A. (1988). Residential crisis services: A review. *Hospital and Community Psychiatry*, **39**, 1095–9.

Szmukler, G. I. (1987). The place of crisis intervention in psychiatry. *Australian and New Zealand Journal of Psychiatry*, **21**, 24–34.

Viney, L. L., Clarke, A. M., Bunn, T. A., and Benjamin, Y. N. (1985a). An evaluation of three crisis intervention programmes for general hospital patients. *British Journal of Medical Psychology*, **58**, 75–86.

Viney, L. L., Benjamin, Y. N., Clarke, A. M., and Bunn, T. A. (1985b). Sex differences in the psychological reactions of medical and surgical patients to crisis intervention counselling: Sauce for the goose may not be sauce for the gander. *Social Science and Medicine*, **20**, 1199–205.

Vingerhoets, A. J. M. and Van Heck, G. L. (1990). Gender, coping and psychosomatic symptoms. *Psychological Medicine*, **20**, 125–35.

Waldron, G. (1984). Crisis intervention: Is it effective? *British Journal of Hospital Medicine*, April, 283–7.

Winter, D. A., Shivakumar, H., Brown, R. J., Roitt, M., Drysdale, W. J., and Jones, S. (1987). Explorations of a crisis intervention service. *British Journal of Psychiatry*, **151**, 232–39.

RECOMMENDED READING

Aguilera, D. C. and Messick, J. M. (1982). *Crisis intervention: theory and methodology*, (4th edn). Mosby, St. Louis, MO. (A concise and readable book; chapters 2, 3, and 5 are particularly useful.)

Caplan, G. (1974). *Support systems and community mental health*. Grune and Stratton, New York. (Chapter 1 contains a helpful account of the concept of support in relation to crisis.)

Hawton, K. and Kirk, J. (1989). Problem-solving. In *Cognitive behaviour therapy for psychiatric problems. A practical guide*, (ed. K. Hawton, P. M. Salkovskis, J. Kirk, and D. M. Clark), pp. 406–26. Oxford University Press. (Contains useful information on behavioural techniques.)

Szmukler, G. I. (1987). The place of crisis intervention in psychiatry. *Australian and New Zealand Journal of Psychiatry*, **21**, 24–34. (Good discussion of the application of crisis intervention to psychiatric disorders.)

Viney, L. L., Clarke, A. M., Bunn, T. A., and Benjamin, Y. N. (1985a). An evaluation of three crisis intervention programmes for general hospital patients. *British Journal of Medical Psychology*, **58**, 75–86. (A study of the effectiveness of crisis intervention with hospital in-patients.)

6

Behavioural psychotherapy

LYNNE DRUMMOND

The chapter begins with an account of the historical background of behavioural psychotherapy which weaves in a series of theoretical strands. The aims of treatment are then considered. The section on selection incorporates a detailed guide on how one conducts a behavioural analysis and formulation. The material on the therapeutic process highlights the technique of exposure, and also includes response prevention, covert sensitization, orgasmic reconditioning, stimulus control, habit reversal, mass practice, and operant strategies. Problems in the course of therapy are then dealt with, and the chapter ends with a brief account of training requirements.

Behavioural psychotherapy is surprisingly difficult to define. Whereas it has often been stated that it is a group of treatments based on the application of learning theory, this is only partly true. Many behavioural treatments have been discovered and refined by trial and error and by clinicians trying to see what works effectively. In many cases, learning theory has had to be modified to incorporate the clinical findings.

It has been suggested that behavioural psychotherapy is the application of common sense. This again is only partially true. Whereas the exposure principle can be seen to be a variant of the common sense approach that if a person has a car accident they should drive again as soon as possible, the importance of the duration of therapeutic exposure is not so commonly recognized. Similarly, some treatments appear to be contrary to a common sense view.

A short definition of behavioural psychotherapy states that it is a collection of treatments which have the central hypothesis that psychological distress results from learned behaviour and that this behaviour can therefore be unlearned (Stern and Drummond 1991). This brief definition can be used to describe most behavioural treatments. However, it would be a mistake to conclude from this that behavioural psychotherapists ignore possible genetic, structural, and biochemical components to the development of psychiatric syndromes. A good behavioural clinician considers the whole patient and his environment in the behavioural formulation and then tries to identify areas where there is potential for change.

Behavioural psychotherapy has been shown to be effective and probably the treatment of choice for phobic disorders including agoraphobia; obsessive-compulsive disorder and sexual dysfunction. It has been demonstrated to be effective for habit disorders including many tics; obesity, bulimia, and anorexia nervosa; sexual deviation; social skills problems including anger control; marital problems and abnormal illness behaviour. It has also been found to play an important part in the treatment and management of a variety of medical problems including hypertension and post-myocardial infarction; in rehabilitation of chronic schizophrenia; in the management of depression; alcohol and drug dependency; and childhood or adult behavioural disturbances.

The mainstay of much behavioural psychotherapy is exposure. Other frequently used treatments include self-imposed response prevention; sexual skills exercises; modelling; stimulus control techniques; role-play and rehearsal; contingency management and reinforcement schedules and covert sensitization. Education of the patient about their condition and the rationale for treatment is usually the first step. Most programmes require the patient to complete homework exercises.

HISTORICAL BACKGROUND

Research on behavioural psychotherapy has developed from several strands. For example, the work of Masters and Johnson (1966, 1970) generated the effective treatment of sexual dysfunction. The techniques used are similar to other behavioural treatments but were devised in parallel to developments in the treatment of anxiety disorders. For simplicity, this section will concentrate on the historical development of behavioural treatment for phobic and obsessive-compulsive disorder.

Behaviour therapy principles go back to earliest times, and can be illustrated by a quotation from John Locke (1693):

If your child shrieks and runs away at the sight of a frog let another catch it and lay it down a good distance from him: at first accustom him to look upon it; when he can do that to come nearer to it and see it leap without emotion; then to touch it lightly when it is held fast in another's hand; and so on until he can come to handle it as confidently as a butterfly or a sparrow. (This quotation is cited by Marks, 1987.)

In 1919, Freud (1919/1955) described the treatment of a boy with a fear of horses using the exposure technique of encouraging him to gradually approach the feared object. Similarly, the French psychologist, Pierre Janet, described an early example of exposure treatment used to treat a patient with obsessive–compulsive disorder (Janet 1903).

The concept of behaviourism and viewing behaviour as due to learned experience became popular at the beginning of the nineteenth century. This movement adopted a philosophical framework that all experience could be explained by behavioural theory. This is, of course, an over-simplistic view; any theory is only a model and can never represent absolute truth. Some early views about children being born *tabula rasa* whose personality is totally determined by learned experience appear excessively limited and naive today. However, some interesting experiments were performed which demonstrated a model for the development of phobias.

In their famous case of Albert, Watson and Rayner (1920) demonstrated that an 11-month-old child with a positive interest in furry animals developed a fear of rats after a steel bar was struck making a loud noise whenever he put out his hand towards a white rat. This case was not replicated, however, and the theory of a straightforward relationship between the genesis of phobias and classical conditioning was modified by other researchers who commented on individual differences in the susceptibility to aversive stimuli (e.g. Pavlov 1927). Later, Eysenck (1957), suggested that individuals who condition easily are more likely to develop phobias. Other workers emphasized that the intensity and amount of reinforcement following any action also has an effect on the degree of conditioning which occurs (Spence *et al.* 1958).

In the initial development of behavioural treatment for phobias, Mowrer's (1950) view of fear acquisition was widely accepted as a model for the evolution of clinical phobias. According to this view, classically conditioned fear leads to avoidance behaviour. Avoidance leads to a reduction of fear and thus the avoidance behaviour is reinforced by diminished anxiety.

This model, however, was challenged by several investigators. First, it was found that many phobic patients could not recall a traumatic experience relating to the onset of the phobia (Buglass *et al.* 1977; Goldstein and Chambless 1978). Secondly, several workers failed to replicate Watson and Rayner's (1920) experiment (English 1929; Thorndike 1935). Thirdly, it did not appear compatible with the gradual onset of phobias often seen in clinical practice (Emmelkamp 1985); finally, it did not explain the common stereotyped patterns of fear-provoking objects and situations. In a series of laboratory-based experiments with adult volunteers, Ohman and his colleagues (Ohman *et al.* 1984) demonstrated that humans are much more likely to be aversively conditioned to phylogenetically old fear-relevant stimuli (e.g. snakes, spiders) than to neutral stimuli (e.g. flowers, mushrooms).

The finding that situations which evoke fears are non-random, led Marks (1969) to propose the concept of pre-potency; this is the tendency for a particular species to attend preferentially to certain stimuli of evolutionary importance rather than other, evolutionary irrelevant, stimuli even when encountered for the first time. Seligman's (1971) concept of preparedness extends this evolutionary model further. Preparedness refers to the idea that certain stimuli are more likely to be associated with each other and with certain responses.

Behavioural psychotherapy was introduced and popularized in the United States by Joseph Wolpe. The treatment used was systematic desensitization (SD), for simple phobias. This is based on the principle of reciprocal inhibition: if a state incompatible with anxiety can be produced then anxiety cannot occur. Relaxation is incompatible with anxiety and was thus used (Wolpe 1958).

Systematic desensitization in phobic disorder was widely investigated. For example, Gelder *et al.* (1967) compared it with individual and group psychotherapy in patients with phobic disorders. SD was consistently more effective than the other two treatments. Although successful, SD is a time-consuming treatment for both patient and therapist.

In vivo exposure methods, originally called flooding (a term largely dropped today), were then investigated (Stampfl and Levis 1967). *In vivo* exposure was pioneered with phobic patients (e.g. Watson and Marks 1971). A variety of such phobias were treated successfully with rapid exposure in real life. Concerns in some therapists that anxious patients would be harmed and other symptoms would appear proved unfounded.

Treatment of agoraphobia by exposure was then investigated (e.g. Mathews *et al.* 1976) and also found to be effective. Over the next decade, exposure treatments were refined and crucial therapeutic factors isolated. For example, the importance of duration of exposure was discovered (Stern and Marks 1973) *In vivo* exposure was also found to be more effective than exposure in imagination (Emmelkamp and Wessels 1975).

Group behavioural treatment of agoraphobia was then examined. Hand *et al.* (1974) compared 'structured' with 'unstructured' groups, and found progress greater in the former. Only the structured group continued to improve after treatment and to three month follow up. Moreover, it required less professional time. However, it is often difficult in practice to compose a group of similar phobic patients at the same time. Also, progress of the group is limited by the rate of progress of the slowest member.

Further development of self-exposure methods has resulted in a diminution of therapist time. Marks *et al.* (1983) showed that brief therapist-aided exposure was a useful adjunct to self-exposure homework instructions. Even the latter alone is a potent treatment for agoraphobia. Current experience supports the use of this approach although involvement of family members in treatment is thought to be beneficial.

Exposure was also investigated in obsessive-compulsive disorder. Marks *et al.* (1975) found treatment effective in three-quarters of patients with long-standing rituals. Exposure was often combined with modelling and self-imposed response prevention. Modelling refers to the therapist's demonstration of the desired behaviour; in self-imposed response prevention the patient is instructed not to ritualize. Both techniques are described in detail in the treatment section. The principles outlined by Janet were refined in a series of studies (Levy and Meyer 1971; Rachman *et al.* 1971, 1973), until the development of an effective therapy for most patients with compulsive behaviour.

Similar optimism was not justified, until the mid 1980s, for patients with obsessive ruminations as the main problem. The only technique available until then was thought stopping which sought to reduce ruminations by aversive techniques. The patient was instructed to ruminate whereupon the therapist would shout loudly. This was repeated several times until the patient had difficulty in concentrating enough to ruminate. The therapist gradually reduced the volume of the shouting until the patient could imagine the shouting without his input. Although this technique helped a few patients it was not generally effective and is virtually obsolete.

A newly developed technique of audio-taped habituation is more effective as demonstrated by both case report (Salkovskis 1983;

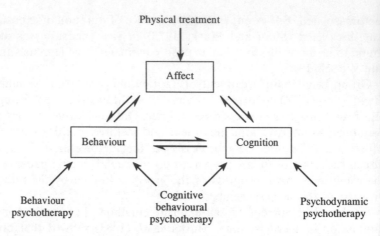

Figure 6.1 The components of psychiatric syndromes and the site of action of the various types of therapy. NB These components interact with each other and thus a treatment acting on affect will also alter behaviour and cognition.

Headland and McDonald 1987), and in a controlled trial (Lovell *et al.* 1994). (Audio-taped habituation is described fully in the treatment section.)

AIMS OF THERAPY

Behavioural psychotherapy aims to alter symptoms by modifying behaviour. These symptoms have three main components, affective, cognitive, and behavioural, and are often associated with coexistent physical symptoms (see Fig. 6.1).

For example, a phobic woman may fear spiders. This leads to extreme anxiety in the vicinity of spiders (affective component); a fear that the spider may crawl on to her body which she worries will result in her 'going mad' due to anxiety (cognitive component). This results in her withdrawing from the feared situation and avoiding any stimuli which remind her of spiders (behavioural component). Theoretically, treatment could be directed at any one of these components. She could be offered anxiolytic drugs to reduce anxiety (affective component), or be given psychoanalytic therapy to explore the roots of her fear (cognitive component), or be encouraged with behavioural treatment to approach her feared object (behavioural component). In reality, these three components interact with each other in such a way that alteration in one affects the others. However, dealing with the behavioural component is often the most efficient option. If the patient with spider phobia is given an anxiolytic drug, she may soon be able to approach the feared object and have fewer fearful thoughts but once the drug is withdrawn, she may quickly relapse. Psychoanalytic therapy would take several months before she feels confident to approach a spider. Behavioural treatment would encourage her from the start to begin confronting the fear-provoking situation and to persist in it long enough for her anxiety to wane. The full treatment would take four to six weeks.

The aim of behavioural treatment is thus to establish more adaptive patterns of behaviour and unlearn previous maladaptive ones which fuel the problem. In the above example, the patient's escape strategy was aggravating the situation. The presence of a spider made her feel extremely anxious. She escaped from the situation by running from the room; this reduced her anxiety. Her escape has thus been reinforced by the lowered anxiety level; this increases the likelihood of escape again which eventually leads to complete avoidance of all situations where spiders may exist.

It is important to take a comprehensive history and perform a complete behavioural assessment to ensure that all aspects of the problem are covered. For example, a 26-year-old man presented with an eight-year history of exposing his genitals to women in the park. Whereas this target problem could be dealt effectively with the aversion technique of covert sensitization, this would still leave him with the risk of relapse. A detailed history revealed that this deviant activity was his only sexual outlet. He therefore needed sexual skills training to encourage him to take up non-deviant sexual fantasies and to seek an appropriate sexual outlet.

SELECTION

Indications

The obvious role for behavioural psychotherapy is for one of the many conditions amenable to this approach. Most of these have been listed in the beginning of this chapter. The list can be extended to include any condition where behavioural analysis points to a patient's behaviour or coping pattern contributing to the disorder.

With most techniques, it is essential that the patient is motivated to change and willing to try the treatment. The only exception is in certain reinforcement regimes (operant programmes) with chronic patients but here ensure that rigorous ethical standards are applied.

CONTRA-INDICATIONS

In most cases where the patient is unwilling or unable to embark on behavioural psychotherapy, then the treatment should be explained in detail. He should be advised to seek help in the future following consideration or if circumstances change.

In the case of alcohol and drug misuse or dependence it is advisable for the patient to undergo detoxification prior to any behavioural treatment because of the risk of state-dependent learning (i.e. skills which are learnt in an intoxicated state often are not present when non-intoxicated). Also, in treating anxiety, alcohol and many drugs can complicate the clinical picture by withdrawal symptoms being indistinguishable from those of anxiety.

Benzodiazepine medication even at prescribed doses may be a contra-indication due to a concern about state-dependent learning and the withdrawal effects which can be experienced with short-acting benzodiazepines, as the blood level of these drugs varies during the day. In fact there is no evidence that state-dependent learning is a problem. However, psychological factors can be important and patients on drugs will often attribute improvement to the drug rather than to their own efforts in therapy. For all these reasons it is advisable to withdraw patients from benzodiazepines prior to behavioural psychotherapy or, in the case of the chronic benzodiazepine user who has extreme difficulty in withdrawing, to reduce the drug to a steady evenly spaced dose of not more than the equivalent of 15 mg of diazepam per day.

Depression is another condition which has to be tackled with caution. Severely depressed patients should be actively treated before commencing behavioural psychotherapy since they do not habituate to the anxiety induced by exposure programmes (Foa 1979). Moreover, they do not learn new skills effectively and tend to construe events negatively. However, when a patient has mild or moderate depression associated with his condition, treatment of the underlying condition usually alleviates the depression as well.

Schizophrenia and other psychotic states also need to be approached carefully. Foa (1979) noted that a few patients with obsessive-compulsive symptoms who failed to respond to exposure had over-valued ideas that their obsessions were correct. Some schizophrenic patients present with bizarre obsessive-compulsive symptoms but do not do well with exposure treatment. However, reinforcement management programmes (operant programmes) are regularly used to rehabilitate chronic schizophrenic patients.

BEHAVIOURAL ANALYSIS

When assessing a patient for suitability for behavioural psychotherapy, a full psychiatric history and mental state examination are necessary. The presence of any contra-indications, such as physical or psychotic illness, should be noted.

Performing a behavioural assessment is not difficult but there may be copious information to obtain especially if the problem is long-standing (for a full account see the assessment chapters in Stern and Drummond 1991). The patient should first be asked to give a brief description of the main problem; further detailed information must then be sought.

Therapists may benefit from using a mnemonic to help them organize their questions so that no information is omitted. The following examples of the two ABCs and the three Ps serve to give a reasonable behavioural analysis.

(1) ABC

The first ABC covers antecedents, behaviours, and beliefs, and consequences. This mnemonic coined by O'Leary and Wilson (1975) reminds the therapist that the antecedents and consequences of a behaviour as well as the patient's beliefs about it can modify the frequency of that behaviour. These factors should be teased out and form part of the formulation since treatment is usually geared to modify them.

(2) ABC

The use of this mnemonic dealing with affect, behaviour, and cognition was discussed on p. 142.

(3) Three Ps

This covers predisposing, precipitating, and perpetuating factors of the problem all of which should be assessed in order to complete the formulation.

Abbreviated assessment (BASIC ID)

It is necessary on occasion to do an abbreviated assessment due to lack of time. It is then useful to apply the plan described by Lazarus (1973) His schema can be remembered by the mnemonic BASIC ID. This represents the major headings in history-taking:

—BEHAVIOUR
—AFFECT
—SENSATIONS
—IMAGERY
—COGNITION
—INTERPERSONAL RELATIONSHIPS
—DRUGS

Most of these have been discussed above. However, physical sensations that accompany symptoms are important as they may fuel the patient's beliefs about the situation. Imagery refers to pictorial thoughts formed in the imagination. It is also important to know about the patient's family and social circumstances and their interpersonal relationships since these may affect the course of therapy. Finally, a full drug history is essential as drugs and their side-effects may impede progress.

It is important to ascertain in every assessment why the patient has presented at this time, and his aims and expectations of treatment.

At the end of the evaluation, the therapist should be able to determine if behavioural treatment is indicated and present the patient with a formulation of their problems and treatment rationale. Baseline measures can then be taken, and if the patient accepts treatment, a plan devised co-operatively.

BEHAVIOURAL FORMULATION

A behavioural formulation is in essence a hypothesis about a disorder, behaviour, or symptom which attempts to identify any predisposing, precipitating, and perpetuating factors. It is not engraved on stone and thus may alter as treatment unfolds and other factors come to light. The formulation should be shared with the patient since it helps them to hear their problem summarized. This is particularly true when the problem seems insurmountable. A short summary can demonstrate

hat it is manageable. Discussing the formulation with the patient also
llows the therapist to ensure that he has understood the nature of the
roblem fully; it also confirms that he has been heard.

The behavioural formulation for a woman with spider phobia might
e presented thus:

You have told me that you have been frightened of spiders for as long as you
an remember. Your mother was similarly frightened. This is not unusual. A
endency to develop phobias is often passed from one generation to the next.
Your mother's fear and avoidance of spiders would have taught you to regard
hem as creatures best avoided. Many children have specific animal fears from
he age of about three. You developed this fear but your mother's reaction to
piders probably contributed to your not overcoming it as you grew to
adolescence.

Once you had this fear, you would always run away if you saw a spider or
even a picture of one in a book or on television. This served to strengthen your
fear. High anxiety is very unpleasant and therefore a reduction in it is like a
eward. In your case, escaping from or avoiding the situation reduced your
anxiety. These behaviours were then 'rewarded' by diminished anxiety. If you
eward any behaviour, you increase the chance of it recurring. Therefore, every
time you escaped from or avoided contact with spiders, you increased your
fear and strengthened your belief that these were the only ways to avoid
unpleasant sensations. You, therefore, became increasingly phobic of spiders
until the present time.

MEASUREMENT OF CHANGE

Measurement of the problem is taken seriously in behavioural
treatment. Each patient is considered as a single-case experiment.
There are several advantages to this type of approach:

(1) In the initial stage it encourages the patient to express his goals;
this prevents the therapist hopelessly trying to pursue a course without
the patient's motivation.

(2) It allows patient and therapist to monitor progress and ensure that
the treatment is working. Failure to progress is recognized early and
the treatment modified appropriately.

(3) As treatment progresses, the patient may have a dim memory of
the severity of the original problem and misjudge the degree of
progress.

(4) The therapist may similarly have a vague recollection about the presenting problem and underestimate or, more commonly overestimate progress.

QUESTIONNAIRES

Although questionnaires are only one of the types of measure used they are commonly administered. For anyone new to behavioural psychotherapy, it is best to become familiar with a few tried and tested questionnaires, of proven reliability and validity. It is also important to ensure that the questionnaire actually measures the target symptoms and behaviours. Although this comment seems overly facile, it is a common error to use a measure of personality traits, for example, when trying to assess a change in the patient's clinical state

OBJECTIVITY AND TYPES OF MEASUREMENT

Some forms of measurement are more objective than others. The use of self-report or therapist–report questionnaires combined with observation by patient, relatives and therapist usually suffice. The list below, which covers the main categories is given in order of increasing objectivity.

(1) *Self-report*. Asking the patient 'How often do you experience panic in a day?' provides a rough guide to the frequency of a behaviour. Self-report can be made of more use with standardized questionnaires or visual analogue scales. Once the patient has completed a questionnaire, an element of self-observation operates and subsequent ratings are often more valid than initial ones.

(2) *Relative's report*.

(3) *Self-observation*. This requires patients to monitor their own behaviour over a period of time. A diary is a commonly applied method.

(4) *Relatives' observation*.

(5) *Impartial professional interview and ratings*. These measures are used in research and involve a professional person not involved with or blind to the patient's treatment.

(6) *Direct observation* using role-play (impartial professional rater).

7) *Direct observation* in vivo. With certain behaviours, the therapist can observe a patient's progress in real life, for example, a patient with obsessive-compulsive fears of contamination may have been unable to touch the door handle but achieve this during treatment.

Reliability of these measure can be increased by setting up a standard 'behavioural avoidance test' which can be performed by the patient repeatedly during treatment and be used to monitor progress. An example of this is a journey for an agoraphobic patient which follows a set route, starting with a walk, continuing with a visit to a small shop and buying an item like a newspaper, then moving on to a bus trip, a large, busy shop, and, eventually a train journey.

8) *Direct observation of result*. The most obvious example is in the treatment of obesity where weight can be directly measured. Unfortunately, such objective criteria are rarely available in clinical practice.

PROCESS

Exposure treatment

Exposure treatment is effective in two-thirds of agoraphobic patients (Mathews *et al.* 1981) and about 80 per cent of these with obsessive-compulsive disorders (Foa and Goldstein 1978; Marks *et al.* 1975). It is also highly effective for specific and social phobias (Marks 1981).

Despite its efficacy for a wide range of psychiatric conditions, there is often concern about using exposure outside of specialist centres. This arises from erroneous views about its applicability, success rate, and time commitment. In fact, behavioural psychotherapy is a remarkably cost-effective and efficient treatment and easily applied in general practice and hospital settings (Marks 1981, 1986; Stern and Drummond 1991). Although training is required, this can be achieved by reading textbooks dealing with technique (e.g. Hawton *et al.* 1989; Stern and Drummond 1991) and obtaining supervision from an experienced therapist.

The most effective exposure method has been shown to be prolonged rather than short duration (Stern and Marks 1973), real life rather than fantasy (Emmelkamp and Wessels 1975) and regularly practised as self-exposure homework tasks (McDonald *et al.* 1978).

Example of exposure treatment

Jill, a 40-year-old married secretary came to the clinic accompanied by
her husband and teenage daughter. She gave a 20-year history of fears
of travelling on her own and staying alone in the house. These
problems had worsened over the previous two years following a house
move some distance away from her family of origin. Her husband, a
factory worker, worked shifts and was often out all night. Jill would
not let her daughter leave the house at such times. She worried that she
was being unreasonable and that this might prevent her daughter
attending university.

A full history of the problem was obtained. Jill, the youngest of a
family of three girls, had always been anxious and shy. At the age of 12
she had felt unwell and fainted during a school assembly. Following
this she had been unwilling to return to school. After a week at home
she had eventually been persuaded to return if her elder sister
accompanied her to the gates and met up with her at break and
lunchtimes. Thereafter, she was always accompanied on the journey to
and from school until she left aged 16.

She started work as a typist and later as a secretary. Since the office
was close to her sister's workplace she was always accompanied. She
avoided travelling on buses or trains for fear she might faint.

Jill married Roy, a friend of her elder brother, at age 21. They both
described their marriage as happy. They had one daughter but had not
had any other children as they felt that this would cause them to
restrict their style of living. Initially they had lived in rented
accommodation near to Jill's parents and two of her siblings. Two
years previously they had bought a house five miles away from their
former residence. To get to work she was required to catch either a bus
or train. She had attempted to get to work on the first day after
moving but had panicked at the bus stop and returned home. Since
that time she had remained off work.

A working hypothesis for the origin and maintenance of Jill's
symptoms was established from the history. The therapist explained thus:

Although you have always been a shy and nervous person, it seems that your
problems really began after you fainted at school. This was an unpleasant
experience which you learned to associate with being away from your family.
Following this episode, you avoided going anywhere alone and therefore
strengthened the belief. You never allowed yourself to discover whether or not
you could be alone without fainting.

Although you managed to cope when you were near to your parents and sisters, the move of house meant that it was no longer convenient for them to accompany you whenever you went out.

Currently, whenever you are in danger of being alone, you take precautions to prevent this. When you went to the bus stop to go to work, you were tense because of your expectation that something dreadful might happen. Due to your tension, you began to notice physical symptoms of anxiety, such as your heart pounding and believed that this was evidence that something terrible was about to happen and you might die.

The next step was to tell Jill and Roy about the nature of anxiety and its treatment. First, the physical and emotional symptoms of anxiety were clarified. Then it was described how avoidance of feared situations led to further avoidance. Thirdly, they were told how anxiety does eventually reduce, even though this may take up to two hours during prolonged exposure to fear-provoking situations. Also, that if this exposure exercise was practised regularly, anxiety gradually waned in both intensity and duration. Finally, they were given the three golden rules for exposure treatment:

(1) Anxiety is unpleasant but does no harm: 'I will not die go mad or lose control'.

(2) Anxiety does eventually diminish: 'It cannot continue indefinitely if I face up to the situation'.

(3) Practice makes perfect: 'The more I repeat a particular exposure exercise the easier it becomes'.

Following this explanation of the rationale of treatment, targets were identified. She chose four specific tasks she wished to perform by the end of treatment which would demonstrate improvement. These were to travel to work alone on the bus during the rush hour; to travel to work alone on the train during the rush hour; to travel alone by bus and underground train into the centre of London and to visit the main shopping areas; and to remain in the flat alone overnight while Roy was on night shift.

Jill decided that it would be easiest for her to start by tackling her problem of walking alone. Roy and her daughter, Louise, agreed to help by acting as 'co-therapists'. All agreed that every evening, when either Louise or Roy arrived home, they were to go out for a walk. Jill was to leave first and walk along a predetermined route; the co-therapist was to wait for five minutes and then follow. They were to take care that the exposure time was long enough for Jill's anxiety to lessen (habituation) (usually between one and two hours). Jill was to record details of the exposure exercises in a diary and to note her anxiety levels at the beginning, middle and end of the task. She would record the level using a 0–8 scale where 0 meant no anxiety and 8 extreme anxiety or panic. If Jill found her anxiety diminishing during the week, she was to go out for a long walk alone.

At the second session the following week, Jill was delighted with her progress. She had managed not only to walk alone but had visited local shops and done some shopping while Louise remained at home. The therapist praised her for this excellent progress. The session was then used to tackle bus travel.

Initially, Jill wanted Roy to sit beside her but eventually agreed to sit at the front of the bus while Roy and the therapist sat at the rear. After a few minutes, Jill became very anxious and complained to the therapist of symptoms of panic. She was gently reminded that this feeling, although unpleasant, would eventually pass, whereas if she gave up, her anxiety might be even worse next time. She returned to her seat and after a further 45 minutes looked more relaxed and cheerful. At the pre-arranged stop, Jill, Roy, and the therapist left the bus. Jill was praised by the therapist who said: 'You have done extremely well. Despite feeling panicky you have managed to face up to your fear and have learned that these frightening and nasty symptoms do eventually lessen.'

On the return journey, Jill sat alone upstairs while husband and therapist sat downstairs. Again, she coped excellently and readily agreed to continue this practice with Roy during the following week. She was to use driver-only buses once her confidence increased and to tackle bus travel alone.

Over the next six sessions, Jill faced the problems of underground train travel, shopping, and being alone in the house. Much of this programme was done by Jill practising at home with Louise and Roy helping out when appropriate. If it was necessary for the therapist to assist in the exposure this was always followed by Jill practising the same exercise daily before the next appointment.

The target of remaining alone at home was difficult to achieve as Louise would always come in at some time even if she did stay out late. Jill was particularly keen to stay alone all night. It was arranged that Louise would spend a week away from home during the school holidays when Roy was due to do a week of night work. On the first night, Jill's sister agreed to be at home and be telephoned if Jill felt overly anxious. Jill was delighted that she managed the task without resorting to the telephone.

By the eighth session all targets of treatment had been achieved. The principles of treatment which Jill had successfully learned and applied were reiterated. The therapist advised her to practise the new behaviours over the following months. Everyone has good and bad days, weeks or months, and the important thing would be for Jill to face up to difficult situations even during the 'bad' times when she felt more anxious. A period of illness which restricted her activities might well lead to a slight increase in fear when she returned to health. Finally, she was congratulated and arrangements made for reviews at one, three, six, and twelve months to ensure that her gains were maintained.

A concern about exposure treatment has been that it requires considerable professional input to accompany a patient into fear-provoking situations. Fortunately, self-exposure instruction can be all that is required for the treatment of many patients with phobic and obsessive-compulsive disorders (Ghosh *et al.* 1988; Marks *et al.* 1988). The efficacy of self-exposure has led to the development of self-help manuals (e.g. Marks 1978). However, few patients can complete a treatment programme successfully without some professional assistance. A professional needs to guide the patient, help to devise targets, monitor progress, offer encouragement and advice in the face of any difficulties.

Self-imposed response prevention

Although exposure is the cornerstone of treatment for obsessive-compulsive disorder, it is not sufficient to overcome the problem as rituals serve to lessen anxiety and prevent habituation occurring. Although compulsions or rituals initially reduce anxiety, they only reduce it minimally and transiently. The limited efficacy of the rituals leads to them being repeated many times. Overall, they serve, therefore, to prolong anxiety and do not allow the anxiety to diminish naturally.

It is thus necessary to ask the patient not to perform rituals. This can be achieved by educating the patient about their effect. Exposure tasks should be graded commencing with those which cause anxiety but at a level which is tolerable without ritualizing. Even with highly motivated patients, slips will occur and they will find themselves performing the rituals occasionally. It is therefore advisable to tell them that this is to be expected but will not interfere with therapy as long as they repeat the exposure task immediately.

An identical approach is taken with the patient seeking reassurance which also interferes with habituation by causing temporary relief from anxiety. It is necessary to educate relatives, friends or professionals who are offering the reassurance so that they respond appropriately. Since relatives have difficulty withholding reassurance it is useful to role-play situations where this is requested and suggest they reply 'Dr X has asked me not to answer questions like that.'

Audio-taped habituation treatment for obsessive ruminations

Audio-taped habituation involves finding out the complete sequence of thoughts in a rumination. It is then found that some of these thoughts cause anxiety and are obsessional in type whereas others are anxiety-reducing or covert rituals. The patient is then asked to record the anxiogenic thoughts on to an audio-tape without the anxiety-reducing words and phrases. A continuous loop tape, as in answering machines, is utilized as this saves the patient having to record the same thoughts repeatedly. The patient is then asked to play the tape back to himself several times a day. The tape is thus an exposure exercise and must be listened to until anxiety is consistently reduced by at least half. As with all exposure methods it must be performed regularly until the ruminations cease to be a problem.

Reduction of undesirable behaviour

Exposure is useful in overcoming anxiety in most forms of anxiety disorder. However, maladaptive behaviour may develop in response to stimuli unrelated to fear and in these cases alternative strategies are needed. The therapist has several options depending on the problem:

(1) eliminating the behaviour using aversive stimuli (only indicated if the behaviour is life-threatening or constitutes a major public nuisance, e.g. covert sensitization);

(2) modifying the stimulus leading to the response (e.g. orgasmic reconditioning);

(3) modifying the response to the stimulus (e.g. stimulus control techniques);

4) replacing the problem behaviour with alternative adaptive responses (e.g. habit reversal);

5) reducing the desirability of the problem behaviour (e.g. mass practice; response cost).

These five categories are not mutually exclusive and a therapist who tries to eliminate a particular behaviour without helping the patient to develop alternative strategies will fail at the task.

Application of covert sensitization in the treatment of sexual deviancy

There are very few indications for aversion therapy. It is infrequently used due to ethical considerations. However, antisocial sexual behaviour resulting in a threat to others requires effective action. Rapid treatment to suppress deviant sexual urges based on aversion principles may be justified.

The form of aversion generally used is covert sensitization. This involves asking the patient, almost always male, to describe two or three aversive scenes and to rate their degree of aversiveness. An aversive scene may be related to the deviant behaviour (e.g. being attacked by fellow prisoners following conviction) or, if no aversive scene connected with the behaviour is forthcoming, can be unrelated (e.g. falling into a vat of vomit). Scripts are then written describing arousing and aversive scenes. The patient is asked to relax and to imagine in detail an arousing scene. Before the patient ends the imagined scene the therapist asks him to change to an aversive scene which is also described in detail. This procedure is repeated five or six times per session. The patient is then instructed to read through the scripts in a similar manner at home. Alternatively, the scripts can be audio-taped and played back at home. It is important to check frequently the anxiety level caused by the aversive scene as habituation can occur, reducing its aversion value. It is useful to change aversive scripts frequently to prevent habituation. As therapy progresses the aversive scene is introduced progressively earlier in the arousing scene until anxiety results as soon as the patient thinks about his deviant fantasy.

The treatment can succeed but clearly requires high motivation. Even in such cases, an effective plan must incorporate elements to increase general personal functioning including sexual.

Application of orgasmic reconditioning in the treatment of sexual deviancy

If a patient has a sexual preference which worries him and his partner but is not inherently dangerous, then less radical treatment is used. In orgasmic reconditioning, originally described by Marquis (1970), the patient is asked to masturbate regularly to his troublesome deviant fantasies but, at the point of orgasmic inevitability, to switch to the desired, 'non-deviant' fantasy. As treatment progresses, the non-deviant stimulus is introduced progressively earlier in the arousal process until masturbation is achieved without a deviant fantasy. Following this, sexual or social skills training is usually needed to ensure that the arousal to non-deviant stimuli persists.

When dealing with distressing sexual urges it is important to set realistic goals. It is not possible, and many would argue not desirable, to change the orientation of an exclusively homosexual person. In this case, counselling to help accept the sexual preference may be indicated. Similarly, if a homosexual paedophile is referred for treatment, it is unrealistic to set the goal of adult heterosexual contact. Adult homosexual orientation is more likely to be achievable.

Application of stimulus control techniques in the treatment of obesity

Obesity is widespread in the Western world and has been resistant to medical, psychodynamic and early behaviourial approaches. The development of behavioural treatments in the 1960s proved more successful (e.g. Stuart 1967). The programme consists of four elements:

(1) Description of the behaviour to be controlled. Patients are asked to keep daily diaries of amount of food ingested, and time and circumstances of eating.

(2) Modification and control of the discriminatory stimuli governing eating. Patients are asked to limit their eating to one room, to use distinctive table settings and to make eating a 'pure' experience unaccompanied by other activities like reading or watching television.

(3) Development of techniques to control the act of eating such as counting each mouthful of food and replacing utensils after each mouthful and leaving some food on the plate at the end of a meal.

(4) Prompt reinforcement of behaviours which delay or control eating.

Although this treatment usually results in weight loss, many patients regain it following the termination. Booster sessions, often run by lay-therapists and available at the person's worksite, have been recommended to prevent such relapse (Stunkard 1977).

Treatment of troublesome habits using habit reversal

Problem behaviour may take the form of bad habits learned in response to a range of stimuli. Azrin and Nunn (1973) pioneered the treatment of habit reversal for a number of habits including tics, nail biting, and neurodermatitis. This treatment has four components:

(1) *Awareness training.* Habits may be performed repeatedly without the patient realizing it. The first step in treatment is to promote awareness by discussing the habit and its trigger factors, and by asking the patient to record its frequency.

(2) *Competing response training.* This involves finding an activity incompatible with the habit and encouraging the patient to perform this whenever the urge to practise the habit occurs. For example, a young woman with facial tics, started the tic by furrowing her forehead and then progressed to grimacing with her whole face and bending her neck. Firm pressure lifting her eyebrows aborted the tic.

(3) *Habit control motivation.* It is important that the patient be encouraged to think about the negative results of the habit and to focus on the improved quality of life resulting from overcoming it.

(4) *Generalization training.* This involves incorporating the competing response into everyday life in a way which is unobtrusive. For example, the woman with facial tics worked at a desk for much of the day. She found she could control the tics by resting her forehead on to her hand and pushing her eyebrows upwards. This manoeuvre was not noticeable to colleagues as she appeared to be resting her head and thinking. She started to wear a hairband which also helped to remind herself not to contract the muscles of her forehead.

Mass practice

Mass practice entails the patient repeating an activity until it becomes boringly repetitive. For example, a man who repeatedly cleared his throat found he was being ridiculed by colleagues. He was instructed to clear his throat continually for 30 minutes three times a day in private but not to engage in the habit at other times. After a week of the exercises, he was unable to clear his throat for the period required and no longer did it at other times.

Response cost

Response cost, based on operant principles, involves having the patient perform a penalty which either consumes time or effort or which is unpleasant whenever target behaviours are performed. Examples include asking the patient to donate a set sum of money to her least favourite charity whenever she uses a swear word, or requiring a child to mop the entire floor following an episode of urinary incontinence.

Applying operant techniques to chronic problems

In the case of long-standing behavioural problems, such as in some institutionalized schizophrenic patients, treatment based on operant conditioning has been used. This has been described as applying 'sticks and carrots' but careful analysis is needed before its application since one person's 'carrot' may be another person's 'stick'. Premack (1959) addressed this aspect by observing that high-frequency preferred activity can be used to reinforce lower-frequency, non-preferred activity. If a child, for instance, spends most of his time playing with toy soldiers, this preferred activity could be used to reinforce the lower-frequency non-preferred activity of helping to wash-up.

The demand for treatment aimed at reducing undesirable behaviour and increasing socially acceptable forms has increased since the 1980s with the closure of psychiatric hospitals and the move towards community care.

Positive reinforcement is the most appropriate and commonly applied type of reinforcement. Negative reinforcement (or punishment) is hardly ever used and only in dangerous or life-threatening situations (due to ethical considerations). Examples of reinforcers are listed below:

Reinforcers which increase specified activities

(A) *Positive reinforcers*

(1) Social approval (e.g. nurse's approval of a patient's improved self-care).

(2) Higher-frequency preferred activities.

(3) Feedback reinforcement (e.g. constructive comments in a social skills group).

(4) Food reinforcers.

(5) Tokens: awarded for certain activities which can be 'spent' on a number of other reinforcers.

(B) *Negative reinforcers*

This entails removal of an aversive event after a specific response is obtained (aversive relief) but it has little place in contemporary treatment. It may be used covertly however in the management of deviant sexual behaviour.

Reinforcers which reduce specified activities

(A) *Punishment*

This refers to applying an aversive stimulus in response to certain behaviours; it should have no role in therapy.

(B) *Response cost*

(1) Penalty involving time and effort in response to certain behaviours.

(2) A positive reinforcer is removed if certain non-desired activities are indulged in, for example, time out (removal of the person from a reinforcing environment for some minutes).

PROBLEMS IN THE COURSE OF THERAPY

Many problems with behavioural psychotherapy can be obviated if a full history and behavioural assessment are done. It is then important to educate the patient about the condition and treatment plan. An integral part is to persuade the patient that the treatment is rational and relevant. Some patients, particularly those who have embarked on other forms of treatment unsuccessfully, may be more difficult to convince. In these cases it is helpful to explain, in lay terms, research findings including those on efficacy. With highly sceptical patients it is worthwhile spending two or three meetings to ensure they are satisfied with the treatment plan. This can be arrived at by coming to a 'bargain' with the patient. For example the therapist might say:

I understand your reluctance to undergo behavioural treatment for your agoraphobia as you have been treated unsuccessfully with several courses of drugs. I am much more confident that you would gain considerable benefit from this treatment. We know that seven in every ten people with agoraphobia improve with this kind of treatment. Before you worry that you may be one of the three in ten who do not, let me tell you that we know the complications which make the treatment less effective and you have none of those. The only remaining factor which determines treatment outcome is how much you want to get better and how doggedly you stick to the task. As you are unsure about this, I would suggest that we try it for two weeks to begin with. If, at the end of this time, you are improving then we should continue; if not we can reconsider.

It is useful to negotiate a number of sessions after which progess is reviewed together. Setting the agenda for the patient's goals during therapy is another important component. This clarifies to both therapist and patient when therapy should end. This agenda, however, should be subject to review.

Despite these measures, not all patients who could be helped by a behavioural approach accept it. Some have adapted their life to the problem for so long that treatment seems worse than the condition itself. For others it is family and friends who desire change whereas they are content to remain as they are. As many as a quarter of patients who could benefit refuse treatment. In these cases, the behavioural assessment can still be useful. For some patients it reveals that family factors influence their decision, and family therapy may be appropriate here. Other patients may have personality difficulties better suited to psychoanalytic psychotherapy. Yet others may be best treated with drugs initially. In all cases, it is important to let patients know they have the right to refuse treatment and that this decision will not jeopardize their receiving behavioural treatment in the future.

A minority of patients undergo behavioural treatment but fail to improve. This should be clear early in treatment as the measures fail to show improvement. The therapist should first ensure that the behavioural assessment and treatment plan were correct and realistic. For example, a woman with obsessive-compulsive disorder failed to respond to exposure treatment for her fears of contamination.

These fears had begun in the wake of her mother's death. Further enquiry revealed that she had failed to mourn her loss. Treatment with guided mourning preceding the exposure treatment was then given with good effect.

Secondly, the therapist should ensure that the treatment is being carried out correctly. This may involve accompanying the patient while the relevant task is performed. Patients may misunderstand instructions. For example, an agoraphobic woman failed to improve on her exposure task of travelling on buses. The therapist accompanied her only to discover that she constantly wore dark glasses and listened to music on a personal tape player to distract herself from the exposure task. Removal of these items led to more anxiety initially but she soon began to show improvement.

Thirdly, other conditions may impede treatment. Foa (1979) examined the reasons for failure in patients with obsessive-compulsive disorder who did not benefit from exposure and response prevention despite full compliance. One group had over-valued ideas that the obsessional fear was rational. Although they demonstrated habituation of anxiety during prolonged exposure, this was not maintained between sessions. The second group of patients were depressed. These patients failed to show any sustained reduction in anxiety during prolonged exposure sessions.

Another reason for failure with obsessive-compulsive disorder is that the patient is performing covert rituals. For example, a man with checking rituals failed to respond but close questioning revealed that whenever he performed an exposure task he would think the words: 'God, please make sure no harm will come'. This was impeding the habituation of his anxiety. He had difficulty stopping this 'prayer' as it came into his mind automatically. Treatment was therefore continued with him wearing a personal tape player on to which he had recorded the phrase 'I have not checked and disaster will occur.' This phrase was repeated continuously during exposure by it being recorded on a loop tape.

TRAINING

The more intensive and prolonged a training the more expensive it is. Costly training should result in a professional with a wider view of problems who is able to perform autonomously. However, this does not necessarily result in good outcome. In a series of studies (reviewed by Marks 1981), psychiatric nurses who underwent a course in behavioural psychotherapy demonstrated that they could treat patients with phobias, obsessive-compulsive rituals, sexual dysfunction, and sexual deviation and obtain at least as good an outcome as did psychologists and psychiatrists. These behavioural nurse-therapists are relatively inexpensive to train.

Even more inexpensive are lay-therapists. They are trained in exposure techniques for certain discrete problems by self-help organizations such as Phobic Action in the United Kingdom.

Many professionals have been concerned about people with limited training offering treatment to psychiatric patients. However, with an estimated six-monthly prevalence of between 5 and 13 per cent for phobic disorder in the adult population of the United States (Myers *et al.* 1984), it is clear that no service could ever provide sufficient resources. Lay-therapists may be able to help those with uncomplicated phobic conditions. Screening is obviously essential to ensure that only suitable patients are treated in this way. This requires general practitioners to be well informed about diagnosis and treatment of phobic disorder. A professional service is also required to whom patients can be referred if lay treatment fails.

With lay-workers and nurse-therapists treating many patients with anxiety disorders it may seem that psychiatrists do not need an in-depth knowledge of behavioural psychotherapy. Nothing could be further from the truth. They are often referred more difficult and complex patients with multiple problems. They are in a position to offer several forms of treatment flexibly. For example, a patient may be referred who has severe depression, obsessive-compulsive disorder, and anorexia nervosa. The psychiatrist is well placed to sort out which symptoms are related to which diagnosis. Treatment would probably start with drug management of the depression. Once it had improved behavioural treatment of the other two conditions would ensue. Even if the psychiatrist feels that these treatments can be performed by another member of the multidisciplinary team, he or she will still need to have full knowledge of the treatments to make an appropriate referral. The psychiatrist may also be needed to assist if the treatment course does not run smoothly.

Training in behavioural psychotherapy can only be obtained through direct experience. There are several handbooks (e.g. Stern and Drummond 1991), as well as many texts about theory and results of treatment (e.g. Marks 1987). The best way to learn is to read a handbook and then treat the simpler cases under supervision of an experienced therapist. The academic texts can then be used to further the trainee's understanding of the techniques used.

CONCLUSION

Behavioural psychotherapy is a highly effective and cost-effective treatment for most of the anxiety disorders, sexual problems, habit disorders, and appetitive disorders. Increasing numbers of conditions are being shown, through controlled trials, to respond to treatment. As well as widening its applicability, research has also focused on more cost-effective ways of treating patients (Ghosh *et al.* 1988).

A major area of interest is to better understand and manage patients who fail to improve. There may be many reasons for this, as discussed earlier. Good results may be obtained by performing a further behavioural analysis and applying other treatments in conjunction with or prior to behavioural psychotherapy (Drummond 1993).

Cognitive therapy is now a popular treatment for many conditions. It can be combined with behavioural psychotherapy if there are appropriate indications. Salkovskis and Warwick (1985), for example, applied cognitive therapy to patients with obsessive-compulsive disorder who failed to respond to behavioural treatment due to over-valued ideas that their obsessions were correct.

In summary, behavioural psychotherapy is widely applicable in psychiatric and medical practice. It is a short-term treatment which often produces marked changes within a matter of weeks. The training needed varies with the setting in which it is to be applied. Attention needs to be paid to treatment failures and to the role of prevention.

REFERENCES

Azrin, N. H. and Nunn, R. G. (1973). Habit reversal: A method of eliminating nervous habits and tics. *Behaviour Research and Therapy*, **11**, 619–28.

Buglass, D., Clarke, J., Henderson, N., Kreitman, N., and Presley, A. S. (1977). A study of agoraphobic housewives. *Psychological Medicine*, **7**, 73–86.

Drummond, L. M. (1993). The treatment of severe, chronic, resistant obsessive-compulsive disorder: An evaluation of an inpatient programme using behavioural psychotherapy in combination with other treatments. *British Journal of Psychiatry*, **163**, 223–9.

Emmelkamp, P. M. G. (1985). Anxiety and fear. In *International Handbook of behavior modification and therapy*, (ed. A. S. Bellack, M. Hersen and A. E. Kazdin), Plenum, New York.

Emmelkamp, P. M. G. and Wessels, H. (1975). Flooding in imagination v flooding *in vivo* in agoraphobics. *Behaviour Research and Therapy*, **13**, 7.

English, H. B. (1929). Three cases of the "conditioned fear response". *Journal of Abnormal and Social Psychiatry*, **34**, 221–5.

Eysenck, H. J. (1957). *Dynamics of anxiety and hysteria*. Routledge & Kegan Paul, London.

Foa, E. B. (1979). Failure in treating obsessive-compulsives. *Behaviour Research and Therapy*, **17**, 169–76.

Foa, E. B. and Goldstein, A. (1978). Continuous exposure and complete response prevention in the treatment of obsessive-compulsive neurosis. *Behavior Therapy*, **9**, 821–9.

Freud, S. (1955). Turnings in the ways of psychoanalytic therapy. In *Standard edition*, Vol. 2. Hogarth, London. (Originally published 1919.)

Gelder, M. G., Marks, I. M., and Wolff, H. H. (1967). Desensitization and psychotherapy in the treatment of phobic states: a controlled enquiry. *British Journal of Psychiatry*, **113**, 53–73.

Ghosh, A., Marks, I. M., and Carr, A. C. (1988). Therapist contact and outcome of self-exposure treatment for phobias: a controlled study. *British Journal of Psychiatry*, **152**, 234–8.

Goldstein, A. J. and Chambless, D. (1978). A reanalysis of agoraphobia. *Behavior Therapy*, **9**, 47–59.

Hand, I., Lamontagne, Y., and Marks, I. M. (1974). Group exposure (flooding) *in vivo* for agoraphobia. *British Journal of Psychiatry*, **124**, 588–602.

Hawton, K., Salkovskis, P. M., Kirk, J., and Clark, D. M. (1989). *Cognitive behavior therapy for psychiatric problems: a practical guide*. Oxford University Press, Oxford.

Headland, K. and McDonald, R. (1987). Rapid audiotaped treatment of obsessional ruminations. *Behavioural Psychotherapy*, **15**, 188–92.

Janet, P. (1903). *Les obsessions et la psychasthenie*. Baillière, Paris.

Lazarus, A. A. (1973). Multimodal behaviour therapy: treating the "Basic ID". *Journal of Nervous and Mental Disorders*, **156**, 404–11.

Levy, R. and Meyer, V. (1971). Ritual prevention in obsessional patients. *Proceedings of the Royal Society of Medicine*, **64**, 115–20.

Locke, J. (1693). *Some thoughts concerning education*. Ward, Lock, London.

Lovell, K., Marks, I. M., Noshirvani, H. and O'Sullivan, G. (1994). Should treatment distinguish anxiogenic from anxiolytic O.C. ruminations? Results of a pilot controlled study and of clinical audit. *Psychotherapy and Psychosomatics*, **61**, 150–5.

Marks, I. M. (1969). *Fears and phobias*. Academic Press, New York.

Marks, I. M. (1981). *Cure and care of neurosis: theory and practice of behavioural psychotherapy*. Wiley, New York.

Marks, I. M. (1987). *Fears, phobias and rituals*. Oxford University Press, Oxford.

Marks, I. M., Hodgson, R. and Rachman, S. (1975). Treatment of chronic OCD 2 years after *in vivo* exposure. *British Journal of Psychiatry*, **127**, 349–64.

Marks, I. M., *et al.* (1983). Imipramine and brief therapist-aided exposure in agoraphobics having self-exposure homework. *Archives of General Psychiatry*, **40**, 153–62.

Marks, I. M., *et al.* (1988). Clomipramine, self-exposure and therapist-aided exposure for obsessive-compulsive rituals. *British Journal of Psychiatry*, **152**, 522–34.

Marquis, J. N. (1970). Orgasmic reconditioning: Changing sexual object choice through controlling masturbation fantasies. *Journal of Behavior Therapy and Experimental Psychiatry*, **1**, 263–70.

Masters, W. H. and Johnson, V. E. (1966). *Human sexual response*. Churchill, London.

Masters, W. H. and Johnson, V. E. (1970). *Human sexual inadequacy*. Churchill, London.

Mathews, A. M., *et al.* (1976). Imaginal flooding v. real exposure in agoraphobics: Outcome. *British Journal of Psychiatry*, **129**, 362–71.

Mathews, A. M., Gelder, M. G. and Johnston, D. W. (1981). *Agoraphobia: nature and treatment*. Guilford, New York.

McDonald, R., Sartory, G., Grey, S. J., Cobb, J., Stern, R., and Marks, I. M. (1978). Effects of self-exposure instructions on agoraphobic outpatients. *Behaviour Research and Therapy*, **17**, 83–5.

Mowrer, O. H. (1950). *Learning theory and personality dynamics*. Arnold, New York.

Myers, J. K., *et al.* (1984). Six month prevalence of psychiatric disorders in three communities. *Archives of General Psychiatry*, **41**, 959–67.

Ohman, A., Dimberg, U. and Ost, L-G. (1984). Animal and social phobias: Biological constraints on learned fear responses. In *Theoretical issues in behavior therapy*, (eds S. Reiss and R. R. Bootzin). Academic Press, New York.

O'Leary, K. D. and Wilson, G. T. (1975). *Behavior therapy: Application and outcome*. Prentice Hall, New Jersey.

Pavlov, I. P. (1927). *Conditioned reflexes*. Academic Press, London.

Premack, D. (1959). Towards empirical behaviour laws: 1. Positive reinforcement. *Psychological Review*, **66**, 219–33.

Rachman, S., Hodgson, R., and Marks, I. M. (1971). Treatment of chronic obsessive-compulsive neurosis. *Behaviour Research and Therapy*, **9**, 237–47.

Rachman, S., Marks, I. M., and Hodgson, R. (1973). The treatment of obsessive-compulsive neurotics by modelling and flooding *in vivo*. *Behaviour Research and Therapy*, **9**, 237–47.

Salkovskis, P. M. (1983). Treatment of an obsessional patient using habituation to audiotaped ruminations. *British Journal of Clinical Psychology*, **22**, 311–13.

Salkovskis, P. M. and Warwick, H. M. C. (1985). Cognitive therapy of obsessive-compulsive disorder: treating treatment failures. *Behavioural Psychotherapy*, **13**, 243–55.

Seligman, M. E. P. (1971). Phobias and preparedness. *Behavior Therapy*, **2**, 307–20.

Spence, K. G., Haggard, P. F., and Ross, L. G. (1958). UCS intensity and the associated (habit) strength of the eyelid CR. *Journal of Experimental Psychology*, **95**, 404–11.

Stampfl, T. J. and Levis, D. G. (1967). Essentials of implosive therapy: a learning theory based psychodynamic behavior therapy. *Journal of Abnormal Psychology*, **72**, 496–503.

Stern, R. S. and Drummond, L. M. (1991). *The practice of behavioural and cognitive psychotherapy*. Cambridge University Press, Cambridge.

Stern, R. S. and Marks, I. M. (1973). Brief and prolonged flooding: A comparison in agoraphobic patients. *Archives of General Psychiatry*, **28**, 270–6.

Stuart, R. B. (1967). Behavioral control of overeating. *Behaviour Research and Therapy*, **1**, 357–65.

Stunkard, A. J. (1977). Obesity and the social environment: Current status and future prospects. *Annals of the New York Academy of Sciences*, **300**, 298–320.

Thorndike, E. L. (1935). *The psychology of wants, interests and attitudes*. Appleton-Century, London.

Watson, J. B. and Rayner, R. (1920). Conditioned emotional reactions. *Journal of Experimental Psychology*, **3**, 1–14.

Watson, J. P. and Marks, I. M. (1971). Relevant and irrelevant fear in flooding—a crossover study of phobic patients. *Behavior Therapy*, **2**, 275–93.

Wolpe, J. (1958). *Psychotherapy by reciprocal inhibition*. Stanford University Press, Stanford.

RECOMMENDED READING

Erwin, E. (1978). *Behavior therapy*. Cambridge University Press. (A readable account of the scientific, philosophical, and ethical foundations of the behavioural approach.)

Foa, E. and Emmelkamp, P. M. (ed.) (1983). *Failures in behavior therapy*. Wiley, New York. (Leading workers in the field examine reasons for therapeutic failure which serves to instruct how one attempts to do an optimal job.)

Marks, I. M. (1978). *Living with fear*. McGraw-Hill, New York. (A self-help book for anxious patients written for a lay audience but full of case histories demonstrating the treatments in practice.)

Marks, I. M. (1981). *Cure and care of neurosis: Theory and Practice of Behavioural Psychotherapy*. Wiley, New York. (Although somewhat out of date, an excellent background to the theoretical and clinical background of behavioural psychotherapy.)

Marks, I. M. (1987). *Fears, phobias, and rituals*. Oxford University Press. (A full account of research in animal and human behaviour related to behavioural psychotherapy as well as a section on syndromes and their treatment and research.)

Stern, R. S. and Drummond, L. M. (1991). *The practice of behavioural and cognitive psychotherapy*. Cambridge University Press. (A practical guide which concentrates on how techniques are performed in practice. Case histories are used to demonstrate these techniques.)

Thorpe, G. L. and Olson, S. L. (1990). *Behavior therapy: concepts, procedures and applications*. Allyn & Bacon, Boston. (Solid introductory text covering basic notions in learning theory and their clinical relevance.)

7

Cognitive psychotherapy

NICHOLAS B. ALLEN

This chapter begins by recognizing the difficulty of providing an exhaustive definition of cognitive therapy while its applications and concepts are diversifying rapidly. The cognitive model of psychopathology and therapy is presented in the context of its historical development, where it can be seen as a distillation of certain themes from experimental psychology, behaviour therapy, and psychodynamic therapy. The seminal work of Aaron Beck and his colleagues is emphasized, and the therapy is presented as a directive and time-limited approach, which focuses on helping patients to gain new skills in managing distressing emotions and other psychological symptoms. Other important features of cognitive therapy include its provision of detailed treatment guidelines, and its commitment to rigorous outcome assessment. The limitations of this approach are also discussed, as are some of the more recent theoretical and technical developments designed to overcome these.

Defining any approach to psychotherapy is difficult because various schools often use different language to describe similar phenomena and techniques. A particular school may also encapsulate a wide variety of emphases, with resultant overlap between approaches. This is particularly the case with cognitive therapy. Although a prototypic version of cognitive therapy can be described, approaches identifying themselves as 'cognitive' range from those emphasizing a highly prescriptive approach, and a focus on behavioural change (e.g. Meichenbaum 1977), to others that highlight less structured and exploratory aspects, and stress conceptual change (e.g. Guidano and Liotti 1983). The reasons for this breadth are most likely due to the stage of development of cognitive therapy (i.e. it is still in a phase of active growth), and to the nature of the central construct invoked, namely cognition.

Dobson and Block (1988) suggest that cognitive-behaviour therapies[1] share three propositions: (1) cognitive activity affects behaviour; (2) cognitive activity may be monitored and altered; and (3) desired behavioural change is achievable through cognitive change. Although this is a sound starting definition, its capacity to describe cognitive therapy relies on the definition of 'cognition'. By and large this definition has been an everyday version of the concept (Teasdale 1993). For instance, Beck describes cognitions as 'any ideation with verbal or pictorial content' (Beck *et al*. 1979*a*), or as 'stream-of-consciousness or automatic thoughts that tend to be in an individual's awareness' (Beck *et al*. 1983). This definition, which emphasizes conscious experience, differs from that of an experimental cognitive psychologist, who regards cognition as any phenomena pertinent to human information-processing, including memory and attention, as well as mechanisms that occur very early in the processes of human perception and are non-conscious (Neisser 1967). Other debates regarding the relationship between cognition and emotion also highlight how the definition of 'cognition' can influence the way in which cognitive phenomena are construed (Lazarus 1982; Zajonc 1980). Thus, depending on the phenomena subsumed under cognition, Dobson and Block's principles could be used to cover almost all psychotherapies involving mentalistic phenomena, including, for instance, psychodynamic and experiential approaches. However, their principles operate best when cognition relates to consciously experienced verbal and pictorial phenomena.

An alternative way to define cognitive therapy is to consider its *modus operandi*. Hawton *et al*. (1989) offer such a process-oriented definition proposing that cognitive-behaviour therapy is typified by its:

—expression of concepts in operational terms;
—empirical validation of treatment;
—specification of treatment in operational terms;
—evaluation of treatment with reliable and objective measures;

[1]The terms 'cognitive therapy' and 'cognitive-behaviour therapy' often cause confusion. In general, the two terms mean the same thing, except that the term 'cognitive-behaviour therapy' makes explicit reference to the fact that techniques derived from behaviour therapy (see Chapter 6) are usually included in the treatment protocol. This should be seen as reflecting a form of technical rather than theoretical eclecticism (i.e. that although behavioural techniques are recognized as effective, the mechanisms by which they achieve change are understood in terms of cognitive constructs and models). For our purposes the terms will be used interchangeably.

—emphasis on the "here and now";
—objective to help patients to bring about desired changes in their lives;
—focus on new learning and changes outside the clinical setting;
—explicit description of therapeutic procedures to the patient;
—collaboration of the patient and therapist to deal with identified problems;
—use of time limits and explicitly agreed goals.

This definition has the advantage over more substantive ones in avoiding the debate about the nature of cognition. Most mainstream approaches, however, include both content- and process-oriented definitions.

THEORETICAL BACKGROUND: AN HISTORICAL CONTEXT

Three traditions, experimental psychology, behaviour therapy, and psychodynamic therapy, have influenced the development of cognitive therapy.

The notion of cognition in experimental psychology goes back to the nineteenth century, when two pioneering psychologists, Wilhelm Wundt (1888) and William James (1890), both defined their subject as the science of mental life. This early research chiefly concerned itself with matters of cognition, such as the processes whereby information was perceived, stored, and used in the mind. The methodology involved subjects trained in introspection examining their cognitive processes during experimental tasks. This phase of research was overtaken by a behaviourist framework during the 1920s, largely due to difficulties in demonstrating the validity of self-report data generated by this introspective methodology, and concerns this would compromise psychology's standing as a legitimate science (MacLeod 1993). Behaviourism offered an alternative in which phenomena had to be observable and objectively quantifiable. This limited the data of experimental psychology to overt behaviour. Although behaviourism employed cognitive constructs to explain observed behaviour (e.g. classical and operant conditioning involving storage and retrieval of information in order to exert an enduring influence on behaviour), these were kept to a minimum, and consideration of subjective phenomena eschewed.

Behaviourist research flourished as investigators conducted controlled experiments designed to examine the role of various processes, especially learning, in determining behaviour. By the 1950s and 1960s, however, psychologists became dissatisfied with the capacity of the model to explain complex behaviour. This was particularly relevant in areas like natural language acquisition, where children learn linguistic skills of such idiosyncrasy and complexity that they are well beyond the capacity of adults to reinforce discriminately (Chomsky 1959; Vygotksy 1962). Other challenges to the paradigm included Bandura's (1977) work on vicarious learning, and Mischel's on delay of gratification (Mischel *et al.* 1972). Even ostensibly simple behaviour such as a reaction time task was shown to contradict predictions from behavioural accounts (e.g. Crossman 1953). Attempts to deal with these aspects without threatening the behaviourist framework included using the notion of 'covert' behaviour to explain the role of thoughts (Homme 1965). George Kelly's (1955) work on personal constructs and Jean Piaget's (1954) studies of child development also influenced interest in cognitive concepts.

An alternative framework, based on information-processing, thus emerged in psychology, linguistics, computer science, neuroscience, and philosophy. This 'cognitive science' (Gardner 1985) utilized information-processing and the computer as the metaphor to explain intelligent behaviour; cognitive psychology began to be accepted as an alternative to behaviourism. Information-processing concepts like parallel and serial processing, limited capacity and multiple channel systems, temporary storage buffers, and selective filters were used to extend the models developed by psychologists (MacLeod 1993). Experimental psychologists were then able to predict more precisely the behavioural performance of subjects during various tasks. This new model has developed to the point where the cognitive approach probably represents the pre-eminent paradigm in contemporary psychology.

As behaviourism in psychological *science* was questioned, its limitations in clinical *practice* were also noted. Important behaviourally oriented therapists not only felt that they were required to ignore important mental phenomena, but some of the disorders they treated entailed symptoms that were inherently cognitive (Dobson and Block 1988). One obvious example is obsessive-compulsive disorder. Although compulsive behaviour lent itself to behavioural analysis, the obsession often went unexplained.

Thus, although the emphasis in traditional behaviour therapies on overt behaviour provided a marked increase in efficacy of treatment, especially those for disorders chiefly defined by their behavioural correlates (i.e. phobic anxiety), the need to extend the application of these therapies created an impetus for a model that could guide treatment of non-behavioural symptoms.

The most influential pioneering work to emerge from behaviourism was that of Donald Meichenbaum (1977). His research on training schizophrenic patients to use 'healthy talk' stimulated his curiosity into the relationship between self-instruction (including thoughts) and behaviour modification. He proposed that these 'covert behaviours' were subject to the same laws of conditioning as overt behaviours, and also reasoned that self-instructions were crucial to the voluntary control of behaviour. Meichenbaum developed self-instructional training (SIT) programmes designed for difficulties related to self-control (e.g. impulsive children). Later, SIT was extended to other disorders like schizophrenia and anxiety. Skills taught in SIT were: (1) problem definition; (2) problem approach; (3) attention-focusing; (4) coping statements; (5) error-correcting options; and (6) self-reinforcement. Although dealing directly with cognitive phenomena, this pioneering endeavour had a behavioural flavour with its emphasis on modelling, graded tasks, and self-reinforcement.

Introducing cognitive phenomena into behaviour therapy was initially treated with suspicion but the work of Meichenbaum and his kind, who presented this change as a logical evolution of behavioural technique and philosophy, did much to allay these concerns. The other crucial development in the acceptance of cognitive approaches was the rigorous assessment of outcome to which the cognitive-behavioural treatments have been subjected, some of which show a superiority of cognitive-behavioural techniques over purely behavioural ones (e.g. Dobson 1989). More explicitly cognitive approaches such as those of Beck (1967) and Ellis (1962) were accepted more hesitantly.

Important questions were also raised by cognitive therapists regarding the psychodynamic model of personality and its associated treatment. In particular, emphases on long-term therapy, the unconscious, detailed scrutiny of personal history, and insight into the transference as the main vehicle for change, were questioned (Beck 1967; Ellis 1962). In addition, some outcome reviews of traditional psychotherapy suggested there was little evidence for their efficacy (Eysenck 1969; Rachman and Wilson 1980).

Roots of cognitive therapy are also detectable in neo-Freudian models: Sullivanian (Arieti 1980), Adlerian (Schulman 1985); logotherapy (Frankl 1985); and Horneyan (Rendon 1985). Indeed, Albert Ellis and Aaron Beck, two central figures in cognitive therapy, were originally trained in psychoanalysis. Ellis (1962) became frustrated with standard psychoanalysis on observing that 'patient after patient would say to me: "Yes, I see exactly what bothers me now and why I am bothered by it; but I nevertheless still am bothered. Now what can I do about that?"' He began to experiment with more active, directive, and short-term treatments. The resultant rational-emotive therapy (RET) regards emotional disturbance in terms of an A-B-C model, where A refers to an activating event, C to the consequence for the person (usually an emotional response), and B refers to the beliefs or cognitive processes that mediate the relationship between A and C. Neurosis comes about through irrational beliefs, whose essence relate to unrealistic or absolute expectations (Ellis 1970). The similarity between these irrational 'musts' (i.e. 'I must be approved of by others') and Karen Horney's notion of 'the tyranny of the shoulds' clearly indicates his own intellectual heritage. By replacing irrational beliefs with more realistic ones, changes in distressing emotion follow. Although RET employs a range of behavioural and emotive techniques, the pre-eminent activity is the logical examination of the patient's beliefs through questioning, challenge, and debate.

Beck noted consistent themes in the conscious ideation of his patients, especially those with depression. His 'cognitive triad of depression' comprises negative views of the self, the world, and the future (Beck 1967). These phenomena, he asserted, were neglected in psychoanalytic treatment in favour of emotional and motivational material. Depressed patients also showed distorted thinking patterns, focusing on negatively construed experiences or explanations for events. Schemata, a term derived from cognitive psychology, are cognitive structures guiding this information-processing. In those vulnerable to emotional disorders, schemata from early life experiences are unrealistic and distorted, facilitating dysphoric responses. Once responses are established, negative schemata continue to exert an effect on information-processing which serves to maintain and exacerbate the emotional state.

Beck's theory is conceptually similar to that of Ellis, and entails similar techniques to those used in RET. Differences relate to their personalities, and to RET's emphasis on more logical-philosophical discussion wedded to the ethos of rational hedonism, compared to

Beck's cognitive therapy which is more deductive, emphasizing gathering evidence for and against particular conclusions.

Cognitive therapy has diversified both in application and range of models, including emphasis on problem-solving skills (e.g. D'Zurilla and Goldfried 1971), coping skills (Meichenbaum 1977), and self-control processes (Rehm 1977). A trend has also emerged for cognitive models to move from 'rationalist' (i.e. promoting more accurate perception, in the belief that inaccurate perception lies at the heart of neurosis), to constructivist models which stress a person's active role in the construction of *any* perceived reality (Mahoney 1991). Thus, the constructivist approach emphasizes the viability rather than the validity of a way of thinking, and a less directive and more exploratory approach to psychotherapy has emerged as a result. Although these developments have been criticized for ignoring the programmatic approach inherited from behaviour therapy, and for losing touch with scientific psychology (MacLeod 1993; Ross 1991), it has been counter-argued that the changes have permitted therapy to be directed to more difficult conditions (Neimeyer 1993).

Among these diverse cognitive approaches, that described by Beck and his colleagues (i.e. Beck *et al.* 1979*a*, 1985, 1990; Wright *et al.* 1993) is most useful in encapsulating the central defining features of cognitive therapy, and has been carefully assessed in a series of outcome studies (Hollon and Najavits 1988). This chapter will therefore focus mainly on Beck's work.

OBJECTIVES

The aims of cognitive therapy are twofold: to reduce distress by teaching skills to recognize, evaluate, and change relevant cognitive processes; and, in later phases, to engender an understanding of themes in maladaptive cognitions in order to modify enduring sets of attitudes and beliefs that are the basis of the patient's vulnerability. The approach to a problem involves the following steps: eliciting automatic thoughts; testing their accuracy and viability; developing realistic alternatives; and identifying and challenging underlying maladaptive schemata (Beck *et al.* 1979*a*).

Three types of cognitive phenomena determine psychopathology, especially emotional disorders: automatic thoughts; cognitive distortions; and schemata. Automatic thoughts, the surface level of

cognition, are the often transitory verbal and pictorial experience
that maintain abnormal mood states. They are automatic in as much
as they emerge spontaneously, and are often difficult to resist. Despite
the ubiquitous nature of automatic thoughts, many people are
unaware of them, and need help to develop the skill of 'thought
catching' before further therapy proceeds. These thoughts show a
specific relationship to the kind of mood states they engender. For
instance, depression relates to thoughts about loss, defeat, rejection,
and hopelessness, anxiety to thoughts of threat and danger, and panic
to a catastrophic interpretation of bodily symptoms (Clark and Beck
1989).

Cognitive distortions refer to misinterpretations of reality that
reinforce negative conclusions. Beck (1967) describes specific kinds of
cognitive distortions, including over-generalizing (a single instance is
taken as an example of a wide range of situations), dichotomous
thinking (only extreme points of view are considered), selective
abstraction (attending solely to negative aspects of a situation),
personalizing (assuming oneself is the cause of an event or of another's
actions), 'should' statements (absolute imperatives are applied to one's
own or another's behaviour), 'catastrophizing' and minimizing
(emphasizing negative and down-playing positive outcomes).

Information about oneself and one's environment is perceived,
stored, and recalled through schemata which are assumed to evolve
during repeated experiences; these help a person to recognize
consistencies so that novel information is linked to current
knowledge efficiently. Since a bias towards schema-congruent
information occurs, psychopathological states result from schemata
that facilitate interpretation of situations in terms of threats to the self,
such as loss, failure, rejection, and danger. These schemata are not
accessible without considerable introspection. Although it is possible
to describe them in verbal terms, such as 'If I am a good person, bad
things will not happen to me', it is not expected that they exert their
influence necessarily through verbal conscious processes. In other
words, the form of schemata are usually deduced on the basis of
recurrent cognitive distortions and automatic thoughts. Once a
schema is activated by a congruent mood state or event, it
dominates perceptions of current and future situations.

In summary, cognitive therapy aims to elicit, evaluate, and modify
negative automatic thoughts, cognitive distortions, and maladaptive
schemata using a range of cognitive, emotive, and behavioural
techniques outlined below.

SELECTION

The first judgement about selection is in terms of diagnosis. Ludgate *et al.* (1993) propose that cognitive therapy is indicated for non-psychotic forms of depression, anxiety disorders, eating disorders, substance abuse, and most personality disorders. The therapy may also be useful as an adjunct to other treatments in psychotic depression, bipolar disorder, schizophrenia, schizo-affective disorder, and mild dementia. It is not suitable for severe dementia, delirium, and moderate to severe mental retardation. These assertions are not based on outcome literature but rather on the premise that in cases where intellectual functioning is severely compromised by organicity application of cognitively oriented techniques is limited.

Many conditions treated by cognitive therapy may also be dealt with by alternative approaches, including medication. For instance, researchers have noted an equivalent effect of cognitive therapy and medication in depression, although cognitive therapy may have superior outcomes at one- and two-year follow-up (Hollon *et al.* 1991). Several controlled trials suggest that cognitive therapy is superior to standard behaviour therapy or medication in generalized anxiety and panic disorder (see Beck 1993), both in short- and long-term follow-up. Studies also support better effects from the cognitive therapy of eating disorders compared to other psychotherapies (Fairburn *et al.* 1991). 'Either-or' type decisions are, however, often unnecessary. Moreover, a synergistic effect from the combination of medication and cognitive therapy treatments is likely in several conditions, particularly depression (e.g. Agras *et al.* 1992; Bowers 1990; Miller *et al.* 1989).

In determining suitability for cognitive therapy on the basis of clinical features, most attention has been paid to depression. There have been some suggestions that antidepressant medication is more effective than cognitive therapy for those with more severe depression (Elkin *et al.* 1989), but other studies fail to replicate this finding (Hollon *et al.* 1992; McLean and Taylor 1992; Thase *et al.* 1991*c*). Indeed Thase *et al.* (1991*a*) reported an uncontrolled trial in which cognitive therapy was effective for a group of unmedicated, 'endogenously' depressed in-patients. Furthermore, cognitive therapy is equally effective across groups with and without endogenous symptoms as indicated by abnormal sleep electroencephalograph (EEG) patterns (Simons and Thase 1992), abnormal dexamethasone suppression results (considered in some cases as a biological marker

for melancholic depression) (McKnight *et al.* 1992), or Research
Diagnostic Criteria endogenous diagnosis (Thase *et al.* 1991*b*). Thus
evidence supports the view that cognitive therapy's efficacy extends
beyond mild and moderate depressions.

A third approach to selection is to consider psychological features
which may enhance benefit from cognitive therapy. Good problem-
solving ability, minimal impairment of learning and memory function,
and high motivation for self-control are examples. In Safran and
Segal's (1990) assessment interview which seeks to determine
suitability for short-term cognitive therapy, selection criteria are that
the patient displays:

—the capacity to access and identify automatic thoughts;
—awareness and differentiation of emotions;
—acceptance of responsibility for change;
—understanding and acceptance of the cognitive rationale;
—capacity to form a therapeutic alliance, as reflected in both
  therapist–patient interaction and past relationships;
—shorter rather than longer duration of problems;
—a low propensity to rigidly use avoidant information processing
  strategies to reduce anxiety;
—ability to maintain a problem focus.

Safran *et al.* (1993) have found that a semi-structured interview to
assess these criteria can predict outcome of short-term cognitive
therapy. Another criterion correlating with good outcome is the
willingness and capacity to complete prescribed homework exercises
(Fennell and Teasdale 1987; Persons *et al.* 1988).

As mentioned above, cognitive therapy is not suitable for those whose
capacity to engage in its logical and empirical procedures is limited.
Organic brain syndromes and acute psychotic states are examples,
although it should be noted that cognitive therapies are increasingly
being seen as relevant to the management of some psychotic symptoms
(Birchwood and Tarrier 1992). Another way to tackle suitability
emerges from research that shows non-responders are more likely to
have severe symptoms (especially cognitive symptoms like
hopelessness), interpersonal problems (e.g. marital discord), and more
difficulties in the therapeutic relationship (Robins and Hayes 1993). On
the other hand, technical procedures have been especially designed with
these patients in mind (Safran and Segal 1990; Young 1990).

Cognitive therapists also typically apply self-report inventories to
assess symptomatology and cognitive processes. Beck's inventories to

assess depression (Beck *et al.* 1979*a*), hopelessness, (Beck *et al.* 1974), suicidal ideation (Beck *et al.* 1979*b*) and anxiety (Beck *et al.* 1988), are commonly used in the initial assessment and during the course of therapy. Other relevant questionnaires include the Automatic Thoughts Questionnaire (Hollon and Kendall 1980) which measures the frequency of thoughts typical of depression, and the Dysfunctional Attitudes Scale (Weissman and Beck 1978) which focuses on dysfunctional beliefs.

As in many forms of psychotherapy, assessment and treatment are iterative processes. Indeed, given cognitive therapy's empirical nature, the patient is encouraged to participate actively in the assessment process, and to collaborate in modifying procedures in the light of new circumstances. Assessment procedures usually involve self-monitoring and are part of homework exercises. Their aim is to establish a clear cognitive-behavioural analysis of the patient's problems. In this respect, the initial interview shares many features with behavioural interviewing (see Chapter 6), by concentrating on description of the problem in terms of its behavioural, cognitive, affective, and physiological components, as well as situational and maintaining factors (Kirk 1989). The customary behavioural emphasis on specific detail (e.g. What? Where? When? How often? With whom? How distressing? How disruptive?) also typifies cognitive-behavioural assessment, as does the emphasis on avoidance behaviours, coping styles, and inner resources. More specific to cognitive therapy assessment is the pivotal focus on conscious thoughts and images, and their role as symptomatic, precipitating, and maintaining factors in dysphoric moods and problem behaviours. These procedures are used in the initial assessment phase, and typically continue throughout the therapeutic process.

PROCESS

The process of cognitive therapy entails both a set of techniques and a particular style of interaction or therapeutic relationship known as 'collaborative empiricism' (Beck *et al.* 1979*a*). The therapist aims to create an atmosphere where resistance and competition between therapist and patient are reduced by a collaborative, task-oriented alliance. The therapist blends empathy with an active and problem-oriented focus. The main tool to maintain this focus is referred to as 'Socratic questioning' (Beck *et al.* 1979*a*), so-called in that it attempts to imitate a philosophical dialogue. Socrates used questions rather than assertions to expose the illogical or inconsistent quality of another person's position. Patients are expected to develop a questioning and curious attitude towards their condition, extending to erecting hypotheses about links between thoughts and feelings, and designing experiments to test these. The therapist's stance is prescriptive in so far as he makes certain assumptions about the phenomena on which to focus, and plays an active role in structuring sessions and setting homework tasks. However, the role is not entirely directive since the therapist looks to the patient to provide crucial information, and to participate actively in gaining an understanding of his problems.

Just as the therapist is expected to be active, so is the patient. He completes homework exercises from the very first session in order to generalize skills acquired in therapy to everyday life. Completion of the exercises is associated with better outcomes, an effect not solely due to differences in motivation or the use of active coping strategies (Burns and Nolen-Hoeksema 1991).

The structure of a typical session reflects this active, problem-focused style. It often begins with a review of homework tasks, followed by the drawing up of an agenda in order of importance. Only a limited number of issues can be covered during a single session. Many patients find it difficult to focus on a distinct topic without straying into other ostensibly relevant problems, but which may not facilitate resolution of the issue at hand. This is not surprising given that most patients experience their situation as a complex tangle of intertwined facets; this contributes to a perception of being 'stuck' and unable to change self-defeating behaviours. A cardinal technique is to inculcate the idea of dealing with one problem at a time, or even to divide it up into subtasks. Accordingly, an important skill for the therapist is to re-direct a patient to the task at hand, while empathically confirming that any related matters raised are pertinent but will be attended to at another time.

The therapist seeks to identify the salient cognitive and behavioural dimensions of the problem. Specifically, he tries to differentiate between objective reality and the patient's idiosyncratic cognitive appraisal of events, and related emotional reactions. Once these elements are clearly delineated, therapist and patient attempt to identify one or two automatic thoughts inherent in the emotional response. With target cognitions mapped out, a range of strategies are deployed to evaluate their veracity and adaptiveness, and to devise more realistic and useful alternatives. At the end of the session the therapist reviews the material covered, seeks the patient's feedback, and sets homework exercises to be completed before the next appointment.

Techniques relate to the aims of therapy: to elicit and test automatic thoughts; provide rational alternatives; and identify and modify underlying dysfunctional schemata. Early on, when symptom reduction is the goal stressed, work focuses on automatic thoughts. It is important to work efficiently to affect prompt symptomatic relief, especially in a condition like depression where motivation is a key factor and the risk of suicide may loom. Therapy is thus more prescriptive, behaviourally focused, and structured in early sessions.

Behavioural techniques (called thus because they emphasize overt behaviour, not because they fail to target cognitive mechanisms) include scheduling activities, graded task assignment, behavioural and cognitive rehearsal, and diversion techniques (Beck *et al.* 1979*a*). Exposure may also be used extensively, especially to overcome anxiety, and is described in detail in Chapter 6. Scheduling involves recording what is done between 9 a.m. and 12 midnight, on an hourly basis. Activities are rated for both mastery (i.e. level of achievement for the patient to do an activity) and pleasure, on 10-point scales. This is usually the first task for patients, especially those with depression, since it helps both the therapist and patient to observe links between activities and mood. It also helps to break down the patient's perception of being in a consistently dysphoric mood, whatever the circumstances. Once these links are established, scheduling is used to lift mood (or at least to alleviate the worst periods), as well as to provide for a sense of achievement when difficult tasks are attempted.

Graded task assignments help patients to achieve difficult goals (e.g. challenging a superior at work) by breaking down the required activity into more achievable subtasks. These assignments are a good 'tonic' for those who typically try to achieve everything at once, or procrastinate. They also help patients unwilling to accept the limitations imposed by their clinical status (i.e. being severely depressed). In cases where problems in concentration, low self-efficacy, or skill deficits interfere with task completion, behavioural and cognitive rehearsal is conducted during the session or as homework in order to increase the capacity to overcome these obstacles. Rehearsal is particularly effective to improve skills for managing anger or interpersonal conflict. Finally, diversion techniques, such as physical activity, social contact, and imagery, are used to achieve temporary relief from dysphoric emotions.

Techniques applied early in therapy also seek to identify and test automatic thoughts. The nature of these is first explained, including their role in maintaining unwanted emotional states and problem behaviours. One explicit way to identify these thoughts is to ask patients what goes through their mind when they experience an unpleasant emotional state or face a difficult situation. Although some recall and report these phenomena readily, a clear recollection may be biased by the *post hoc* nature of the task. Various strategies are therefore deployed to examine the relationship between automatic thoughts and problematic behaviour and emotions as realistically as possible. For instance, a mood change during the session is an ideal opportunity to inquire about accompanying thoughts (e.g. a depressed patient who becomes upset while reflecting on a past rejection, or the anxious patient apprehensive about the consultation itself). Imagery also helps to recall the full emotional context of a situation in more detail than is afforded by verbal account alone. The therapist must work with the patient to paint as vivid a picture as possible, while the latter shares associated thoughts and feelings. Role-playing can also provide a more vital set of cues in order to recall cognitive–emotive links.

The 'downward arrow' technique (Burns 1980) is a method to explore the relationship between conscious cognitions and dysfunctional assumptions. The therapist repeatedly asks 'So what if that is true, what does that mean?' (with appropriate variations in phrasing) to thoughts a patient associates with a dysphoric state. This is particularly pertinent when automatic thoughts are not as potent as the emotional response engendered by them. Insight into a basic fear, such as of loneliness, failure, subordination, or being overwhelmed by one's own emotions, often ensues. The technique also enables hypothesis development about dysfunctional schemata that underlie vulnerability.

Another strategy commonly utilized to assess negative automatic thoughts is self-monitoring such as the daily record of dysfunctional thoughts (Beck *et al.* 1979a). Patients are required to recognize unpleasant emotions by recording their occurrence, the situation or thought that triggered them, and associated automatic thoughts. Patients complete this record sheet during, or as close to, actual experiences as they are able in the hope that the quality of information gained will be superior when recorded *in vivo* rather than when recalled during a session. The next step is to test the accuracy and adaptiveness of negative thoughts. Much time is devoted to this and to developing ational alternatives. Socratic questioning is used to probe thoughts related to problematic emotions and behaviour. These questions are: 1) What is the evidence to support the thought? (2) Are there any alternative interpretations? (3) Am I totally to blame for this negative event, and can I do anything about it? and (4) What if my interpretation is true? How will I manage then? (Thase and Beck 1993). These questions aim to establish to what degree particular thoughts are biased or exaggerated, and if they do reflect a real difficulty or skill deficit, how the patient can best cope with a 'worst-case scenario'.

The final step in dealing with negative automatic thoughts is to develop rational alternatives. The therapist leads a problem-solving exercise to test current thoughts and alternatives by posing the above questions. The daily record of dysfunctional thoughts is used extensively at this point, first during, and then between sessions, at times of distress. The record asks the patient to consider realistic alternatives to specific negative automatic thoughts, and to re-rate their emotional state and level of belief in the original thoughts. The therapist guides this process initially in the anticipation that the patient will eventually apply the procedure in the 'heat of the moment'. When facing an emotionally demanding situation she first records her thoughts *in vivo*, and then collaboratively works on developing alternatives during a session. A phase follows in which the patient is encouraged to become progressively more independent at this task, until she is able to apply it during the most difficult episodes between sessions.

On occasion, evolution of realistic cognitions prompts further negative automatic thoughts which, ironically, make it seem that realistic thoughts are emotionally aversive. For instance, a patient responding to the thought: 'Because a person only spoke to me briefly, he must be angry with me' with a realistic response 'If he were really angry with me he probably would have expressed it more obviously' may be reminded of previous occasions when people expressed anger towards him, and of his perceived inability to cope with this experience. These second-order automatic thoughts are dealt with directly to ensure they do not hinder therapy. With progress the patient is encouraged to 'internalize' these new skills by relying less on recording techniques, such as the daily record of dysfunctional thoughts, and more on mental self-monitoring.

During therapy, consistent themes in the negative automatic thoughts that a patient experiences in a number of circumstances usually emerge. These themes are indicative of dysfunctional assumptions underlying these phenomena. All the above procedure are relevant to detect these. Autobiographical techniques are also applied to examine the evolution of these assumptions (Beck *et al* 1979*a*). This process may begin from as early as the first few session to a later point after a measure of symptomatic control has been achieved. Techniques used to bring about change in basic attitude resemble those used with automatic thoughts in that they employ a logical, philosophical, and empirical examination. However, the process is slower, involving more exploration and reflection than modifying thoughts.

Conducting 'behavioural experiments' in which a patient acts in accordance with an alternative to a customary dysfunctional assumption provide experiential as well as logical evidence that he need not be bound by these maladaptive beliefs. For instance, in a patient living by the rule: 'If I disagree with someone, even in the smallest way, he will reject me,' an experiment in which he voices polite disagreement with others in order to find that this is not necessarily followed by rejection, may provide crucial evidence for an alternative viewpoint.

TERMINATION

Cognitive therapy was conceived as short-term and time-limited. Explicit goals and timetables for achieving them are therefore set. Termination is usually not as complex as for more open-ended treatment, but is still addressed throughout, by emphasizing that indefinite treatment is unnecessary. Indeed, the therapist's objective is to impart knowledge and techniques of therapy in order that the patient may generalize gains to future problems and to those not fully addressed during treatment. Dependence on the therapist is not only discouraged, but patients are expected to become more self-reliant as therapy proceeds.

Nevertheless, poorly handled termination is problematic, interfering with the capacity to maintain the process of change. As it approaches, patients may express concern about relapse or the capacity to apply cognitive techniques without therapeutic support (e.g. 'I'll forget what I've learned' or 'I won't be able to discipline myself when therapy ends'). These thoughts are approached similarly to other negative thoughts dealt with in therapy. It is helpful to emphasize a patient's good use of treatment by recalling illustrative achievements. Role-plays where the therapist presents worst-case scenarios, with accompanying negative thoughts and interpretations, and the patient plays the therapist's role by guiding the problem-solving process and proposing more realistic alternatives, also help in the termination phase. An additional option is to offer a 'booster session' to review progress about a month after the final meeting.

PROBLEMS ENCOUNTERED DURING THERAPY

Several problems may be encountered, therapist or patient-based, although a blend of the two is most common. The chief caveat for the therapist is to be careful not to lose sight of the individual patient while focusing energetically on his problems and techniques to assist with these. The risk here is that his resources and assets may be missed, and thus not appropriately harnessed.

In the face of what can be intense hopelessness in the patient's interpretation of a situation, the therapist must maintain optimism and a solution orientation. This can be difficult when hopeless scenarios are presented that are ostensibly convincing; at these times it is important that the therapist re-emphasize fundamental problem-solving principles, and/or deploys new tactics. Many patients, while apparently rejecting optimism, later report that this was pivotal in stemming the tide of hopelessness. To this end, the therapist also learns to deal with her own negative thoughts, particularly regarding tardy progress or lack of gratitude. Thoughts like 'If all my patients do not get better I must be an incompetent therapist' or 'After all my efforts this patient should show me more gratitude' exemplify dysfunctional interpretations. The therapist's recognition of these thoughts reduces any corresponding frustration, making it easier to maintain the optimistic, empathic, and action-oriented attitude that facilitates the therapeutic process. Patients may also harbour counter-therapeutic beliefs, ranging from 'Maybe I want to be depressed' to 'I am too disorganized to do homework tasks' (Beck *et al.* 1979*a*). If left unchecked they can impede progress; thus they require direct attention using the same techniques described earlier.

Short-term forms of cognitive therapy may not be suitable for all patients; for instance assumptions made may not apply to those with personality disorder (Young 1990). Assumptions such that patients: (1) have access to feelings, thoughts, and images with brief training; (2) have an identifiable problem on which to focus; (3) are motivated to complete homework and learn self-control strategies; (4) engage collaboratively after a few sessions; as well as that (5) difficulties in the therapeutic relationship are not major; and (6) all cognitions can be altered through empirical analysis, logical discourse, and gradual practice, may not apply. Young (1990) proposes particular modifications for personality disorder, as part of his so-called 'schema-focused cognitive therapy'. This approach resembles aspects of psychodynamic therapies inasmuch as involving more confrontation regarding cognitive and behavioural avoidance of emotion and making more explicit use of the therapeutic relationship. It is also typically of longer duration in order to overcome resistance and highlight the early origins of beliefs.

Attempts to apply cognitive therapy to a wider range of clinical problems has in fact resulted in several technical modifications. Apart from Young's approach, other developments also highlight interpersonal processes (Safran and Segal 1990), the role of emotion (Greenberg and Safran 1987), and 'core' versus 'peripheral' schemata (Guidano and Liotti 1983). Core schemata are those that relate to an individual's sense of reality, identity, value, and control; it is proposed that these schemata will be more fundamental, and therefore more difficult to change, than schemata peripheral to these issues. However, if change is achieved in these core schemata, the change is expected to be more profound. Clearly, such concepts are vital if cognitive therapy is to grapple with the thorny issue of change in personality. A particularly interesting development is Linehan's (1993) dialectical behaviour therapy treatment for the borderline patient. This combines training in 'mindfulness' (a term borrowed from Buddhism to describe a non-judgemental awareness of one's experience), interpersonal effectiveness, emotional regulation, and tolerance of distress, with exposure to disturbing memories, and training in self-validation. This procedure, applied both individually and in a group, is effective in helping parasuicidal women meeting criteria for borderline personality disorder (Linehan *et al.* 1991). Obviously, even these initiatives may not help some patients who may be better served by another approach altogether; indeed the cognitive therapist needs to recognize his limits and refer patients on appropriately.

TRAINING

Despite the structured nature of cognitive therapy, its practitioners need to cultivate adequate non-specific skills, such as the capacity for genuineness, empathy, and understanding, given their prominent role n all psychological treatment (Mahoney 1991). Indeed, a synergistic effect of fundamental clinical skills and specific cognitive interventions is likely (Persons and Burns 1985). The therapist must also necessarily understand the cognitive model of psychopathology, its specific applications to different disorders, and the full range of techniques.

Cognitive therapy has been operationalized in the form of pragmatic and clear accounts. Beck's manuals shine as clear and comprehensive (Beck *et al*. 1979*a*, 1985, 1990, 1993; Wright *et al*. 1993). Other helpful guides are those of Hawton *et al*. (1989) and Barlow (1993). The most effective route to competence is to combine reading, observation of experienced therapists, and supervised clinical experience. This includes training experiences in conducting both individual and group sessions. Although personal therapy is not usually a required part of training, many programmes involve exercises applying cognitive-behavioural techniques to one's own difficulties. Specialized training centres are set up in many countries to provide such programmes; indeed, training in cognitive therapy is now a common component of basic programmes in clinical psychology, psychiatry, and social work.

CONCLUSION

Cognitive therapy is a relatively brief, active, directive, and empirically-based form of psychotherapy. It emphasizes collaborative problem-solving by focusing on how cognitive phenomena maintain emotional distress and self-defeating behaviours. It embodies clear technical guidelines, and has, arguably, been evaluated in a greater number of methodologically sound studies than any other form of psychotherapy. It maintains an active dialogue with basic sciences, especially social and cognitive psychology, artificial intelligence, and neuroscience. Cognitive therapy constantly seeks to extend its area of application, modifying techniques to suit new patient groups where appropriate. The model has also played a leading role in the psychotherapy integration movement. According to Beck (1991), cognitive therapy is integrative since cognitive change underlies all effective treatment; cognitive therapy can therefore be used as a framework to incorporate a range of therapeutic techniques. As the model has evolved, it has assimilated important concepts and methods from many traditions in an effort to define effective therapies for an increasingly wide range of clinical problems. Whether this turns out to be hubris (of which the history of psychotherapy is replete) or a genuine leap forward in understanding behaviour change, is best left to history to judge. The capacity of cognitive therapy to take its own advice and maintain a close contact with empirical science, in terms of process and outcome research, as well as basic sciences relevant to human behaviour, will determine its fate in large measure.

REFERENCES

Agras, W. S., *et al.* (1992). Pharmacological and cognitive behavioural treatments for bulimia nervosa: A controlled comparison. *American Journal of Psychiatry*, **149**, 82–7.

Arieti, S. (1980). Cognition in psychoanalysis. *Journal of the American Academy of Psychoanalysis*, **8**, 3–23.

Bandura, A. (1977). Self efficacy: Toward a unifying theory of behaviour change. *Psychological Review*, **84**, 191–215.

Barlow, D. H. (1993). *Clinical handbook of psychological disorders*, (2nd edn). Guilford, New York.

Beck, A. T. (1967). *Depression: Clinical, experimental and theoretical aspects.* Harper & Row, New York.

Beck, A. T. (1991). Cognitive therapy as *the* integrative psychotherapy. *Journal of Psychotherapy Integration*, **3**, 191–8.

Beck, A. T. (1993). Cognitive therapy: Past, present, and future. *Journal of Consulting and Clinical Psychology*, **64**, 194–8.

Beck, A. T., Weissman, A., Lester, D., and Trexler, L. (1974). The measurement of pessimism: The Hopelessness Scale. *Journal of Consulting and Clinical Psychology*, **42**, 861–5.

Beck, A. T., Rush, A. J., Shaw, B. F., and Emery, G. (1979*a*). *Cognitive therapy of depression.* Wiley, New York.

Beck, A. T., Kovacs, M., and Weissman, A. (1979*b*). Assessment of suicidal intention: The Scale for Suicidal Ideation. *Journal of Consulting and Clinical Psychology*, **47**, 343–52.

Beck, A. T., Epstein, N., and Harrison, R. (1983). Cognitions, attitudes and personality dimensions in depression. *British Journal of Cognitive Psychotherapy*, **1**, 1–16.

Beck, A. T., Emery, G., and Greenberg, R. L. (1985). *Anxiety disorders and phobias: A cognitive perspective.* Basic Books, New York.

Beck, A. T., Epstein, N., Brown, G., and Steer, R. A. (1988). An inventory for measuring clinical anxiety: Psychometric properties. *Journal of Consulting and Clinical Psychology*, **56**, 893–7.

Beck, A. T., *et al.* (1990). *Cognitive therapy of personality disorders.* Guilford, New York.

Beck, A. T., Wright, F. D., Newman, C. F., and Liese, B. S. (1993). *Cognitive therapy of drug abuse.* Guilford, New York.

Birchwood, M. and Tarrier, N. (1992). *Innovations in the psychological management of schizophrenia.* Wiley, London.

Bowers, W. A. (1990). Treatment of depressed inpatients: Cognitive therapy plus medication, and medication alone. *British Journal of Psychiatry*, **156**, 73–8.

Burns, D. D. (1980). *Feeling good: The new mood therapy*. Morrow, New York.

Burns, D. D. and Nolen-Hoeksema, S. (1991). Coping styles, homework compliance, and the effectiveness of cognitive behavioural therapy. *Journal of Consulting and Clinical Psychology*, **59**, 305–11.

Chomsky, N. (1959). Review of B. F. Skinner's *Verbal behaviour*. *Language*, **35**, 26–58.

Clark, D. A. and Beck, A. T. (1989). Cognitive theory and therapy of anxiety and depression. In *Anxiety and depression: Distinctive and overlapping features*, (ed. P. C. Kendall and D. Watson). Academic Press, San Diego.

Crossman, E. R. F. W. (1953). Entropy and choice time: The effect of frequency unbalance on choice responses. *Quarterly Journal of Experimental Psychology*, **5**, 41–51.

Dobson, K. S. (1989). A meta-analysis of the efficacy of cognitive therapy for depression. *Journal of Consulting and Clinical Psychology*, **57**, 414–19.

Dobson, K. S. and Block, L. (1988). Historical and philosophical bases of the cognitive behaviour therapies. In *Handbook of cognitive-behavioural therapies*, (ed K.S. Dobson). Hutchinson, London.

D'Zurilla, T. J., and Goldfried, M. R. (1971). Problem solving and behaviour modification. *Journal of Abnormal Psychology*, **78**, 107–26.

Elkin, I., *et al.* (1989). National Institute of Mental Health treatment of depression collaborative research program:1. General effectiveness of treatments. *Archives of General Psychiatry*, **46**, 971–82.

Ellis, A. (1962). *Reason and emotion in psychotherapy*. Citadel, Secaucus, NJ.

Ellis, A. (1970). *The essence of rational psychotherapy: A comprehensive approach to treatment*. Institute for Rational Living, New York.

Eysenck, H. J. (1969). *The effects of psychotherapy*. Science House, New York.

Fairburn, C. G., *et al.* (1991). Three psychological treatments for bulimia nervosa. *Archives of General Psychiatry*, **48**, 463–9.

Fennell, M. J. V. and Teasdale, J. D. (1987). Cognitive therapy for depression: Individual differences and the process of change. *Cognitive Therapy and Research*, **11**, 253–71.

Frankl, V. (1985). Cognition and logotherapy. In *Cognition and psychotherapy*, (ed. M. Mahoney and A. Freeman). Plenum, New York.

Gardner, H. (1985). *The mind's new science: A history of the cognitive revolution*. Basic Books, New York.

Greenburg, L. S. and Safran, J. D. (1987). *Emotion in psychotherapy*. Guilford, New York.

Guidano, V. F. and Liotti, G. (1983). *Cognitive processes and emotional disorders*. Guilford, New York.

Hawton, K., Salkovskis, P. M., Kirk J., and Clark, D. M. (ed.) (1989). *Cognitive behaviour therapy for psychiatric problems: A practical guide*. Oxford University Press, Oxford.

Hollon, S. D. and Kendall, P. C. (1980). Cognitive self statements in depression: Development of an Automatic Thoughts Questionnaire. *Cognitive Therapy and Research*, **4**, 383–95.

Hollon, S. D. and Najavits, L. (1988). Review of empirical studies on cognitive therapy. In *Review of psychiatry*, (ed. A. J. Frances and R. E. Hales). American Psychiatric Press, Washington, DC.

Hollon, S. D., Shelton, R. C., and Loosen, P. T. (1991). Cognitive therapy and pharmacotherapy for depression. *Journal of Consulting and Clinical Psychology*, **59**, 88–99.

Hollon, S. D., *et al.* (1992). Cognitive therapy and pharmacotherapy for depression: Singly and in combination. *Archives of General Psychiatry*, **49**, 774–81.

Homme, L. E. (1965). Perspectives in psychology: XXIV. Control of coverants, the operants of the mind. *Psychological Reports*, **15**, 501–11.

James, W. (1890). *The principles of psychology*. Dover, New York.

Kelly, G. A. (1955). *The psychology of personal constructs*. Norton, New York.

Kirk, J. (1989). Cognitive-behavioural assessment. In *Cognitive behaviour therapy for psychiatric problems: A practical guide*. (ed. K. Hawton, P. Salkovskis, J. Kirk, and D. Clark). Oxford University Press, Oxford.

Lazarus, R. S. (1982). Thoughts on the relations between emotion and cognition. *American Psychologist*, **37**, 1019–24.

Linehan, M. M. (1993). *Cognitive-behavioural treatment of borderline personality disorder*. Guilford, New York.

Linehan, M. M., Armstrong, H. E., Suarez, A., Allman, D., and Heard, H. L. (1991). Cognitive-behavioural treatment of chronically parasuicidal borderline patients. *Archives of General Psychiatry*, **48**, 1060–4.

Ludgate, J. W., Wright, J. H., Bowers, W. A. and Camp, G. F. (1993). Individual cognitive therapy with inpatients. In *Cognitive therapy with inpatients: Developing a cognitive milieu*, (ed. J. H. Wright, M. E. Thase, A. T. Beck and J. W. Ludgate). Guilford, New York.

MacLeod, C. (1993). Cognition in clinical psychology: Measures, methods or models? *Behaviour Change*, **10**, 169–95.

Mahoney, M. J. (1991). *Human change processes*. Basic Books, New York.

McKnight, D. L., Nelson-Grey, R. O., and Bernhill, J. (1992). Dexamethasone suppression test and response to cognitive therapy and antidepressant medication. *Behaviour Therapy*, **23**, 99–111.

McLean, P. and Taylor, S. (1992). Severity of unipolar depression and choice of treatment. *Behaviour Research and Therapy*, **30**, 443–51.

Meichenbaum, D. H. (1977). *Cognitive behaviour modification*. Plenum, New York.

Miller, I. W., Norman, W. H., Keitner, G. I., Bishop, S. B., and Dow, M. (1989). Cognitive behavioural treatment of depressed inpatients. *Behaviour Therapy*, **20**, 25–47.

Mischel, W., Ebbesen, E. B., and Zeiss, A. (1972). Cognitive and attentional mechanisms in delay of gratification. *Journal of Personality and Social Psychology*, **21**, 204–18.

Neimeyer, R. A. (1993). An appraisal of constructivist psychotherapies. *Journal of Consulting and Clinical Psychology*, **61**, 221–34.

Neisser, U. (1967). *Cognitive psychology*. Appleton-Century-Crofts, New York.

Persons, J. B. and Burns, D. D. (1985). Mechanisms of action of cognitive therapy: The relative contributions of technical and interpersonal interventions. *Cognitive Therapy and Research*, **9**, 539–51.

Persons, J. B., Burns, D. D., and Perloff, J. M. (1988). Predictors of drop out and outcome in cognitive therapy for depression in a private practice setting. *Cognitive Therapy and Research*, **12**, 557–75.

Piaget, J. (1954). *The construction of reality in the child*. Basic Books, New York.

Rachman, S. J. and Wilson, G. T. (1971). *The effects of psychological therapy*, (2nd edn). Pergamon, Oxford.

Rehm, L. (1977). A self control model of depression. *Behaviour Therapy*, **8**, 787–804.

Rendon, M. (1985). Cognition and psychoanalysis: A Horneyan perspective. In *Cognition and Psychotherapy* (ed. M. Mahoney and A. Freeman). Plenum, New York.

Robins, C. J., and Hayes, A. M. (1993). An appraisal of cognitive therapy. *Journal of Consulting and Clinical Psychology*, **61**, 205–14.

Ross, A. (1991). Growth without progress. *Contemporary Psychology*, **36**, 743–4.

Safran, J. D., and Segal, Z. V. (1990). *Interpersonal process in cognitive therapy*. Basic Books, New York.

Safran, J. D., Segal, Z. V., Vallis, T. M., Shaw, B. F., and Samstag, L. W. (1993). Assessing patient suitability for short-term cognitive therapy with an interpersonal focus. *Cognitive Therapy and Research*, **17**, 23–38.

Schulman, B. H. (1985). Cognitive therapy and the individual psychology of Alfred Adler. In *Cognition and Psychotherapy* (ed. M. Mahoney and A. Freeman). Plenum, New York.

Simons, A. D. and Thase, M. E. (1992). Biological markers, treatment outcome, and one year follow up in endogenous depression: Electroencephalographic sleep studies and response to cognitive therapy. *Journal of Consulting and Clinical Psychology*, **60**, 392–401.

Teasdale, J. D. (1993). Emotion and two kinds of meaning: cognitive therapy and applied cognitive science. *Behaviour Research and Therapy*, **31**, 339–54.

Thase, M. E. and Beck, A. T. (1993). An overview of cognitive therapy. In *Cognitive therapy with inpatients: Developing a cognitive milieu.* (ed. J. H. Wright, M. E. Thase, A. T. Beck, and J. W. Ludgate). Guilford, New York.

Thase, M. E., Bowler, K., and Harden, T. (1991a). Cognitive behaviour of endogenous depression: Part 2. Preliminary findings in 16 unmedicated inpatients. *Behaviour Therapy*, **22**, 469–78.

Thase, M. E., Simons, A. D., Cahalane, J., and McGreary, J. (1991b). Cognitive behaviour therapy of endogenous depression: Part 1: An outpatient clinical replication series. *Behaviour Therapy*, **22**, 457–68.

Thase, M. E., Simons, A. D., Cahalane, J., McGreary, J., and Harden, T (1991c). Severity of depression and response to cognitive behaviour therapy. *American Journal of Psychiatry*, **148**, 784–9.

Vygotsky, L. S. (1962) *Thought and language*. MIT Press, Cambridge, MA.

Weissman, A. N., and Beck, A. T. (1978). *Development and validation of the Dysfunctional Attitude Scale: A preliminary investigation*. Paper presented at the annual meeting of the American Psychological Association, Toronto, Canada.

Wright, J. H., Thase, M. E., Beck, A. T., and Ludgate, J. W. (1993). *Cognitive therapy with inpatients: Developing a cognitive milieu*. Guilford, New York.

Wundt, W. (1888). Selbstbeobachtung und innere Wahrnehmung. *Philosphische Studien*, **4**, 292–309.

Young, J. E. (1990). *Cognitive therapy for personality disorders: A schema focused approach*. Professional Resource Exchange, Sarasota, FL.

Zajonc, R. (1980). Feeling and thinking: Preferences need no inferences. *American Psychologist*, **35**, 151–75.

RECOMMENDED READING

Barlow, D. H. (1993). *Clinical handbook of psychological disorders* (2nd edn). Guilford, New York. (The second edition of this practical manual, with chapters on most of the major applications of cognitive-behavioural therapy, is a real improvement on an already excellent volume. Its contents are very up to date, and the chapters are all written by experts in their field.)

Beck, A. T., Emery, G., and Greenberg, R. L. (1985). *Anxiety disorders and phobias: A cognitive perspective*. Basic Books, New York. (Beck's treatment manual for anxiety disorders represents not only various innovations in technique, such as the imagery-based interventions, but also an increasingly sophisticated cognitive theory of emotional disorders.)

Beck, A. T., Rush, A. J., Shaw, B. F., and Emery, G. (1979). *Cognitive therapy of depression*. Wiley, New York. (This is the classic 'how to do it' cognitive therapy treatment manual; clear, comprehensive and readable. A good place to start if you want a detailed account of the cognitive therapy process.)

Birchwood, M. and Tarrier, N. (1992). *Innovations in the psychological management of schizophrenia*. Wiley, London. (This book includes descriptions of the application of some cognitive therapy principles to the management of psychotic symptoms.)

Brewin, C. R. (1988). *Cognitive foundations of clinical psychology*. Erlbaum, Hove, UK. (A clear, brief introduction to the relationship of basic psychological research to cognitive models of psychopathology.)

Guidano, V. F. and Liotti, G. (1983). *Cognitive processes and emotional disorders*. Guilford, New York. (One of the early accounts of a constructivist approach to cognitive therapy; notable for its integration of attachment theory principles.)

Hawton K., Salkovskis P. M., Kirk J., and Clark D. M. (1989). *Cognitive behaviour therapy for psychiatric problems: A practical guide.* Oxford University Press. (An edited book with excellent practical chapters on treatment of a range of psychiatric conditions; it includes chapters on marital problems, cognitive behavioural assessment, chronic psychiatric handicaps, and problem solving, as well as the usual fare.)

Linehan, M. M. (1993). *Cognitive-behavioural treatment of borderline personality disorder.* Guilford, New York. (Linehan's innovative work with these challenging patients represents one of the more exciting developments of this therapy. It is described in detail in this volume.)

Mahoney, M. J. (1991). *Human change processes.* Basic Books, New York. (Mahoney's book paints a broad, at times exhilarating intellectual canvas. It describes the historical and philosophical underpinnings of the constructivist approach to cognitive therapy, as well as various innovations in technique.)

Wright, J. H., Thase, M. E., Beck, A. T., and Ludgate, J. W. (1993). *Cognitive therapy with inpatients: Developing a cognitive milieu.* Guilford, New York. (Another practical manual aimed at integration of cognitive therapy into the in-patient setting. Of great value to those working with more severe disorders.)

Young, J. E. (1990). *Cognitive therapy for personality disorders: A schema focused approach.* Professional Resource Exchange, Sarasota, FL. (Young's slim volume is still one of the best accounts of the adjustments required to standard cognitive techniques when working with patients with long-standing personality-based difficulties.)

8

Couple therapy

MICHAEL CROWE

Michael Crowe introduces the chapter with a brief account of change in marriage as an institution. Following a section on theoretical models he presents an approach which combines principal components from behavioural and systems theory and incorporates the useful concept of a hierarchy of levels of intervention. The next section deals with couple therapy in practice and is illustrated with several clinical vignettes. The chapter ends with comments on training and research findings.

The 1990s are not an easy decade for the institution of marriage, especially in Western societies. Pressures exist which tend both to idealize and to undermine couple relationships, and it may be that these contradictory forces contribute to the demand for couple therapy (Crowe and Ridley 1990). There is, simultaneously, an interest in exploring the nature of couple interaction and a parallel process emphasizing the fragility of such relationships and the need for 'self-actualization'. Marriage itself is becoming less popular, having reached a peak in the 1960s. Added to this, many unofficial pairings exist, some of which result in children and are marriages in all but name. Although we do not know the rate of breakup of these common law relationships it is likely that it is no lower than the divorce rate of one in three formal marriages. These common law relationships mean that marriage and divorce statistics since the 1980s are only approximate.

In the modern world many forces are at work to lessen the importance of marriage. Many women seek to combine the satisfaction of a career with the rearing of children. Although men have increasingly responded to the challenge of sharing household and family responsibilities, considerable tension still typifies many a relationship as to the equitable division of duties (Oakley 1974). More women are opting to become single parents. On the other hand, children of divorced parents do less well at school and in employment and suffer depression, low self-esteem, and neurotic symptoms more commonly than those with parents remaining together (Dominian 1968). Problems for children increase further when the custodial parent remarries and a 'reconstituted or blended family' is created (Robinson 1991). Effects on divorcing partners are also mainly negative, with increased alcoholism, depression, heart disease, cancer, accidents, and suicide in the first year.

In the light of these findings a good argument can be made to do what we can to reduce the divorce rate. Helping couples to stay together, however, is not the sole purpose of therapy. It can also be effective to deal with many of the diverse problems that affect partners in a relationship. For example, a wife's depression may be exacerbated by her husband's lack of empathy; if the husband can be helped to understand her better the depression may be relieved. In another instance, a jealous man may make his wife even more distressed than himself: the couple may be able to decrease the jealousy and its effect on them both by improving their communication and mutual understanding.

APPROACHES TO TREATMENT

A wide range of theoretical models of marriage and marital problems has been expounded, by psychoanalytic, behavioural, rational–emotive, cognitive, and systems-oriented practitioners.

A central concept in the psychoanalytic position, ably reviewed by Daniell (1985) and Meissner (1978), is the inner (often unconscious) world of the two partners determining the nature of their interaction and their responses to changing circumstances. It is as though each partner has an internal blueprint of both the relationship and their partner's personality, which in disturbed marriages usually bears very little resemblance to what more objective observers perceive. Therapy aims to help the partners to become aware of these inner worlds and their origins enabling them to reduce misunderstandings through insight, and to get in touch with their own feelings and those of their partner. Transference to the therapist is usually interpreted. An important focus is understanding the infantile feelings underlying the marital relationship and the 'repetition-compulsion', which leads to the person treating his/her partner similarly to the way he/she felt about the opposite-sexed parent. A principal outcome is liberation of the relationship from past adverse influences and a corresponding diminution of problems. Therapy is relatively extended and the pace of change gradual, but the improvement may be enduring (Crowe 1978).

The behavioural approach (behavioural marital therapy or BMT), in contrast, relies on current observed and reported behaviour. The rather simple premise is that the troubled couple have reached either a very low level of mutual positive reinforcement or are using overly coercive methods to control each other's behaviour. Stuart (1980) and Jacobson and Margolin (1979) emphasize the need for sensible negotiation of rights and duties and work on everyday tasks in this pursuit. Two main types of therapeutic activity take place, reciprocity negotiation and communication training. In the former, the couple request changes in behaviour on each side and negotiate how this can be achieved through mutually agreed tasks. In communication training the couple are encouraged to speak directly and unambiguously to each other about feelings, plans, or perceptions, and to feed back what they have heard and understood. Origins or deeper meanings of behaviour are downplayed, the emphasis being more on possible change in the interaction in the here and now.

Although the behavioural and psychoanalytic models appear incompatible, they can be partly reconciled by regarding them as concentrating on different levels of the mind. Thus, psychoanalytic concepts such as the inner world of the partners, their shared fantasies, and the need for personal insight and mutual understanding are not negated by the behaviourist's notions of mutual reinforcement of desired behaviour and the need to negotiate everyday exchanges. Segraves (1982) has devised a combined psychodynamic–behavioural approach in which the underlying cause of the couple's problems is assumed to be their conflicting internal fantasies (or blueprints) of themselves and each other. Intervention, however, is directed at both helping them to understand these and to increase reality-based communication in order to improve their ability to negotiate.

Aaron Beck (1988) has applied his cognitive-behavioural scheme to the problems of couples, identifying in their communication misunderstandings, generalizations, and focus on negative aspects of a problem, typical of the thinking of depressed patients. His approach involves the same therapeutic processes which have been successful in treating depression: challenging assumptions; reducing expectations; relaxing absolute rules; and focusing on the positive rather than the negative (see also Chapters 6 and 7).

In a similar way the rational–emotive approach of Albert Ellis has been adapted to relationship problems (Dryden 1985a). A distinction is made between marital 'dissatisfaction' and 'disturbance'. Dissatisfactions are dealt with by negotiation as in the behavioural model, whereas disturbances need a more elaborate approach, reducing the exaggeration of problems by, for example, outlawing words like 'intolerable' and replacing them with less extreme terms like 'difficult to put up with'. There is an analysis of repetitive cycles of cognitive and behavioural disturbance, in which each partner attributes negative or hostile intentions to the other. These distortions, dealt with in both individual and conjoint sessions, are examined to promote understanding and, in turn, to modify miscommunication.

The systems approach to couple therapy derives partly from concepts developed by therapists such as Minuchin (1974) and Haley (1980) in their work with families, and partly from a more detailed understanding of the couple's interaction such as that of Sluzki (1978). The approach is particularly suitable for couples because it addresses the relationship as such, in addition to the two partners who comprise it.

A central concept here is enmeshment, an excessive involvement of one person in what is essentially the private business of another. It is most common in relationships between parents and their growing children; often the hardest task for parents is to 'let go' and allow the child to separate and individuate. This type of enmeshment is also seen in couple relationships where one partner wants to be more intimate than the other. The concept of intimacy can relate to many aspects of life including sexual, physical, emotional, and 'operational' (Crowe and Ridley 1990): the latter referring to sharing of plans and information about each other. A conflict may arise between partners on how close or distant they wish to be in respect to one or more of these spheres. Systemic therapy attempts to clarify the degree of optimal distance.

Another key concept is homeostasis—the tendency for relationships to remain in the same configuration no matter what external factors or changes may impinge on them. Negative feedback systems are assumed to operate which restore the relationship to the status quo following an event or change that could tend to alter its nature. In some couples, however, symptoms in one partner may be the sole means to restore the status quo; if not the relationship may become too unstable and perhaps break down.

Underlying all systems thinking is the concept of circular causality. In a relationship things do not occur necessarily because one partner 'causes' them but rather as the result of a complex cycle of interaction in which both partners actively participate. Moreover, a person's actions within a relationship stem not from a single cause, either in the immediate or remote past, but as the product of a continuing chain of causation in which both partners are initiators and recipients. Thus, when approaching a couple problem, systems therapists do not focus on one of the protagonists (e.g. through medication or individual psychotherapy), but pursue, instead, change in which both partners contribute actively to facing and solving the problem. Failing that, the status quo is 'reframed' as being of mutual benefit to the couple and the suggestion is made that they should not attempt to change (paradoxical injunction).

The behavioural-systems approach

The approach selected for more detailed consideration in this chapter is referred to as behavioural-systems couple therapy (BSCT, see Crowe and Ridley 1990) in that it combines concepts from these two salient theoretical models. The behavioural dimension, similar to that of Stuart (1980) and Jacobson and Margolin (1979), consists of the relatively straightforward methods of reciprocity negotiation and communication training. The systems dimension is more complicated, divisible into systems thinking, so-called structural moves during the session, tasks and timetables, and the use of paradox.

Given the multiple therapeutic options as outlined in the previous section (and more could be added to the list), it would be futile to try to cover them all in this chapter. For a more detailed coverage of the other approaches to couple therapy, the reader is referred to Dryden (1985*b*). The focus here is therefore on one model, useful to the trainee for its relative straightforwardness, and which serves well as a foundation on which to add other dimensions with increasing clinical experience.

The various components of BSCT can be incorporated at any time in the therapy session although tasks, time-tables, and paradox are usually reserved for the 'message' at the end, and are linked to homework assignments to be carried out between sessions. Negotiation, communication training and structural moves, in contrast, are applied in the course of the session in order to alter the interaction *in vivo*.

In order to facilitate therapists' understanding and use of the BSCT approach, we have developed the 'hierarchy of alternate levels of intervention' (ALI hierarchy). This links each type of intervention to a specific clinical situation and makes it easier for the therapist to select an appropriate level at which to work.

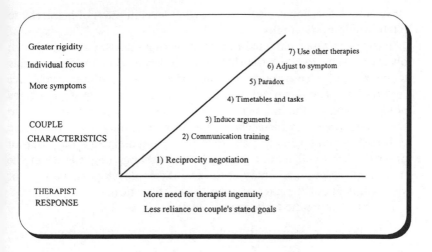

Figure 8.1 The hierarchy of alternate levels of intervention (ALI) (after Crowe and Ridley 1990).

Figure 8.1 shows the ALI hierarchy in diagrammatic form, the vertical axis representing the couple's presenting problems, the horizontal axis covering the therapist's potential interventions. As symptoms or complaints about the behaviour of a partner become more prominent, or as the system seems to be more rigid, the therapist moves from a behavioural, problem-solving approach to a more systems-oriented one.

BSCT is generally short term involving 5 to 10 sessions over a period of 3 to 6 months. Before the couple is seen, each partner completes a questionnaire detailing family history, previous medical or psychiatric problems, present and/or previous marriages and children, and current emotional state. Preparing to see a couple includes studying the written material and any referral letter, and devising a formulation that could explain the nature of the presenting problems. This may involve, for example, the couple's stage in the family life cycle (e.g. birth of first child, 'empty nest'), a recent major life event such as retirement, or the diagnosis of a serious illness in a partner. Hypotheses are not necessarily 'true' explanations of the cause of problems but rather a means of informing hunches and framing strategies. A decision is also made at what level in the ALI hierarchy to pitch initial interventions.

Therapy is best conducted in a room with a one-way screen with an observing team to assist the therapist. However, it is quite acceptable to work in a conventional consulting room without such live supervision. The main advantage of the screen is in training, as novices observe the immediate experience of therapy and try to emulate it when they themselves come to work under live supervision. A further advantage lies in the therapist being assisted by a group of observers who will be less biased by the feelings engendered in the treatment room, and may between them develop a variety of viewpoints about the partners and their interaction.

Several therapeutic tasks pertain to the first session:

(1) developing rapport with both partners, without favouring either;

(2) remaining in control;

(3) maintaining momentum; and

(4) maximizing opportunities for the couple to experience a change in their interaction.

A useful move in the first few minutes is to ask the partners to face and talk to each other rather than to the therapist—so-called 'decentring' (Minuchin 1974). Maintaining this configuration during the session is helpful inasmuch as it enables the therapist to observe the couple's interactional pattern and allows them to negotiate directly about aspects of their joint lives on which they need to achieve a compromise. Decentring also makes it possible to encourage arguments on everyday issues which in turn helps to reduce inhibition and to strengthen the less assertive partner. However, it is not necessary to maintain this position throughout. Indeed, some moves such as circular questioning (see below) require the therapist to be the centre of communication.

It may be difficult in any event to preserve the decentred position since the couple will often try to break out to talk directly to the therapist instead of to each other. The therapist will also be tempted to intervene. One method to participate and still remain decentred is to request the partners to ask each other questions which the therapist regards as salient. For example, one might say: 'You seem to differ on this; I wonder if you could ask your wife to advance her views so that you can discover what those differences are'. Again, if a partner turns to the therapist he or she might say: 'Could you first see what your partner thinks about that?' In this way the session continues in a decentred fashion, the couple encouraged to communicate directly rather than through the therapist.

Another consideration is a balance between lightness and seriousness. Partners are tempted to dismiss each other's concerns as 'neurotic' or as 'over-reactive'. The therapist should draw them away from these positions and urge them to treat each other respectfully. It is also useful to promote any lightness manifest in the communication, especially if humorous or playful. Messages offered at the end of a session also can afford to be relatively 'light' even when they convey a distressing idea.

That the focus should be the relationship, not symptoms or problems of one partner, is pivotal. It is, therefore, essential to avoid any undue attention on individual complaints. Although it may seem unsympathetic the therapist needs to interrupt such a series of complaints and refocus the discussion on to the relationship. In a similar vein, too detailed a history-taking is best avoided. In fact, a great deal of information would have been obtained via the questionnaire; it is usually best to relate historical issues to current problems, and not to spend excessive time elucidating events from the remote past.

The couple can delay grappling with their problems in a variety of ways. Intractable arguments about genuine, critical issues, such as an extramarital affair or the imminence of divorce, may dominate their thoughts. These have to be handled with respect. However, when they occupy session after session, they may have to be put aside, by indicating, for example, that the main task is to improve the current interaction and thus enable more informed decisions about other relevant matters.

Another impediment to progress is a partner persisting with extensive monologues, the other allowing, even encouraging this to occur. The reticent partner is often the one with a psychiatric illness or label; the other feels the responsiblity to act as spokesperson in order to help them both as well as the therapist. This can be done with the best of intentions, perhaps to provide the therapist with a clear idea of what transpires at home, but ultimately proves counter-productive, both in the one-sidedness of information given and in limiting opportunuties for interaction in the session. One way to overcome this is to emphasize ways in which the ostensibly 'sick' partner can teach or otherwise help the more 'competent' one.

The therapist's style of therapy may also slow down momentum. It is, of course, essential to manifest appropriate empathy to both partners but when this becomes an end in itself, rather than a means to change interaction progress may be inhibited. Decentring or posing circular questions (see below) are indicated to overcome this, so increasing interplay between the partners and refocusing the discourse on here-and-now interaction. Both aspects are more easily achieved if live supervision is used and the therapist given feedback *in vivo*.

In this model, partners need to communicate openly with each other. Some are adept at doing this but at an intellectual level only. Their interchange is akin to a committee meeting; items which are not part of the agreed agenda, such as feelings of sadness or anger, are suppressed or ignored. In other couples, there is a discrepancy between, say, a husband who is logical and self-controlled and his wife who readily expresses feelings. In both scenarios it is necessary to increase flexibility in emotional expression. Thus, in the 'committee meeting' couple, any expression of emotion is a change and an improvement, and if accompanied by understanding even better. In the 'discrepant' couple the logical partner is encouraged to be more expressive (perhaps with the partner's assistance) and the overly expressive partner possibly to be relatively restrained.

The technique of circular questioning, mentioned above, derives from the systems model and is particularly useful in couples manifesting resistance to change. This resistance is detectable in, *inter alia*, a difficulty in construing problems in relationship terms, a focus on individual behaviour and a demand for a 'medical' solution. The therapist assumes an active role, deliberately asking questions of one partner about the other, following the answer with another question of the second partner about the first, and so on. A sequence of interaction ensues which can then be directly examined. Couples are less defended in this mode of communication than when talking about themselves. Other forms of circular questioning involve a comparison between what went on at different periods in the relationship and discussion of hypothetical scenarios in the future (e.g. the consequences of separation). Whatever the form, the purpose is to elicit information which can then be applied to therapeutic purpose.

SPECIFIC TECHNIQUES

(1) Reciprocity negotiation

Returning to the ALI hierarchy (see Fig. 8.1), interventions used at the first level are reciprocity negotiation and problem-solving. These are the simplest ways of helping couples to begin to manage their difficulties. The partners state their complaints in everyday terms; the therapist then helps them to think about how to change their interaction in order to ensure that each gets what he or she wants from the other.

The theory behind reciprocity negotiation is partly operant conditioning and partly the social exchange theory of Thibault and Kelley (1959). The assumption is that satisfaction in marital and similar relationships depends on each partner receiving positive reactions to their behaviour from the other, or in other words 'maximum rewards for minimum cost'. A corollary is that each partner in a well-functioning relationship is prepared to do things which the other finds rewarding as long as reciprocation takes place. Couples in difficulties either reward each other infrequently or the rewards are unequally distributed. In either case, a lower than ideal level of reward in the relationship occurs; a tendency for the partners to use negative or coercive tactics to motivate the other follows. This negative approach to influence the partner is ineffective, especially in distressed couples (Weiss 1978). Moreover, distressed couples show little mutual positive reinforcement, much aversive interaction, and inadequate problem-solving (Schindler and Vollmer 1984).

Reciprocity negotiation is a staged process. The initial step is a complaint; this is then translated into a wish for alternative behaviour which is conceived of as a task. The task becomes part of the couple's homework between sessions. Both partners are given tasks, the product of reciprocal negotiation. The following case illustrates the typical process.

Caroline claims her husband Douglas always keeps her in the dark about his life, friends, and plans. Douglas does not appreciate that she needs to know about these aspects. She says: 'You never talk, you have your head under the bonnet of the car, or you are out with your mates, or watching football . . .' She is brought back to the point by the therapist here because she is digressing and being negative. The therapist then clarifies whether Douglas is willing to share more with her and if so when this would be convenient. It is helpful to specify how long it would be sensible to expect them to converse at one sitting, and then to plan such a 'talk session' at regular intervals. In this case, in which conversation has not been part of their repertoire, it is a good idea to experiment during the session and to proffer relevant advice about communication in order to make it more likely that the session at home will be rewarding for them both. It is customary to have the other partner 'lodge' a complaint too. In this case Douglas wants the two of them to socialize more often. The therapist seizes on this as a potential reciprocal task, suggesting

they negotiate an evening out at fortnightly intervals. The couple is responsible
for determining the arrangement although the therapist may suggest that this
features in their 'talk' session.

Several criteria should be met to facilitate the transition from
complaint to task. The wishes must be specific, replicable, positive,
practicable, and acceptable to both partners. It is usual to concentrate
on everyday matters rather than exotic tasks such as arranging an
overseas holiday. Ideally, the tasks can be carried out daily. Even if, as
often occurs, the tasks are not implemented as planned, the idea of
reciprocity negotiation itself may enable the couple to think more
positively.

(2) Communication training

The next strategy in the ALI hierarchy is training in communication.
The couple are asked to converse with each other in a decentred way
and their mode of communication observed by the therapist. Many
communication problems can be noted, including those outlined
above, namely monologues, rehearsing old arguments, failing to
understand the other person's feelings, and interacting at an
intellectual level only. Many other forms of faulty communication
can be modified; a summary of these is given below.

Since Virginia Satir's (1964) pioneering contribution on family
communication, other workers (e.g. O'Leary and Turkewitz 1978;
Olson et al. 1983) have taken the subject further by developing
communication training programmes. Olson, in particular, has
emphasized positive communication skills, such as empathy,
reflective listening, and supportive comments, in enabling couples
and families to share their changing needs. These contrast with
negative forms of communication like double binds and criticism that
minimize the ability to share feelings.

Problems of communication encountered in couple therapy include:

—lack of empathy;
—inability to express emotion;
—failing to listen;
—monologues with no break for feedback;
—one partner is the spokesman and the other silent;

—mind-reading (i.e. partner A knows better than B what is in B's mind);
—wandering off the topic;
—continual criticism; and
—the sting in the tail (i.e. a positive comment followed by criticism).

Communication training is a more demanding therapy than reciprocity negotiation. Like the latter, it depends on a well-motivated couple; but it also requires greater understanding on their part. They have to be more constructive in their comments and to speak in a way that is new for them.

The therapist first decentres himself, and instructs the couple to converse about an everyday topic. A problem of communication soon emerges. The couple then begin again using a different approach. This may involve: encouraging more mutual feedback; one partner avoiding 'mind-reading'; or pointing out that one partner is inattentive to the other's emotional message. Through these diverse methods, partners are helped to: speak for themselves, using the 'I' position; communicate feelings to each other; show empathy; use a tone of voice congruent with what is being said; speak briefly and await an answer; stick to the topic; and attend to both verbal and non-verbal levels of communication.

The therapist remains neutral with respect to the partners since the target of the work is the relationship. The therapist is the ally of both partners even in the face of one or other trying to form a unilateral alliance. It is perhaps harder to remain neutral in this pursuit than in reciprocity negotiation because of the more intrusive nature of the interventions.

An example illustrates the point: Joe, a professional man, attempted to help his wife Sandy avoid panicking about hosting dinners. He gave impressive advice (although failing to look at her), saying there was no need to worry as long as she had food prepared exactly when the wine would have been opened for the requisite two hours. He did not notice her quiet crying until the therapist pointed it out. Although Joe then became concerned and comforted her, he needed help to understand that his demands were stringent, and that she had good reason to panic if he became impatient over the issue of the 'wine'. It was critical that the therapist did not side with Sandy even though Joe seemed unreasonable. By remaining neutral the therapist managed to continue the therapy successfully. Indeed, Joe was later able to express his own sense of insecurity and to seek Sandy's understanding.

(3) Structural moves

These assume various forms of which the most common is to encourage argument in a couple. This is especially pertinent in those who are inhibited or avoid differences because of one partner's sensitivity to conflict. The problem may be a partner's sexual reluctance or depression. The more dominant partner, usually confident verbally and more at ease than the other, may effortlessly take the spokesperson role. The other partner is either reticent for much of the time or spends considerable energy diplomatically trying to placate the other and so reduce conflict.

One strategy is to have them argue over something trivial; for example, whether the toilet roll should be placed with the paper hanging down against the wall or away from it! This must be a genuine difference and not merely a therapist task. However, an issue that is too serious, such as education of the children or religion, is avoided because such couples may be reluctant to argue about them.

On identifying an issue about which they can disagree, the therapist encourages them to discuss it without inhibition and urges the submissive partner to participate with conviction (which may be quite foreign to him or her). It does not matter how the argument ends; the goal is to give them the experience of a heated exchange. The discussion may end with either partner giving in but, more satisfactorily, they may 'agree to differ', perhaps a new experience where one partner habitually submits. If the exercise has proceeded effectively, a homework task may be set, to argue about another trivial matter for a limited time, and, as in the session, to end by agreeing to differ.

Another intervention providing a novel experience is reversed role-play. Here they address an issue on which they have contrary opinions but assume the other's position, physically and attitudinally. The exercise promotes mutual understanding, especially through adopting the other's viewpoint.

A third form of intervention is 'sculpting', in which the partners position themselves to express their perceptions of their relationship. For example, a husband who feels downtrodden might position his wife on a chair with himself kneeling on the floor and her hand on his head. She, however, might place them both standing, embracing, and looking into each other's eyes. This contrast in perceptions then provides a lively topic to explore and forms the basis for homework.

In all *in vivo* interventions the chief goal is to alter the couple's experience of their relationship. They thus gain 'experiential' insight nto each other and into themselves, laying the foundation for subsequent change.

4) Timetables and tasks

Much work is done between sessions. At the end of a session the herapist offers a message to the couple in the form of a brief résumé of major themes plus a homework task. This is either behavioural (e.g. arising from reciprocity negotiation) or may arise from systemic understanding of the couple. Behavioural tasks have been described above; systemic ones often centre around a timetable are devised to deal with out-of-control behaviour. For example, in a couple containing a jealous husband, the couple is asked to discuss the accusations for an hour at a set time and at no other time. If the subject is raised at another time the partner is instructed to reply that he or she will only talk about it at the arranged hour.

A time-tabled task can be applied in a variety of comparable situations. This may be the case in a couple in which the man is more eager about sex that the woman (Crowe and Ridley 1986). The couple reach a compromise on the preferred frequency of intercourse, and then agree on a suitable schedule. Crude as this approach may seem, it can satisfy both partners in that the enthusiastic one is assured he will have predictable relations, whereas the less keen other can relax when sex is prohibited and prepare for when it is planned.

Timetables can be arranged for many types of behaviour. For example, if a couple repeatedly argue over dinner they are encouraged to arrange an argument every morning over breakfast. Timetables are also useful to reduce the labelling applied to a partner's behaviour. Thus, in the case of the couple with a jealous partner, timetabling discussion about this is not only aimed at reducing the time it absorbs but also at legitimizing the activity as worthy of attention, thus helping to modify the labelling of the jealous partner as pathological.

Other tasks may be more straightforward and encompass the idea of 'having fun'. In couples, especially those in mid-life, who live dull lives, they may arrange an evening out.

A frequently used timetable is the 'talk' one whereby the couple arrange a time, perhaps two or three times a week, in which they sit together without distraction for some 20 minutes to discuss a topic. This may be simply to discuss the news of the day, to debate a planned activity, or to exchange feelings about something important like their son's schooling.

Although sexual therapy is dealt with in Chapter 9, it should be mentioned that many relationship problems have both a sexual and a non-sexual dimension. Where the sexual difficulty is predominantly motivational rather than technical, couple therapy is commonly suitable as the overall treatment. In such a case, tasks like non-genital sensate focusing (Masters and Johnson 1970) to get the couple back into the habit of physical contact without the pressure of intercourse—may be part of the repertoire of tasks deployed.

(5) Paradoxical interventions

In the event of the above range of interventions proving ineffective paradoxical injunctions derived from systems theory, especially the work of Selvini Palazzoli *et al.* (1978), have a recognized role. The technique is of particular utility in the rigid couple and where one or both partners present resolutely with many individual symptoms which seem to reflect a troubled relationship.

Paradox is always applied carefully, in a sympathetic and caring way. A common form is 'prescribing the symptom', that is, advising the couple that it is best 'for the time being' to persist with the problematical behaviour in one partner and the reciprocal behaviour in the other. They are offered a plausible but challenging rationale for this, which matches a team's systemic appraisal of the relational dynamics.

An example may clarify these ideas. A professional couple in their forties had had a tense relationship for many years characterized by conflicts and power struggles; these had worsened since the wife (Betty) had resumed full-time teaching. The husband (Miles) had ostensibly approved of the move but they had begun to fight about the domestic chores with Miles advising Betty on washing clothes, clearing the kitchen, and the like. Betty, believing she was performing satisfactorily, resented his interference. Reciprocity negotiation and division of the activities between them was ineffective. By the fifth session the therapist began to despair, especially because they were so polite and reasonable with each other.

The observing team suggested a paradox in which the therapist would put himself down and prescribe the problem:

'My colleagues have criticized me for naïvely leading you on to believe that an easy solution to your problems exists. In fact, they now think that following the departure of the children you need arguments to enliven your relationship.

Therefore, you should go on, Miles, picking Betty up on all that she does, and, Betty, you should resist his advice and go your own way. You will then avoid the boredom of the 'empty nest' and play out a parent–child scenario which, despite its painful aspects, is better than the realization you are middle-aged.

This intervention exerted an immediate effect. First, they commended the therapist for his diligence and asserted that earlier therapy had not been wasted. Secondly, they accepted the team's view and appreciated they had been trying too hard for an ideal relationship, and resolved instead to be less critical of each other.

When a paradox is offered it matters little whether it is obeyed or not. Rather, it is the understanding the couple gains that liberates them from the vicious circle they are in; namely, that they enjoy a degree of control over the situation; that they are responsible for creating the circumstances they purportedly dislike; and that the therapist does not seemingly impose a solution.

A paradox has four major elements: (1) positive connotation; (2) a description of the 'symptom' in one partner and reciprocal behaviour in the other; (3) a prescription of both symptom and reciprocal behaviour; and (4) a systemic reason for continuing both.

There are limits to the behaviours which can be prescribed in a paradox. For example, self-harm, violent behaviour, law-breaking, or irresponsible acts are contra-indicated. However, it might be appropriate to prescribe that one partner should try to be depressed and the other act as carer. Paradox is best kept in reserve until other techniques have proved ineffective or the couple are so entrenched in their pathological interaction that no intervention whatsoever makes a difference (see the ALI hierarchy, Fig. 8.1).

TRAINING

In both BSCT and other approaches supervision of clinical practice is important. Live supervision is feasible via a one-way screen—an ideal way to train, especially if the sessions are also video-taped. However, audio-taping is a reasonable substitute if the couple do not consent to video-taping. The therapist is thus able to discuss the recorded session with a supervisor and other trainees in order to revisit his interventions. More traditional methods of supervision are also desirable in order to examine problems that derive more from the therapist himself than from the couple. In this context, one-to-one supervision is most appropriate. A mix of group and individual, and of live–video and traditional supervision is the ideal.

Other theoretical models incorporate their own training recommendations, but a balance of methods is used in all. The psychoanalytic approach sometimes uses an interesting combination of therapy and supervision in which two therapists see the partners individually and come together for joint supervision—as if the therapists represent a surrogate marriage and the lessons of supervision are conveyed to the couple second hand (Daniell 1985). In behavioural couple therapy more emphasis is placed on technique than on transference and therapist feelings, but his personal style may be a pertinent focus. Additionally, in all good supervision the ethical dimension is covered to ensure that couples are not exploited by the therapist in any way, even subtly. This aspect pertains especially in private practice, which lacks the inbuilt peer groups typical of hospital and clinic practice and of training institutions (see Chapter 13).

Factual knowledge needs to be acquired, although the emphasis on it varies between schools. In psychoanalytic courses there may be a requirement for personal therapy whereas this is far less common in behavioural or systems training. In any course it is advantageous to become familiar with the sociology of marriage, and, given multicultural societies, the contribution of ethnicity, religion and the like to couple problems.

In behavioural-systems couple therapy (BSCT) training, understanding behavioural and systemic aspects is crucial but the trainee also acquires knowledge of the strengths of other models, and indications for referral. Much use is made of role-play, with trainees in small groups acting roles of partners and therapist. They practise techniques such as decentring and circular questioning, and devise direct and paradoxical messages, often video-taped so that they can be dissected later. Exercises provide experience of feeling specific emotions like helplessness. Role-play is also used to appreciate, *inter alia*, ethnic differences, gender issues, non-threatening exploration of sexual themes, and the role of psychiatric disorder.

Trainees observe therapy as a member of a team, move on to work with experienced colleagues in co-therapy and ultimately see couples under live supervision. Ideally, they should treat about six couples alone or in co-therapy, but will also have observed many more as part of a live supervision structure.

RESEARCH

All therapies depend for their long-term acceptability on the demonstration of efficacy (and also cost-efficacy). Much outcome research has been done, especially on behavioural marital therapy (BMT), but also increasingly on other models. Reports on BMT produced in the 1970s, as reviewed by Azrin *et al.* (1973), showed improvement compared to controls. Crowe (1978) found significantly greater change in sexual adjustment and 'target problems' with BMT compared to a control condition (supportive). An insight-oriented approach was intermediate in effect, and at follow-up both this and the behavioural approach were superior to the control. A pertinent subsidiary finding was the supportive approach's contribution to improvement on some outcome measures (suggesting non-specific effects as argued by Frank in Chapter 1).

Later studies, reviewed by Jacobson *et al.* (1984), again point to BMT's effectiveness. Emmelkamp *et al.* (1984), for instance, found BMT as effective as systems therapy. In studies, examined by Boddington and Lavender (1995), the efficacy of BMT has been confirmed. In associated analyses, components of treatment have been looked at in terms of outcome. Baucom *et al.* (1990), for example, found only minor differences between traditional BMT and combinations of it with cognitive restructuring or 'emotional expressiveness' training.

An interesting result emerged in a study of insight-oriented therapy. Snyder and Wills (1989) found equivalent improvement at the end of therapy in couples who had received BMT and those who had participated in insight-oriented work; both groups did better than a waiting-list control. However, at follow-up, more BMT couples were divorced compared to couples in insight-oriented therapies. BSCT has not been subject to controlled trials but considerable improvement has been noted by Boddington *et al.*

CONCLUSION

Various types of couple therapy have been outlined and a detailed account of the behavioural systems approach proffered. It is by no means clear whether BSCT or similar forms of couple therapy are more effective than others. Comparative studies suggest equal honours. When active therapies are compared with a control condition, the active therapy has usually emerged as superior.

A familiar dispute between therapists preferring an active approach and those favouring an insight-oriented model revolves around the criticism that only the latter deals with internal conflicts, producing enduring gains; a converse contention is that such a model is unncessarily lengthy and fails to yield behavioural change. Neither claim is probably valid. Insight-oriented therapy certainly leads to change in marital adjustment (Crowe 1978; Snyder and Wills 1989) whereas behavioural marital therapy is associated with positive change maintained 18 months later (Crowe 1978; Baucom *et al.* 1990). The question boils down to cost-effectiveness; active therapies are briefer than their insight-oriented counterparts. However, as relatively less research has been done on the latter several questions remain to be clarified.

Therapy for couples, whatever the model, is proving to be a valid and effective way to tackle not only relationship problems but also those of a psychiatric nature such as depression and jealousy perpetuated by marital or other relational factors. It has the added advantage of avoiding the labelling of many forms of behaviour as 'psychiatric', thereby reducing perceived stigma.

It seems Utopian to suppose that all relationship problems can be prevented or successfully treated, but if it becomes feasible to reduce some of the substantial, associated distress in both adults and their children, a useful purpose will have been served.

REFERENCES

Azrin, N. H., Naster, B. J., and Jones, R. (1973). Reciprocity counselling: a rapid learning based procedure for marital counselling. *Behaviour Research and Therapy*, **11**, 365–82.

Baucom, D. H., Sayer, S. L., and Sher, T. (1990). Supplementing behavioural marital therapy with cognitive restructuring and emotional expressiveness training: an outcome investigation. *Journal of Consulting and Clinical Psychology*, **58**, 636–45.

Beck, A. T. (1988). *Love is never enough.* Harper & Row, New York.

Boddington, S. J. A. and Lavender, A. (1995). Treatment models for couples therapy: a review of the outcome literature and the Dodo's verdict. *Sexual and Marital Therapy*, **10**, 69–81.

Boddington, S., Lavender, A., and Crowe, M. Therapy with couples: an evaluation of the behavioural-systems approach. Unpublished data.

Crowe, M. J. (1978). Conjoint marital therapy: a controlled outcome study. *Psychological Medicine*, **8**, 623–36.

Crowe, M. J. and Ridley, J. (1986). The negotiated timetable: a new approach to marital conflicts involving male demands and female reluctance for sex. *Sexual and Marital Therapy*, **1**, 157–73.

Crowe, M. and Ridley, J. (1990). *Therapy with couples. A behavioural-systems approach to marital and sexual problems*. Blackwell, Oxford.

Daniell, D. (1985). Marital therapy, the psychodynamic approach. In *Marital therapy in Britain*, Vol. 1 (ed. W. Dryden). Harper & Row, London.

Dominian, J. (1968). *Marital breakdown*. Penguin, Harmondsworth.

Dryden, W. (1985a). Marital therapy, a rational emotive approach. In *Marital therapy in Britain*, Vol. 1 (ed. W. Dryden). Harper & Row, London.

Dryden, W. (ed.) (1985b). *Marital therapy in Britain*, Vol. 1 and 2. Harper & Row, London.

Emmelkamp, P. M. G., van der Helm, M. MacGillavry, D., and van Zanten, B. (1984). Marital therapy with clinically distressed couples: a comparative evaluation of system-theoretic, contingency contracting and communication skills approaches. In *Marital interaction: analysis and modification* (ed. K. Hahlweg and N. Jacobson). Guilford, New York.

Haley, J. (1980). *Leaving home*. McGraw Hill, New York.

Jacobson, N. S. and Margolin, G. (1979). *Marital therapy: strategies based on social learning and behavioral exchange principles*. Brunner/Mazel, New York.

Jacobson, N. S., Follett, W. C., Revenstorf, D., Baucom, D. H., Hahlweg, K., and Margolin, G. (1984). Variability in outcome and clinical significance of behavioral marital therapy: a reanalysis of the outcome data. *Journal of Consulting and Clinical Psychology*, **52**, 497–504.

Masters, W. H. and Johnson, V. E. (1970). *Human sexual inadequacy*. Little, Brown, Boston.

Meissner, W. W. (1978). The conceptualisation of marriage and family dynamics from a psychoanalytic perspective. In *Marriage and marital therapy*, (ed. T. J. Paolino and B. S. McCrady). Brunner/Mazel, New York.

Minuchin, S. (1974). *Families and family therapy*. Tavistock, London.

Oakley, A. (1974). *The sociology of housework*. Blackwell, Oxford.

O'Leary, K. D. and Turkewitz, H. (1978). The treatment of marital disorders from a behavioural perspective. In *Marriage and marital therapy*, (ed. T. J. Paolino and B. S. McCrady). Brunner/Mazel, New York.

Olson, D. H., McCubbin, H. I., Barnes, H., Larsen, A., Muxen, M., and Wilson, M. (1983). *Families: what makes them work*. Sage, Los Angeles.

Robinson, M. (1991). *Family transformation through divorce and remarriage*. Tavistock, London.

Satir, V. (1964). *Conjoint family therapy*. Science and Behavior Books, Palo Alto, CA.

Schindler, L. and Vollmer, M. (1984). Cognitive prospectus in behavioural marital therapy: some proposals for bridging theory, research and practice. In *Marital interaction*, (ed. K. Hahlweg and N. S. Jacobson). Guilford, New York.

Segraves, R. T. (1982). *Marital therapy: a combined psychodynamic-behavioural approach.* Plenum Press, New York.

Selvini Palazzoli, M., Boscolo, L., Cecchin, G., and Prata, G. (1978). *Paradox and counterparadox.* Aronson, New York.

Sluzki, C. E. (1978). Marital therapy from a systems perspective. In *Marriage and marital therapy*, (ed. T. J. Paolino and B. S. McCrady). Brunner/Mazel New York.

Snyder, D. K. and Wills, R. M. (1989). Behavioural vs. insight-oriented marital therapy: effects on individual and interspousal functioning. *Journal of Consulting and Clinical Psychology*, **57**, 39–46.

Stuart, R. B. (1980). *Helping couples change.* Guilford, New York.

Thibault, J. W. and Kelley, H. H. (1959). *The social psychology of groups* Wiley, New York.

Weiss, R. L. (1978). The conception of marriage from a behavioral perspective. In *Marriage and marital therapy*, (ed. T. J. Paolino and B. S McCrady). Brunner/Mazel, New York.

RECOMMENDED READING

Bancroft, J. (1989). *Human sexuality and its problems.* Churchill Livingstone, Edinburgh. (An excellent all-round textbook for sexual problems and their treatment.)

Clulow, C. (1985). *Marital therapy: an inside view.* Aberdeen University Press, Aberdeen. (A good guide to the psychodynamic approach to marital therapy.)

Crowe, M. and Ridley, J. (1990). *Therapy with couples: a behavioural systems approach to marital and sexual problems.* Blackwell, Oxford. (A clear and practical account of the behavioural-systems approach to couple therapy, with many case examples.)

Dryden, W. (1985). *Marital therapy in Britain*, Vols 1 and 2. Harper & Row, London. (A good guide to the various marital therapy approaches, with case examples of each.)

Robinson, M. (1991). *Family transformation through divorce and remarriage.* Tavistock/Routledge, London. (A well-researched discussion of divorce, remarriage, and step-families.)

9

Sex therapy

JOHN BANCROFT

In this chapter, John Bancroft deals with the treatment of the couple who present with sexual dysfunction. Following an account of the evolution of sex therapy he describes the therapeutic methods—both behavioural and psychotherapeutic components. The therapist's role in the latter is especially emphasized. Three clinical examples follow to illustrate aspects of the therapy. The chapter ends with a section on some practical considerations.

The modern approach to sex therapy began in 1970 with the publication of Masters and Johnson's (1970) *Human sexual inadequacy*. Their approach was essentially empirical; they espoused no theoretical model. Nevertheless, they filled a vacuum for therapists who had lacked a comprehensive and systematic approach to sexual problems. In 1975, Kaplan's book, *The new sex therapy*, appeared, combining Masters and Johnson's ideas with an admixture of psychoanalytic concepts, and a much more flexible, less structured approach. Both books have remained highly influential. In Europe, the most important text on sex therapy has been Arentewicz and Schmidt's (1983) *The treatment of sexual disorders*. They used a modification of the Masters and Johnson approach, emphasising behavioural aspects.

After 25 years of 'modern sex therapy' we can look back on a series of major changes. Schmidt (1994) has described the changes as having three phases which reflect changes in attitudes to sexual behaviour and relationships between men and women. In the first, therapists adopted a liberal approach to help patients escape from socially determined inhibitions, and to allow free expression of their sexuality. This gave way to greater recognition of the extent to which sexual dysfunction served as a defence against deeper anxieties and interpersonal conflicts. Schmidt suggests that contemporary therapists are reimposing fresh norms for how men and women should interact sexually; sexual

etiquette for the modern politically correct couple! This analysis ma
fit the German situation better than that in the rest of Europe and i
the United States; there had initially been much more emphasis o
behaviour and less on psychotherapy in the German approach. Bu
there has undoubtedly been change and reformulation. Schmidt's thir
phase can be seen as an interesting but incompatible mixture of th
impact of feminist thinking which has challenged assumptions abou
what is 'sexually normal' for women, and an extraordinary process o
medicalization of male sexuality, in which surgeons, in particular, hav
highlighted the physical nature of erectile dysfunction, or impotence a
they prefer to call it. Psychological aspects have been increasingl
ignored and men have been urged to seek physical solutions in wha
Tiefer (1986) has dubbed the 'pursuit of the perfect penis'.

This may have left many sex therapists confused. Whereas in th
1970s they were heralded as agents of sexual liberation, they are now
often accused of reinforcing social stereotypes of male sexua
domination. Whereas they previously embarked on treatment witl
confidence, they are now uncertain of the possible role of physica
factors, particularly concerning male sexual dysfunction. They also
have to contend with another extraordinary change; it is now
commonplace for patients, particularly women, to reveal earlier
experiences of sexual abuse, presenting the therapist with a
background of sexual conflict, guilt, and aversion which appears
much more complex than was the case in the early, optimistic days of
sex therapy. How best to tackle these traumas, how, indeed, to
evaluate their impact, present the therapist with new and largely
unresolved challenges.

Also embedded in Schmidt's schema are differences in how sexual
problems are conceptualized. Masters and Johnson categorized female
problems as either orgasmic dysfunction, vaginismus, or dyspareunia;
and male ones as erectile dysfunction, premature ejaculation, or
ejaculatory incompetence. There was virtually no focus on sexual
desire, and the emphasis on physiological function allowed no scope
for categorizing problems in terms of the couple's interaction, in spite
of the fact that this has always been the main focus of Masters and
Johnson's therapy. Periodically, we hear discussion of whether the
frequency of specific dysfunctions has altered. In fact, prevalence, in
large part, reflects how therapists urge their patients to formulate their
problems.

There is a paradox here. In the first edition of this book, the
treatment presented in this chapter was out of line with the framework

prevailing at that time. How, for example, did the 'sensate focus' approach of Masters and Johnson meet the needs of the woman with orgasmic dysfunction or the man with erectile failure? Ironically, as concepts of sexual dysfunction have changed, the relevance of the basic structure of sex therapy has, if anything, increased, providing as it does an excellent framework to explore the variety of both interpersonal and intrapersonal issues that may arise. It remains less predictable in its effects on the sexual responses *per se* as has been discussed more fully elsewhere (Bancroft 1996). However, it is a clear example of psychotherapy providing a model of intervention which is applicable to a range of problems. Its basic elements are:

(1) Clearly defined tasks are given and the patient (or couple) asked to attempt them before the next session.

(2) Those attempts and any difficulties encountered are examined in detail.

(3) Attitudes, feelings, and conflicts that make those behavioural tasks difficult are identified.

(4) Those attitudes, etc., are modified or resolved so that achievement of the behavioural tasks becomes possible.

(5) The next behavioural tasks are set, and so on.

A basic feature is that the patient or couple always have something *to do* between sessions. Usually, tasks are small steps towards the final goals, although they may involve keeping records or otherwise monitoring behaviour as part of the analysis necessary for treatment.

In applying this model to sexual problems, the emphasis has been on the couple and their sexual relationship. The same model, however, can also be applied to the individual although this requires a more detailed analysis of the difficulty before embarking on treatment. With the couple, in contrast, requirements are universal, involving patterns of communication, self-protection, and self-assertion, which justify a relatively standard approach, at least in the early phase of therapy, when issues relevant to the specific couple become apparent. For this reason, couple therapy is easier than individual therapy and hence will form our focus. For the novice, gaining experience in couple therapy is the best first step. Attention will also be paid to individual therapy, however, since a proportion of patients seek help without sexual partners. Problems associated with sexual preference, gender identity, and deviant forms of sexual behaviour will not be considered. The reader is referred elsewhere for discussion of these issues (Bancroft 1989).

Goals of sex therapy can be defined as:

(a) Helping the person to accept and feel comfortable with his or her sexuality.

(b) Helping the couple to establish a condition of trust and emotional security during sexual interaction.

(c) Helping the couple to explore ways to enhance the enjoyment and intimacy of their lovemaking.

These goals seem vague when compared with the specific ones patients bring with them—improving erections, delaying ejaculation, achieving orgasm. This is because focusing on such specific goals, which may reflect the social norms for sexual functioning, is commonly a large part of the problem. The aim is therefore to encourage them to 'wipe the slate clean', leave preconceptions of sexual normality behind them, and discover what is rewarding for them as a couple. Needless to say, by establishing such goals, the therapist reveals his own values about sexuality. Therapists have their priorities; it is important that they do not deceive themselves into concluding they are neutral. Indeed, the extent to which the therapist's values conflict with the patient's or couple's may raise ethical issues; these are discussed in depth elsewhere (Bancroft 1991).

TREATMENT METHODS

Before considering specific interventions, other therapeutic principles need to be understood by the therapist and made explicit to the couple at the outset.

Initial assessment: its purpose and limitations

Many health professionals, particularly psychiatrists and psychologists, are taught to take a thorough history before embarking on treatment. Masters and Johnson (1970) adopted a similar line, emphasizing the importance of initial assessment and the ensuing 'round table' discussion when the therapist presented an analysis of the origin and cause of the couple's problems. This emphasis is not necessarily appropriate for a number of reasons. First, demonstration of the therapist's skills in analysing the problem, whether valid or not, serves to 'de-skill' the patient or couple at a time when they should be encouraged to 'problem-solve'. Secondly, particularly with sexual problems, it is unrealistic to expect the patient to feel secure enough, either with therapist or partner, to reveal sensitive material at this early stage. The initial history cannot, therefore, be relied on. Thirdly, the uncovering of the full gamut of the person's sexual history, with its embarrassing and confidential themes, without knowing the information needed to help the patient, raises serious ethical questions. The patient may well believe that disclosure is essential in order to obtain help. In fact, it may not be so; unless this type of information is necessary for the therapist to carry out his work, it should not be sought. Fortunately, a strength of this approach is that by setting appropriate behavioural goals, the chance of identifying and uncovering issues relevant to progress is much enhanced (see Bancroft 1991).

Assessment and history-taking are obviously necessary but their aims need to be clear. Unless the nature of the sexual difficulty is accurately established, the appropriateness of sex therapy cannot be ascertained. While it is true that sex therapy can help when sexual dysfunction has an organic basis, it is not useful to embark on therapy unaware of the organic dimension; the result may be to raise unrealistic expectations of change, disillusionment, and loss of self-esteem.

It is also important to determine whether both partners want their sexual relationship to improve; this may only become clear by offering sex therapy. When confronted with the explicit option of working to improve the sexual relationship, one or other may appreciate more clearly that this is not what they seek. Depression may affect a person to the extent that he or she is unable to engage effectively; treatment may be needed for the mood disorder initially.

Sex therapy relies mainly on sessions with both partners. Once therapy is underway the partners may be seen individually, but cautiously and only when necessary. Hence, initial assessment is an important time for the therapist to talk with each partner individually, also providing an opportunity to promote rapport. The best way to achieve this may be for the person to focus in detail on an important past sexual experience in order that the therapist may empathize with his or her reaction and interpretation of that event. Once rapport is established with each partner individually it will put the therapist in good stead when engaging with them together.

The responsibility for change lies with the patient or couple

Sex therapy is not a process where responsibility lies with the therapist, as in the treatment of acute physical illness. Expert help is provided

but the person or couple have responsibility to exploit that help. This
is an 'adult–adult' type of relationship in which the patient must be
prepared to attempt the recommended tasks. (This issue has been
developed further in Chapter 5). It is necessary to make this point
explicit at the outset and return to it repeatedly, either because of
patients' previous expectations of medical care or their tendency to slip
into a passive-dependent relationship with professionals. Failure of
patients to accept responsibility leads to poor outcome.

Consistent with this relationship is the need to agree on frequency
and timing of sessions, and the opportunity for the patient or couple to
carry out assignments, free from major distractions such as moving
house, changing jobs, or having mother-in-law to stay! It may be
appropriate to delay treatment until a period free of such distractions.

The approach includes an educational component

The objective of sex therapy is the patient or couple learning principles
of interacting that not only improve their current situation but can
also be used if similar problems are encountered in the future.
Behavioural improvement alone is insufficient. The patient should
understand how the improvement has occurred. In this respect it is
useful for the couple to experience a 'set-back' before termination so
that they have the opportunity to reapply principles learned earlier. In
this way they can gain confidence that in the event of further set-backs
they would cope without seeking professional help.

It is, nevertheless, important to realize that there is more to sex
therapy than education. In a proportion of cases the therapist need
only set behavioural goals, instruct the couple in principles of
communication, and provide information on anatomical and
physiological aspects of sex—here sex therapy is at its simplest.
More commonly, however, difficulties are encountered in carrying out
tasks, reflecting long-standing conflict or anxiety. Helping the patient
to overcome such difficulties requires particular skills; these will be
considered later.

Two dimensions of treatment will therefore be covered, behavioural
and psychotherapeutic.

(1) The behavioural component

The behavioural component commences almost immediately, without
waiting until a detailed history is taken. Limited physical contact, for

example, can be suggested whatever the nature of the problem allowing therapist and couple to learn from difficulties encountered. There is no quicker way of finding out relevant relationship issues than giving the couple a collaborative task. If, on the other hand, these present no difficulty, nothing is lost and the couple progresses to the next stage.

Treatment is a parallel process of change and discovery. It is essential to emphasize this effect of carefully combining selected behavioural goals with analysis of difficulties encountered in carrying them out. Some behaviourally oriented therapists regard these difficulties as irritants, impeding progress. They are misled, because their recognition and resolution is at the heart of the process.

That we can use a standard programme, at least in the early stage, makes this form of treatment much easier to practise for the inexperienced therapist than an individually tailored method. Resistance to change, however, will vary and be idiosyncratic; this aspect presents the greatest challenge to the therapist. A clearly defined behavioural framework, however, gives the therapist confidence and a secure base on which to operate. As experience is gained, greater flexibility is applied. And whereas the programme is relatively comprehensive in many cases, 'time out' may be needed to resolve obstacles to change as underlying problems and conflicts are identified. Often, principles of behavioural psychotherapy can be used to tackle such problems. In other cases, different approaches are indicated (these are considered below). Throughout, however, the nature of the patient–therapist relationship is crucial particularly its 'adult–adult' quality.

Let us now look at this programme in detail; it is divisible into six stages regardless of the sexual dysfunction.

Stage 1

Each partner is asked to practise 'self-asserting' and 'self-protecting'; that is, making clear what 'I' like, prefer, or find unpleasant or threatening. Beginning a statement with 'I would like . . .' or 'I feel hurt because . . .' instead of the more usual 'shall we . . .?' or 'why don't you . . .?' is often difficult. The customary method of communication, regarded as unselfish, is to think or guess and then aim to carry out what the partner would like rather than putting one's own wishes first. This frequently goes awry, and because of reluctance to hurt the partner, misunderstandings remain concealed and persist. Providing both partners are able to state their own wishes, there is no cause for resentment and differences are resolvable through open negotiation. The therapist advises the couple to try this style of communication in relatively trivial, non-sexual situations before using it during the sexual tasks (e.g. 'I would like a cup of tea, would you?'). The emphasis is on the word 'I'. This principle is incorporated into the entire programme.

The sexual goal in Stage 1 consists of '*touching your partner without genital contact and for your own pleasure*'. An explicit agreement is made to ban attempts at intercourse and genital or breast contact in order to reduce performance anxiety and allow both partners to feel safe. It is an effective way to test trust. Breaking the ban or reluctance to maintain it provides valuable information for the therapist as will be illustrated below. The couple are instructed to have no more than three sessions of lovemaking before their next appointment to avoid too much happening; only a limited agenda can be properly covered at each meeting. The couple are responsible for deciding when those sessions occur, and obviously the more spontaneous the better. But they are specifically asked to alternate in who suggests a session and to clarify who will initiate first. On these occasions, the person who has 'invited' begins by touching the partner's body, other than out-of-bounds areas, in whatever way is pleasurable; the objective is for the toucher to enjoy the experience. The partner being touched has only to 'self-protect' (i.e. to say stop if anything unpleasant is felt). Roles are reversed, the person who has been touched now does the touching. They should not expect to get strongly aroused by this, although they sometimes do. The goal is simply to enjoy the process in a relaxed way. This stage is often difficult for couples (especially men) to grasp as they are so conditioned to think of touching as a way of *giving* rather than *receiving* pleasure. This may lead to recognition of deeply held attitudes such as 'you should only enjoy sex if you are giving pleasure to someone else'—which may be central to the overall problem.

The therapist ensures, by careful inquiry, that these behavioural steps have been carried out with both partners feeling relaxed and secure, before proceeding to Stage 2.

Stage 2

'*Touching your partner without genital contact, for your own, AND your partner's pleasure.*' Sessions continue as before with the couple alternating as initiator, and active touching carried out by only one person at a time. Now, however, the person being touched gives feedback of what is enjoyable as well as what is unpleasant. The toucher can use this information to give as well as to receive pleasure. The ban on genital contact persists.

Sometimes, a partner expresses concern that the intercourse ban will lead to unresolved sexual arousal and frustration. Reassurance is given that frustration of this kind only arises if one is not clear what to expect (i.e. if the possibility of advancing to intercourse or genital stimulation remains). Explicit acceptance of limits on these activities obviates this. However, if after a session either partner is left aroused and in need of orgasm, then it is acceptable for them to masturbate individually but not as a pair.

At an appropriate stage during the first two or three sessions the therapist describes basic points about the anatomy and physiology of sexual response in both sexes, emphasizing commonly misunderstood aspects which often underlie dysfunction. This 'lecture' is given no matter how sophisticated the couple since it is rare for them to be fully aware of all points the therapist will cover. This is also an opportunity to establish a suitable vocabulary that can be used for discussion and reporting back during the genital stage (Stage 3).

Stage 3

Touching with genital contact. The same principles of alternating in touching apply but genital areas and breasts can now be included. The positions adopted for this purpose should be discussed and the couple encouraged to explore and decide on those that suit them. Careful questions about their reactions to different positions may reveal important feelings and attitudes.

Communicating what is enjoyable about the touching often presents difficulties in this stage. The therapist emphasizes that pleasure will vary, making it important for the couple to maintain open communication. They should not assume that because their partner enjoyed a particular type of stimulation on one occasion, it will always be enjoyed to the same extent. Their only goal is to relax and enjoy the experience. The partner being caressed may or may not become sexually aroused; the occurrence of ejaculation or orgasm does not matter and need not signify an end to the session.

The couple have been warned about the 'spectator role' from the start—becoming a detached observer of oneself or one's partner rather than an active participant. Detachment generates performance anxiety and interferes with normal sexual response. One useful method is to concentrate on the local sensations experienced while touching or being touched (i.e. 'lend oneself to the sensations'). If insufficient, the person carries out a relaxation procedure; if that fails, the partner is informed that a problem has arisen and a temporary halt to the session is requested. The session is resumed after a short period of conversation or other activity.

When premature ejaculation is a problem, the couple are introduced at this stage to the 'stop-start' (Kaplan 1975) or 'squeeze' (Masters and Johnson 1970) techniques and asked to incorporate either of them into the touching sessions (see references for details of these techniques). In the case of vaginismus, gradual vaginal dilatation with finger or graded dilators is used. The timing of these techniques and whether they should be carried out individually or conjointly vary (Kaplan 1975) although Masters and Johnson (1970) adhere to a fixed procedure. This will be discussed in relation to individual therapy.

Stage 4

Simultaneous touching with genital contact. Touching is now done by both partners simultaneously. They need to be comfortable with preceding stages before moving on to this one. Difficulties related to taking initiative and assertiveness are often clarified at this point.

Stages 5 and 6

Vaginal containment. Once genital and body touching is progressing well and the male is achieving a reasonably firm erection (or has started to gain control over ejaculation during manual stimulation), the couple moves to vaginal containment. Although initially there was a ban on intercourse, the couple has been discouraged from regarding lovemaking as divided into foreplay and intercourse. Until now, they have experienced a range of physical contact over which they were able to set and accept limits. Now, during a touching session, the woman in the female superior position introduces the penis into her vagina. This not only makes it easier for her to guide the penis but also allows her partner to remain in a 'non-demand position' with the woman in control and able to stop or withdraw whenever she wants. At first, the couple are instructed to try vaginal containment for short periods without other movement or pelvic thrusting, simply concentrating on the sensations of the 'penis being contained' or the 'vagina being filled'. The duration is gradually prolonged. The stage merges into Stage 6 when movement and pelvic thrusting are allowed although initially for short periods only. Again, one is trying to break down the 'big divide' between foreplay and intercourse which, if present, provokes anxiety whenever the step from one to the other is anticipated. Instead, a continuum of behavioural steps is involved merging into intercourse.

The couple are encouraged to practise stopping at any point at the request of either partner to counter the common notion that loveplay once begun must continue until its physiological conclusion, with no escape *en route*. The confidence that either partner can say 'stop' at any stage without incurring anger or hurt in the other is a basic feature of a secure sexual relationship. With confidence, the need to say stop seldom arises. The couple are also advised to experiment with different positions and methods of touching to discover what satisfies and provides variety.

(2) The psychotherapeutic component

Setting behavioural tasks is relatively easy, especially when working with couples. Helping them overcome obstacles to carrying them out is the crux. By planning specific tasks, the therapist 'gives permission' and implicitly counters negative attitudes or fears they may harbour. In some couples, the setting of agreed limits and provision of basic information by a third person may so diminish performance anxiety that normal sexual responses occur. In these cases the couple must learn how they overcame the problem and not remain dependent on an expert. Otherwise, relapse is likely to occur. It is paradoxically reassuring to encounter difficulties during therapy since this signifies that relevant tasks are being tackled.

A discerning therapist recognises a range of intra- and interpersonal problems in the course of treatment. One advantage of sex therapy is that attention can be focused on those, and on fears or attitudes which obstruct achievement of agreed goals. The therapist thus avoids being side-tracked into other less relevant areas. Although factors hindering progress are varied, certain themes, categorized under four headings, occur commonly: (1) misunderstandings about treatment and its aims; (2) ignorance or incorrect expectations about sex; (3) negative or inhibiting sexual attitudes; and (4) relationship problems, especially unresolved resentment and conflict.

Interpersonal problems (e.g. unresolved anger and insecurity in the relationship) tend to emerge during early stages of the behavioural programme, before genital touching begins. Thereafter, intrapersonal issues are more likely, reflecting anxiety, guilt, and conflict around sexuality acquired earlier in life, and usually before the current relationship began. This is the time when previously unexpressed concerns about childhood sexual abuse are most likely to be revealed.

(a) *Misunderstandings about the treatment*

Before the couple applies the therapist's behavioural recommendations, it is reasonable to ensure that they understand their purpose and accept their rationale. This is explained in suitable terms for a particular couple; there is no place for mystique. Difficulty in understanding and acceptance may stem from failure to clarify adequately or from a negative therapeutic relationship. In some cases, the treatment style conflicts with personal values about sex. Commonly, a couple complain that they dislike the lack of spontaneity involved—the feeling that the therapist not only instructs them but looks over their shoulder at what should be an intimate affair. Although understandable, it should be gently pointed out that they are in this position because they have a problem, that intervention is intended as a temporary bridge between the present unsatisfactory situation and a new mutually rewarding sexual relationship. It is worth adding that although the therapist assumes an authoritative role initially in setting limits and suggesting behavioural steps, this will be transferred to the couple as treatment evolves. Therapists need to remind themselves repeatedly of this key point.

Difficulty in accepting the approach may reflect reluctance in one or both partners for the treatment to succeed. At an unconscious level, they seek failure to justify either ending the relationship, accepting a non-sexual one, or engaging in an extramarital affair.

Accepting limits, especially on genital touching and intercourse, is commonly problematic and discussion of such problems is often fruitful. Although failure to understand the rationale behind the limits may be responsible, other factors are more often involved. An example is incorporated in the illustrations below. The limits may be rejected by one or other partner (more often the woman) as an act of sabotage because sexual progress is too rapid and the prospect of 'cure' looms before underlying issues have been exposed and dealt with. Sabotage typically reflects the woman's resentment at being sexually used. This 'bartering' aspect of sex is relevant all too commonly.

(b) *Ignorance or incorrect notions about sex*

Patients' misunderstandings about sex are numerous and only a few will be mentioned. A widely held notion is that an erection indicates advanced sexual arousal and the need for intercourse, at a time when the woman may only be starting to respond. Erection is obvious to both partners whereas internal vaginal lubrication, the equivalent female physiological response, may pass unnoticed. Both occur, however, with similar speed and often as the initial response to sexual stimulation. The belief that if an erection subsides it cannot return also needs to be corrected.

Another widespread assumption is that 'normal sex' involves simultaneous orgasm; this leads to considerable performance anxiety. A belief that a woman should experience orgasm from vaginal intercourse alone and that failure to do so or reliance on clitoral stimulation indicates abnormality needs to be dispelled. The therapist stresses that only a small proportion of women on a minority of occasions achieve orgasm without clitoral stimulation, either by themselves or their partner.

(c) *Negative sexual attitudes*

These are usually acquired during childhood or adolescence and precede the current relationship. Common examples are: 'It is wrong for nice women to take the initiative or to be active during lovemaking'; 'It is only acceptable to experience sexual pleasure when you are giving it to your loved one'; 'Sex is unpleasantly messy because of vaginal fluid and semen' (often felt by people who are fastidious about cleanliness); 'One should never lose control of oneself' (either because it is wrong to do so or frightening). Many more examples could be provided.

Negative attitudes following childhood sexual abuse are particularly difficult to deal with. The abuse may have been sufficiently traumatic and frightening resulting in an understandable aversion or fear of sexual contact. The sense of betrayal, by someone in a position of trust, may make it difficult for the abused person to feel emotional security in a subsequent relationship, necessary for sexual fulfilment. Another form of damage results from the tendency to deny that a child has sexual feelings. The explicit assumption by the adult world that the child was sexually unresponsive and only frightened by the experience may create confusion in a child who, at some stage of the interaction with the adult, was aware of pleasurable feelings. This may lead to a sense of being not only 'sexually abnormal' but also responsible. The incorporation of this belief makes a sexual response difficult to accept later in life. The abused person is often anxious that her partner in adult life will blame or reject her if she discusses the abuse.

(d) *Problems in the relationship*

The distinction between this and the preceding category is not clear-cut as sexual attitudes are commonly reflected in the choice of partner. However, common unresolved problems stem from the couple's difficulty to adapt to one another. By far the most important is veiled resentment, related to the earlier discussed bartering aspect in a relationship. This may give rise to 'post-marital decline' in which sex, formerly exciting and enjoyable, loses its interest for the woman and to a lesser extent the man. A similar decline is commonly seen after childbirth when complex contributory factors are at work.

A sense of relational security is a key to the realization of sexual pleasure. Being 'sexually abandoned' involves letting down our defences such that we can be hurt or rejected. By the same token, to expose oneself defencelessly in the presence of another person and to survive emotionally unscathed has a binding effect. Thus, insecurity is likely to impair sexual enjoyment. This insecurity may reflect a fear of rejection or sexual betrayal; infidelity has particularly deleterious effects in this respect.

What does the therapist do?

Having dealt with problems that may interfere with the behavioural programme, let us consider the therapist's role and tasks to resolve them. This aspect was previously neglected but developments in cognitive therapy provide a framework (e.g. Hawton *et al.* 1989). The therapist's objectives are: helping the couple to understand specific difficulties encountered during the behavioural programme; and taking active steps to help resolve them.

Facilitating understanding

Understanding why one has difficulty in carrying out a particular task is often followed by its diminution. In psychotherapy, understanding leads to reappraisal of the problem and of associated beliefs and values. Female patients are often reluctant to initiate lovemaking, linked to the feeling that such initiation reflects improper enthusiasm. This, in turn, makes them vulnerable to the partner's refusal which is then seen as further evidence of the behaviour's unacceptability. Men are conditioned differently; rejection of their advances is much less threatening to their self-esteem.

By re-examining these assumptions, acknowledging that it is appropriate in an established relationship for the woman to take initiatives, and accepting that both partners may decline at any time, 'cognitive restructuring' follows. This allows the previously unsettling behaviour to be dealt with readily. The process may continue covertly, and between sessions. What can the therapist do to facilitate it?

(a) Setting further tasks may help to focus on the specific problem. Identifying differences between one's reaction to two subtly different tasks is particularly useful. Why, for example, is it easier to show a partner what is found unpleasant than to convey what is pleasurable?

(b) Encourage examination and appropriate labelling of feelings experienced at the time of difficulty (e.g. fear, guilt, disgust, or anger)

(c) Encourage the couple to find an explanation for their difficulty.

Therapists should produce likely hypotheses and evidence for and against but it is more effective if the couple are helped to provide the best explanation rather than have it offered by therapists who may unwittingly have a need to demonstrate their skills. This is unlikely to occur until the couple experience a need to understand a particular difficulty, which often does not happen when the difficulty is first encountered. The therapist can facilitate this by exposing the couple to the same difficulties by repeating homework assignments.

'Socratic questioning' may help; the therapist, with an explanation in mind, poses questions encouraging the couple to view the situation in a particular way. In the event of failure, the therapist offers as a 'last resort' explanations, preferably more than one, so that the couple are provided with options.

The 'cognitive restructuring' inherent in this process may suffice to remove obstacles to behavioural change. But if not, the therapist has to turn to other strategies.

Direct steps to resolve the difficulty

The therapist's tactics can be considered under four headings:

(a) *Making explicit the patient's commitment to specific changes.* At the outset, as already mentioned, treatment goals are purposely vague.

But, as obstacles are encountered, it is necessary to establish explicitly whether the couple want to surmount them (e.g. does the woman want to be able to initiate?) Does the man who finds his partner's genitalia repellant want to overcome that feeling? In other words, is the obstacle a 'resistance' regarded by the patient as a nuisance i.e. ego-alien or is it consistent with his or her value system and therefore something that is not proper to change? Obtaining commitment of this kind is the next appropriate step.

(b) *Setting further behavioural steps designed to tackle the difficulty.* Often problems stem from fears of a 'phobic' kind. A graded approach can then be used. A woman who fears vaginal entry is asked to insert her own finger a short distance, for a brief time. Such small steps do not overwhelm the patient with anxiety, and encourage her to 'stay with' the anxious feelings until they start to subside.

(c) *Reality confrontation.* Anxiety can be challenged cognitively. When it is ego-syntonic and the patient has no obvious wish to overcome a resistance, the therapist considers how incompatible this is with the aims of treatment. Thus, a suggestion that masturbation may help to achieve orgasm or overcome inhibition may be rejected on the grounds that it is an unacceptable behaviour. If the patient seeks help with the partner, then an alternative approach should be offered. If, on the other hand, a patient objects to touching his or her partner's genitals, the incompatibility of such an attitude with treatment goals is emphasized.

Patients may need to be confronted with other inconsistencies between belief and action or between their understanding and the facts. Thus, the view that 'normal' women experience orgasm from vaginal intercourse has to be challenged. Giving permission, often a crucial role, may involve the therapist pointing out inconsistencies between the values of patient and therapist.

(d) *Facilitating the expression of emotion.* Negative emotions play a part in establishing or maintaining sexual dysfunction. The first step in coping with these is to label them correctly. Resentment within the relationship is common; more often than not, its appropriate expression is required before it resolves. The therapist assists in three ways: (1) educates the couple about ways that unexpressed emotions adversely affect them and about benefits of appropriate expression; (2) helps the couple to identify instances where difficulties arise; and (3) encourages the couple to work out adaptive ways to communicate feelings.

A final general series of points on the psychotherapeutic component follows. A common reason for reluctance in a couple to carry out an assignment is inadequate understanding of its purpose or lack of confidence in the therapist and his approach. These aspects are particularly pertinent in the initial stages before a sound alliance has been forged. The rationale of therapy needs to be clarified more than once. It is usually better understood after the first trials of the behavioural assignments. The couple are told that treatment recommendations are based on common sense, not magic. The therapist carefully explains why an assignment is necessary and the patient encouraged to clarify any ambiguity or uncertainty. This not only allows the patient to express doubts about therapy, but also to highlight its educational function.

Other non-specific features of relevance include reassurance, promoting hope, showing warmth and empathy, reinforcing specific behaviour by responding to it with pleasure or praise, and 'inoculating against failure' by preparing the couple for possible set-backs so that when they do arise, they will not be overly discouraged but rather make constructive use of them.

These strategies have no special mystique. Obviously, there is considerable scope for expertise, and therapists will vary not only in their initial aptitude but also in their capacity to learn from experience. Therapists from different backgrounds may find that earlier training and experience can be relevant in dealing with the psychotherapeutic component, provided, that is, the 'adult–adult' quality of the patient–therapist relationship is maintained.

Individual therapy

Whatever the advantages of couple therapy, circumstances may only allow working with the individual; it may even be the most suitable option. This obviously applies to those without partners, and to others who have partners but where the latter are unwilling to participate. Such refusal presents a problem since it implies a negative relationship which may be central. Individual treatment is only indicated if there is a clear-cut goal which does not depend on the co-operation or even involvement of a partner. For example, the person with inhibited sexual attitudes or who feels uncomfortable with his or her body and sexual responses comes into this category. Other examples include vaginismus (the woman is unable to allow anything to enter her vagina such as tampons, her own or the doctor's examining finger) and the inability to experience orgasm during masturbation in either men or women. Sometimes, when erectile difficulties or premature ejaculation are marked, even during masturbation, individual therapy may be worthwhile.

Should we work with such a person when the partner is prepared to co-operate in couple therapy? This is a point on which we should keep an open mind. With vaginismus, there may be women, especially those with marked phobic features or personality problems, in whom individual therapy may precede or even obviate the need for couple therapy.

It is also worth considering the long tradition of treating non-consummation due to vaginismus by working with the woman alone. This was introduced under the initial guidance of Michael Balint (Tunnadine *et al.* 1981). The emphasis is on vaginal examination and the woman's emotional reactions to it. Only female doctors participate and a major theme is the 'giving permission' by an authoritative figure.

Having decided to work with a person rather than a couple, the behavioural programme is likely to be more varied. However, in many cases, goals of treatment are related to 'increasing comfort with one's body' and self-touching and exploration comparable to Stages 1, 2, and 3 of couple therapy. Sexual aids like vibrators may assist, particularly in helping women to experience orgasm for the first time. Their place in couple therapy remains less certain.

More varied in their needs and taxing of the therapist are patients whose principal problem lies in the area of 'socio-sexual approach behaviour' (i.e. difficulty in initiating and maintaining the early phase of a sexual or potentially sexual relationship). The therapist lacks the advantage of seeing the patient interact with a partner that is provided during couple therapy. Careful and time-consuming 'behavioural analysis' of recent attempts at dating or courting is required in order to identify likely reasons for failure. It is advantageous for the patient to be involved actively and at the earliest opportunity. Even though several sessions of careful history-taking may be necessary before a programme is devised, it is possible to launch therapy without delay with 'self-touching programmes' or by setting a task to monitor behaviour between sessions. Eventually, a programme of approach behaviours can be devised. Thus, a male patient may be asked to decide whom he will approach during the next week, and the nature of the approach (e.g. invitation to join him for lunch in the canteen or go ут for a drink). There is once again a need to limit the type and degree эf behaviour attempted. Since agreement of the as yet uninvolved эartner is not obtainable, strategies enabling the patient to set limits without loss of face may have to be worked out and rehearsed.

The therapist informs the patient what he or she can expect in such situations and, as important, what may be expected of them, and how their behaviour may be interpreted by the partner. There are obvious advantages in having either the same-sex therapist—who models the experienced male or female—or an opposite-sex therapist who offers insight into what can be expected by the partner. When a therapist of either sex is available, the patient's needs are considered in the choice. Anxiety about the other sex or the likelihood that the opposite-sex parent played a role in reinforcing negative attitudes, point to the need for an opposite-sex therapist.

Whereas the behavioural programme in individual therapy requires more planning, psychotherapeutic tactics are similar to those in couple therapy. Obvious differences in the one-to-one relationship do exist; extra care, for instance, should be taken to avoid dependency.

CLINICAL ILLUSTRATIONS

Three clinical examples follow to bring the above concepts to life and to show their application.

Jane and Bob

Jane and Bob, married for three years and both 25 years old, had stopped all sexual activity following a brief period when Jane was unable to touch Bob's genitals. She described a strong feeling of disgust but could explain it no further. The therapist asked what she thought disgust meant and eventually suggested it might be a mixture of attraction and repulsion (an interesting idea, with therapeutic value). Jane was then requested to define the difference between touching Bob's penis, and other parts of his body she was prepared to touch. After an unconvincing attempt to explain the difference in terms of texture and shape, she was asked what it meant to be disgusted by something Bob found pleasurable. She then expressed the fear he would lose control if she made him aroused. Bob expressed surprise at Jane's lack of trust.

Following this session, Jane began to touch Bob's penis, although initially she felt mildly nauseous while doing so. Over the following two weeks she began to enjoy her own genitals being touched, a new experience, and described feeling aroused. She was, however, still reluctant to touch Bob's penis more than briefly. Jane was asked why she was now able to enjoy being touched but hesitant to give Bob his pleasure. She reiterated the theme of loss of control, indicating that she felt confident she herself would not lose control but expected Bob to do so when he approached orgasm. What did this loss of control mean to her and, what consequences did she fear? She described the break in communication that occurs when partners are approaching and experiencing orgasm. The break constituted a threat to her; she needed to feel she remained in contact. She was invited to describe other situations where a similar break in communication might occur—such as Bob falling asleep. This did not concern her because she knew she could wake him if necessary. Asked how the time scale of Bob going to sleep compared with his reaching orgasm, she acknowledged with surprise that the orgasmic 'time out' was relatively short, and appeared reassured.

Mary and Peter

Mary and Peter, an unmarried couple, had been living together for four years. Mary complained that she experienced orgasm during masturbation but not during intercourse. Peter doubted that he could accept the ban on genital touching and intercourse. The rationale of therapy was carefully explained; he expressed partial understanding but noted that he might become sexually aroused during a session and could not be held responsible for what might ensue; once aroused he expected to have intercourse. Why would he be unable to control himself? He attributed this to his 'normal maleness', in that men when sexually aroused were not responsible for their actions. Would this apply in any situation (i.e. would he be in danger of raping his partner if he became aroused?) Peter admitted this was unlikely. What had occurred during courting days, before they started to have intercourse? He conceded he had then been able to accept limits.

Asked if she would lose control were she to become aroused, Mary replied negatively. Both were confronted with the stereotypes of the controlled woman and the uncontrolled, animal-like man and were asked to consider the evidence for these. They were then offered a reasoned argument that the stereotypes were to a large extent imposed ɔy societal forces rather than biologically determined. Peter was asked f he preferred to see himself as an 'uncontrolled sexual animal' and lid he feel more masculine as a result. What did the issue of control nean to Mary? She described how, because of her insecurity during lovemaking, she was unable to let go. Could this be relevant to her ɔrgasmic difficulty? Peter felt that it probably was. The importance of feeling safe in a sexual relationship was highlighted and Peter agreed to accept the limits of Stage 1.

Richard and Susan

Richard and Susan had been married for two years. Both 23, they had had a courtship since 17 with intercourse beginning soon thereafter. Sex was initially enjoyable for both although Richard, coming from a strictly religious family, had felt somewhat guilty. A year before they married, Richard's parents had expressed shock upon discovering that they were living together. Richard decided they would stop having intercourse until marriage. Although Susan hoped he would change his mind, Richard persisted. When they resumed intercourse after marriage Susan was no longer responsive.

During Stages 1, 2, and 3 Susan repeatedly described how she resented touching Richard because he enjoyed it and became aroused whereas she did not. At the same time she depicted herself as a failure and felt reluctant to initiate sessions because she would only fail yet again. The couple had obvious problems in dealing with resentment. Susan was able to show anger about certain issues but not about others whereas Richard rarely expressed anger at all. He feared that if he did Susan would be intensely distressed; it was easier to conceal his feelings. The male therapist, concluding that Susan's unresolved resentment was a result of Richard's pre-marital 'rejection' of her sexuality, encouraged her to express this but she doggedly denied anger; in fact, the experience had made her feel inadequate, not angry. At the same time she continued to make provocative comments about resenting Richard's pleasure. Asked how he felt about Susan's sentiments, Richard denied being hurt but conceded he was puzzled.

The therapist eventually decided, in the light of the couple's block in expressing anger and resultant impasse in treatment, to share his own reactions—his exasperation with Susan's mixed message of denial of anger together with her provocative remarks and her declining to try out new behaviour on the grounds she would inevitably fail. The therapist remarked that he would feel angry if he were in Richard's position. The atmosphere became tense with Susan visibly, although not verbally, angry.

Susan stated at the next appointment that she had not wanted to practise any of the assignments since the previous session. She had found the last occasion humiliating and had ceased thinking about treatment. Richard was more expressive, sharing his concern that the therapist had been hard on Susan. The therapist then explained that contrary to Susan's own conclusion he did not see her as a failure but felt frustrated with her attitude. He had felt the need to express his feelings but had worried later that he may have acted too harshly. He was delighted and relieved she had returned. He suggested a similarity between Susan's reaction to the previous session—feeling angry, regarding herself as a failure, and opting out of the programme—and her feelings about Richard's withdrawal from pre-marital sex. By the end of the session the tension was much reduced. The therapist pointed out that although there had been a risk of a break in the therapeutic relationship everyone had weathered the crisis and felt more relaxed and secure. At the next meeting, Susan reported pleasurable involvement in Stage 3 and was able to disclose how hurt she had felt before the marriage.

In this case, the therapist not only provided a model of emotional expression but also revealed himself as a 'genuine' and 'feeling' person with concern for the couple, an obviously important therapist feature. As this case shows, the timing and handling of such an intervention can be difficult, with the associated risk of provoking drop-out. It is usually unwise for therapists to reveal their own anger or other negative feelings until reasonable progress has been made in establishing a therapeutic alliance.

SOME PRACTICAL CONSIDERATIONS

Couple therapy varies in duration but requires an average 12 sessions spread over four to five months. The therapist flexibly adjusts to the needs of the particular case. It is appropriate to start treatment weekly and to extend the interval between sessions when major issues like unexpressed resentment, communication problems, or undue passivity have been dealt with effectively. The last two or three sessions are usually spaced out over a few months so that the couple have an opportunity to consolidate progress and cope with any set-back before terminating.

Progress is slow or absent with some couples; the therapist is then uncertain for how long to persist. If reasonable progress has not been accomplished by about session 18, it is unlikely to occur with further treatment of this kind. In any event, it is advisable to avoid open-ended contracts. A specified number of sessions should be agreed on at the outset with the proviso that when they are completed progress will be assessed and a decision made on whether to continue and for how long. In cases with reasonable prospects, an initial contract of 10 sessions with scope for a further two to four is sensible.

One advantage of this approach is evidence of progress and the couple's ability to make use of therapy in the first four sessions. Where the therapist is uncertain about prospects at the outset (e.g. when one partner is ambivalent about the relationship or where overt hostility makes collaboration unlikely), a limited contract of three or four sessions is advisable. Such a couple are told that further treatment will depend on evidence of progress during those sessions. People who drop out usually do so around the third or fourth session (Bancroft and Coles 1976).

The duration of each session varies. When progress is satisfactory and no obstacles encountered, 30 minutes are sufficient; frequently, a longer period is needed. When appointments have to be time-limited, it is preferable to allow an hour.

Should one or two therapists be involved? Masters and Johnson (1970) advocated a dual-therapist team. This obviously requires substantial justification on economic grounds. Although superior results using two therapists rather than one have not been shown (Bancroft 1989), advantages are obvious: both male and female points of view are represented and apparent collusion of therapist and one partner more easily avoided. Moreover, it is possible for one therapist to remain more objective while the other is more directly involved. Against this, the co-therapist relationship is not necessarily easy, making the choice of a colleague crucial. Proper use of the arrangement requires time outside sessions for adequate discussion. Co-therapy is a valuable training model provided that the more experienced therapist takes care not to monopolize the sessions. So, it is reasonable to practise sex therapy with one or two therapists as opportunities present themselves or as preference dictates.

In the case of individual therapy, it is more difficult to lay down practical guidelines since objectives and the nature of the therapist's involvement vary more greatly. However, similar principles apply.

TRAINING

Because of its 'psychosomatic' nature sexual dysfunction has causa
factors of a medical type in a substantial proportion of cases. For thi
reason, sex therapy is best provided in a setting with access to medica
expertise. Once these medical aspects have been clarified, however
features of a suitable therapist are determined more by personality
experience, and training than by a particular professional background
Doctors, psychologists, social workers, nurses, and marriage guidance
counsellors have all proved effective therapists.

Training often starts with the co-therapist format described above
In addition, regular supervision groups in which continuing case
management is discussed are invaluable. In such sessions, 'role-
playing', in which the therapist takes the role of the patient, can be
particularly illuminating.

CONCLUSION

Sex therapy is indicated for problems of wide-ranging complexity. At
one extreme, a simple behavioural programme with little therapist
intervention will suffice; at the other, considerable psychotherapeutic
skills are required. Most cases fall between these extremes. In all cases,
however, the basic framework is similar, this of undoubted advantage
to the novice.

REFERENCES

Arentewicz, G. and Schmidt, G. (1983). *The treatment of sexual disorders*.
Basic Books, New York.
Bancroft, J. (1989). *Human sexuality and its problems*, (2nd edn). Churchill
Livingstone, Edinburgh.
Bancroft, J. (1991). Ethical aspects of sexuality and sex therapy. In *Psychiatric
ethics*, (2nd edn), (ed. S. Bloch and P. Chodoff), pp. 215–42. Oxford
University Press.
Bancroft, J. (1996). Sex therapy: the strengths and limitations of a cognitive-
behavioural approach. In *Cognitive-behavioural therapy: Science and
practice*, (ed. C. Fairburn and D. Clarke). Oxford University Press, Oxford.
Bancroft, J. and Coles, L. (1976). Three years experience in a sexual problems
clinic. *British Medical Journal*, i, 1575–7.
Hawton, K., Salkovskis, P. M., Kirk, J., and Clark, D. M. (1989). *Cognitive
behaviour therapy for psychiatric problems: A practical guide*. Oxford
University Press.
Kaplan, H. S. (1975). *The new sex therapy*. Baillière Tindall, London.

Masters, W. H. and Johnson, V. E. (1970). *Human sexual inadequacy*. Churchill, London.

Schmidt, G. (1994). *Symposium on sex therapy*. European Association of Sexology Conference, Copenhagen, June 1994.

Tiefer, L. (1986). In pursuit of the perfect penis. The medicalisation of male sexuality. *American Behavioral Scientist*, **29**, 579–99.

Tunnadine, L. P. D. , Morrow, C. S., and Hutchinson, F. D. (1981). Sex problems in practice. Training and referral. Institute of Psychosexual Medicine, Margaret Pyke Centre, and Brook Advisory Centres. *British Medical Journal*, **282**, 1669–72.

RECOMMENDED READING

Bancroft, J. (1989). *Human sexuality and its problems*. (2nd edn). Churchill Livingstone, Edinburgh. (A comprehensive text covering all aspects of sexual behaviour, problems, and treatment.)

Hawton, K. (1985). *Sex therapy: a practical guide*. Oxford University Press, Oxford. (A useful, concise and practical text.)

Hawton, K. (1992). Sex therapy research: has it withered on the vine? *Annual Review of Sex Research*, **3**, 49–72. (A useful review of outcome studies of sex therapy.)

Hawton, K. (1995). Treatment of sexual dysfunctions by sex therapy and other approaches. *British Journal of Psychiatry*, **167**, 307–14. (A review of the literature on the application and outcome of therapies for sexual dysfunction.)

Kaplan, H. S. (1975). *The new sex therapy*. Baillière Tindall, London. (A balanced and eclectic account; particularly recommended are chapters on psychological causes and basic principles of treatment.)

Leiblum, S. R. and Rosen, R. C. (ed.) (1989). *Principles and practice of sex therapy*. (2nd edn). (A multi-author text covering most aspects of modern treatment.)

Masters, W. H. and Johnson, V. E. (1970). *Human sexual inadequacy*. Churchill, London. (A classic text, albeit a little dated, on the various forms of sexual dysfunction.)

10

Family therapy

ARNON BENTOVIM

Family therapy has continued to expand enormously since the last edition of this book. In this chapter, Arnon Bentovim describes the form of family therapy used when the child or adolescent is the referred patient. Following an account of principal theoretical models used he highlights the importance of assessment and suggests three useful frameworks within which it can be done. The process of therapy—its beginning, planning, interventions, and ending—is dissected out, with an accompanying clinical illustration. Problems that arise in the course of treatment are then covered. The final section deals with training.

Family therapy is a psychotherapeutic endeavour that seeks to alter interactions between family members and aims, at the same time, to improve the functioning of an individual member, for instance, a child referred and identified as the patient (Bentovim and Kinston 1978). The approach usually involves working with the family as a group although it can proceed with a single member or a subgroup of the family.

Family therapy is practised by a range of professionals, in diverse contexts like child and family psychiatric departments, social services units, paediatric departments, and day and residential units. Although beyond the remit of this chapter it should be borne in mind that a family approach can also be deployed in circumstances where a family member other than young offspring is the referred patient (Bloch *et al.* 1991).

HISTORICAL PERSPECTIVE

Freud (1909/1977) was among the first to include a parent in the psychotherapy of a child. He worked indirectly with 'Little Hans'' phobic problems by communicating with the boy's father and also seeing them together. The subsequent development of the psychoanalytic treatment of children followed the model with dults—intensive individual psychotherapy (Hug-Hellmuth 1921). A ater innovation was the use of play material to enhance communication between therapist and child; Melanie Klein's (1948) contribution in this regard was particularly important. Classically, the child was seen four or five times a week and the main emphasis was on ntrapsychic life.

A new pattern of treatment emerged with the evolution of the child guidance clinic in the 1920s and 1930s—weekly sessions with the child n conjunction with regular casework with one or other parent. This constituted the standard approach until the 1950s. Then, interest in creating the family as a group was stimulated by studies of communication patterns in families containing a schizophrenic member (Bateson *et al.* 1956; Lidz 1973). Several research groups began to examine the role of family factors in the genesis of schizophrenia, and of psychiatric disorders of childhood. The therapeutic implications of their findings soon followed, culminating in the publication of Ackerman's (1958) *The psychodynamics of family life*. This volume, the first systematic account of psychotherapy of the family, was based on traditional psychoanalytic concepts. Other approaches to family therapy followed, some analytically derived, others incorporating new models. Important examples are the work of Haley (1963, 1971), Minuchin (1974), Minuchin and Fishman (1981), and the Milan systemic approach (Palazzoli *et al.* 1978), to which we return later.

MODELS OF FAMILY THERAPY

Given the lack of a unified theory of family development and corresponding dysfunction it is not surprising that several models of family therapy have been elaborated. Useful overviews of these are provided by Gorell Barnes (1994) and Bentovim and Kinston (1991). Only brief mention can be made of the more important ones here; the interested reader is referred to the Recommended Reading.

Whatever the model, non-specific factors in family work warrant brief mention. Gurman *et al.* (1986) have identified ingredients common to all models of family therapy: helping the family to view their presenting problem in a new light; transforming their attitude of blaming an individual member to an appreciation that problems are interactional and thus tied to the way they function as a family; modifying communication between family members; creating alternative modes of problem-solving, whether directly or indirectly;

modifying the degree of distress associated with symptomatic behaviour, and, more generally, optimizing the position of boundaries between members; and, establishing appropriate hierarchies.

(1) Psychodynamic

Many pioneering family therapists were originally psychoanalysts who transferred their traditional concepts from treatment of the individual to that of the family (Ackerman 1958). In the psychodynamic mode the therapist's task is mainly to interpret, and through the therapeutic relationship, bring family members' unconscious thoughts, feelings and experiences into awareness, especially assisting them to appreciate associations between past and present. The fundamental goals are insight, integration, and adaptive functioning. A family's current behaviour may, for example, relate to an underlying, continuing conflict stemming from a common traumatic experience. When the family repress this aspect of their history, they are helped to see relevant connections (Lieberman 1980; Byng-Hall 1973, 1982). Attention is paid both to members as individuals with their early attachment patterns (Byng-Hall 1991) and to the family group with its typical modes of functioning (Zinner and Shapiro 1974).

(2) Systems, structural and strategic approaches

(a) *Systems*

Concepts that underlie the rubric of general systems theory were originally developed by Von Bertalanffy (1962) in response to a dissatisfaction with reductionism which saw events confined to cause and effect chains. Such thinking is embedded in psychodynamic models which see past events as causal of subsequent ways of behaving. An alternative is to study the pattern of organization of biological systems. The family is construed similarly as a system (Jackson and Weakland 1961; Watzlawick *et al.* 1969). Observation of the family relies on the premise that a system is an organized arrangement of elements, a network of interdependent, co-ordinated parts functioning as a unit. A particular family, therefore, develops typical patterns of being and relating, which are transferred by its members to other social contexts (Main *et al.* 1985). The therapist analyses these patterns by treating the family as a group, including the

eferred child; he observes what transpires between members and
ormulates ideas about possible links between patterns and presenting
roblems. He then conveys his understanding to the family in such a
vay that can convert their newly acquired knowledge into positive
hanges of attitude and behaviour.

The approach can be reinforced by an array of useful techniques, for
xample, family 'sculpting', in which physical scupltures are created to
nap and explore relationships between members. Similarly, producing
. family tree illuminates not only genealogical patterns but also
urrent ways of relating. Those techniques have the distinct advantage
of incorporating children into therapy beyond mere talking.

b) *Structural*

Minuchin (1974) was the innovator of the structural approach, a
particular application of systems theory. His ideas stemmed from an
awareness that psychological problems in children were often linked to
marked social stress, such as immigration and poverty, and
environmental problems generally rather than to the early history of
the family alone.

This led to an approach addressing such problems. Families are
helped to develop communication and social skills. Action techniques
like enactment of a conflict or emotional entanglement are applied.
The therapist is active, his role akin to a director of a play. Immediate
supervision is available through the use of a one-way screen; direct
communication to the therapist during a session helps him to intensify
his effectiveness as a change-promoting agent. Minuchin and his
colleagues (Minuchin 1974) have deployed their methods for
behavioural problems and psychosomatic states such as diabetes,
asthma, and anorexia nervosa. The aim here is to restructure a family
whose rigid patterns both trigger and maintain damaging patterns,
even potentially life-threatening states.

(c) *Strategic*

The strategic therapist (Watzlawick *et al.* 1967, 1974) perceives the fact
of the complaint about a child as the problem, rather than construing
the problem as the target of treatment. Complaints or symptoms arise
through failure to deal with critical life transitions or stressful life
events. Thus, a particular problem, instead of being managed
effectively, leads to a 'solution' which in turn constitutes the
problem. The child who sleeps poorly as a result of a stressful event
at school, may develop severe separation anxiety if parents take him

into their bed to comfort him and then fail to have him return to his own room.

The therapeutic task then focuses on the different 'solutions' tried by the family. One variant is *solution focused therapy* which attempts to discover an exception to the problematic pattern (De Shazer *et al* 1986). Further strategic thinking, for example, Haley (1963, 1971 1977) and Madanes (1991) acknowledge the centrality and power of the symptom, and the part it plays in stabilizing family life. Members are helped to understand how this has evolved, and how the family may be regulated afresh or its collective identity reorganized. It is crucial in this model, therefore, to consider consequences of change even to the point of using paradoxical messages that caution is wise lest change occurs too precipitously with potentially adverse repercussions. This enables the family to discover their own solution, which is positively connoted by the therapist. Play, stories and metaphors like a 'Mr Temper' or a figure who takes control of the child's life are useful methods, the therapist helping the family to locate exceptions to a dominating theme in order to create a new reality (White 1984, 1986).

(3) Integrating psychodynamic and systems models

The most sturdy bridge between psychodynamic and systems models has been erected by the Milan group (Palazzoli *et al*. 1978, 1980). They have attempted to link understanding of unconscious processes which control family relationships with a systems approach of changing covert rules in the family's pattern of communication. Behaviour is seen as working to preserve family stability and coherence. The Milan group have developed a highly organized and influential method characterized by the studious formulation of a hypothesis that might explain the problem, and an observing team placed behind a one-way screen. The hypothesis is systemetically explored through posing questions that recognize the 'circularity' of cause and effect and influence of members on one another and on the therapist. The therapist maintains a position of strict neutrality, careful to use his observer's role to explore different ways the problem can be construed.

Integrated approaches have become progessively more common as therapists combine various effective ways of working (Bentovim and Kinston 1991). Attempts are also being made to treat a diverse set of clinical problems like the traumatic effects of physical and sexual abuse (Bentovim *et al*. 1988) and ramifications of divorce, single parenting or lended families; moreover, ethnic and cultural perspectives are taken into ccount. The effect of practising family therapy on the therapist has also een examined; one view is to note equivalents of transference/counter-ransference patterns of individual therapy.

Although a therapist may develop a preference for a particular model (for many assorted reasons), it is salutary to bear in mind the quivalence of available models in terms of efficacy. Comprehensive eviews of outcome research show that many models are effective with n average three-quarters of treated families improving (Gurman and Kniskern 1981; Gurman *et al.* 1986). The level of effectiveness has een found with a diverse variety of clinical problems.

ASSESSMENT

Family therapy is used in many clinical settings related to children and adolescents, both with those living in a biological family or in the case where family care is shared with professional agencies (e.g. child care). It is now feasible to categorize those problems where family therapy is particularly pertinent.

Where family violence or sexual abuse have occurred, family therapy is contra-indicated initially since the child is unlikely to express feelings in the presence of the perpetrator. A multi-modal approach is indicated in these cases with individual or group work for children or parents, and a family approach used later when rehabilitation of the child and parents is contemplated (Bentovim *et al.* 1988).

In conditions like infantile autism, intellectual handicap and disability in which biological factors predominate, a family approach is unlikely to be relevant, at least in the first instance. But a psycho-educational approach where the family is encouraged to deploy their resources to the maximum benefit of the child is significant as part of an integrated approach.

A framework for assessment

In assessing whether a family is suitable to be treated as a group the therapist will find it advantageous to consider three frameworks: the family life cycle; the three-generational model of family life; and family function in the here and now; these are now outlined.

(1) *The family life-cycle* (Carter and McGoldrick 1980)

The family has a typical life cycle comprising a predictable series o
stages:

(a) Pre-parenthood—two people select one another as partners and
progress through courtship, engagement, and marriage (the las
not necessarily legalised since the 1990s).

(b) Early parenthood—the family consists of an infant or toddler, and
later, perhaps a second infant.

(c) The oldest child is between two and a half years and school age
and may be attending a play-group or nursery school.

(d) The oldest child has begun school and later proceeds to early
secondary school but is still pre-adolescent.

(e) The oldest child has entered adolescence but not yet left home.

(f) The phase between the oldest child's departure from home until
that of the youngest.

(g) All children have now left home and one or both parents are still
working.

(h) The phase between the retirement of the parent/s and their deaths.

Demands and challenges confront one or more family members at
every stage: for instance, the wife becomes pregnant, the husband
becomes a father, the toddler has his first experience of a new sibling
or of relating to persons other than his parents, the child has his first
school experience with demands for learning and relating to peers, the
child enters adolescence and encounters his sexuality and need for
independence, the older adolescent experiments in heterosexual
relationships, the parents relate anew following the departure of
their children from home, and deal with them as young adults. At the
same time as individual members face these various transitions, the
family as a whole must change and grow in order to negotiate each
stage of the cycle effectively.

(2) *The three-generational model of family life*

The second framework concerns the families of origin of the two
parents. Knowledge of these families can illuminate many of the
current family's problems. For instance, the choice of spouse and
nature of the marital relationship may have been determined by either

or both partners' attempts to resolve a conflict which could not be satisfactorily dealt with in their own families. Experiences of the two parents in their families of origin, such as a domineering or rejecting father or an over-protective mother, may lead to a particular 'script' of child rearing in the current family (Byng-Hall 1986). Thus parents who were unduly protected as children may replicate this pattern or adopt an entirely contrary approach so as to avoid giving their children an experience they themselves found undesirable.

In some families, a 'myth' is handed down from generation to generation from which no member can apparently escape. The myth (e.g. 'Ill-luck has always dogged the Browns' or 'The Smiths have been an argumentative lot for generations'), is shared by the family as if they were one 'ego mass' (Bowen 1966), or a single psychic entity (Zinner and Shapiro 1974). Family members are not perceived by one another as separate persons with their own unique qualities but only as elements within the mass. In this way the current family automatically stamps on itself a specific seal inherited through myths, beliefs, and stories, which contribute in large measure to their problems and to the manner in which they are perceived and reacted to. The myths, beliefs, and stories, constructed through repeated conversations and narratives, may be appreciated when families talk together in a fresh way and may then be modified by 'counter-stories' and new information.

(3) *Family function in the here and now*

The third framework pertinent to assessment is the style in which the family typically functions in the here and now to meet each member's needs for psychological survival and growth, in the context of their ethnic background (McGoldrick *et al*. 1982). In a well-functioning family the following are provided: a setting for all members to fulfil their potential; a model for socialization transferable to the outside world; parental models for sexual identification; and clear boundaries demarcating the generations such that children respect the leadership role of the parents with all its implications (Bloch *et al*. 1994). This provision of boundaries suggests that a family consists of various subsystems each of which is bound by a set of rules. The parental subsystem, for example, entails the responsibility of making certain types of decisions for the child subsystem. Other subsystems, apart from the obvious generational one, occur in terms of sex, age, values, and interests. We return to this topic later.

Family function (and its associated problems) can be convenientl;
considered under six headings which describe the language of famil;
therapy (Loader *et al.* 1981; Bentovim and Kinston 1991).

(a) *Communication and exchange of information*—the famil;
communicate with one another both verbally and non-verbally, th
latter often exerting the greater impact. Communication varie:
considerably in terms of whether it actually occurs or not, how
clear, how open and direct, and how responsive family members are to
one another. Often, an incongruity between what is stated and what i
expressed non-verbally is an obvious indicator of family dysfunction

(b) *Emotional state*—expression of a variety of feelings is a salient face
of family function. Some families are highly restricted in their range o
a single emotion like anger predominates. In others, there is virtua
absence of emotional expression with a resultant sense of deadness or
emptiness. Feelings may be expressed by particular members but fail to
elicit an appropriate response from the rest of the family.

(c) *Atmosphere*—expression of emotions contributes with other
factors to the family climate. Every family has a distinctive
atmosphere: chaotic, panicky, over-excited, apathetic, critical,
aggressive, lively, humorous, gay, ironic—the list is infinite. Of
course, many of those listed may occur in a family at different times
but commonly a constellation tends to predominate.

(d) *Cohesiveness*—a family has its own unique sense of solidarity,
belongingness, and loyalty—a sense of members working together to
ensure their continuing life and to enhance their welfare. Cohesiveness
is threatened when alliances form which exclude some members, when
discord develops between two or more members, when a child or
parent is scapegoated for a problem that the whole family should
share, and when members behave vainly and ignore the well-being of
the group.

(e) *Boundaries*—as mentioned earlier the family consists of subsystems
divided by boundaries. In a well-functioning family these are
permeable enough to facilitate easy communication between
subsystems but yet sufficiently intact to allow their autonomy. The
family also respects the rules that govern relationships between
subsystems and the internal process of each of them.

In some families these boundaries do not exist and members are
completely enmeshed. For example, an adolescent child facing an

exciting challenge which should be his alone may be robbed of the experience by parents who fail to maintain adequate distance between themselves and the adolescent. In other families, the boundaries are so rigid that the members act as totally separate persons who merely happen to share the same household.

(f) *Family operations*—the family faces many tasks in managing its day-to-day affairs: to resolve conflict, to make decisions, to face problems, and to deal with the changes inherent in the family life cycle. Families vary considerably in the way they handle these tasks. For instance, the family may deal with a conflict effectively, avoid it, make do with inadequate solutions, or allow a child to play an inappropriately prominent role.

CLINICAL ASSESSMENT

We now turn to the actual task of assessment. The therapist's aims in assessing a child who is the referred patient and his family are: to appreciate the problem in terms of the child presenting it; to understand the origins of this problem and the role that the family may have played in its genesis and maintenance; to determine the changes required in child and family for the relief of the problem and for improved family life; and to motivate the family to accept the need for change and to negotiate a therapeutic contract.

Unlike the individual patient who usually seeks help, members of families are commonly requested by the therapist to attend. Indeed, they may well express surprise, and even show reluctance. Thus, the therapist's first objective is to encourage the whole family to participate; and we are referring to assessment only at this stage. Referring agencies, teachers, and general practitioners among them, need to broach the subject with the family tactfully and with a measure of hopefulness. In some cases, the family may require a home visit or telephone contact to explain carefully what they can expect in treatment and to deal with any actual or potential resistance.

When a therapist invites a family to attend for assessment she should stress the inherent advantages of this move. She should offer a convenient time; families are usually more willing to come after school hours. The content and style of the letter require detailed consideration. It is also obviously crucial to seek the family's consent if video is customarily used or observing therapists are

present; they should have the opportunity to discuss these matter.
fully.

THE PROCESS OF THERAPY

The first session

The therapy room should be comfortable and private, chairs placed in
a circle, and ample play material available. Sufficient time, commonly
two hours, is set aside for this occasion. Therapist and co-therapists
need to exchange ideas about the presenting problem and family
history (whatever is known at this early stage). Formulating a
hypothesis to guide the initial session is an advantageous discipline.
An hour with the family is followed by a period of consultation
between the therapist and observers and a brief concluding phase with
the family comprising feedback and the launch, if apt, of the
therapeutic programme.

Since parents classically dominate this first session the therapist
needs to promote participation of the children; they usually feel
overawed, inhibited, and anxious. Posing neutral questions about
name, age, and school paves the way for a more emotionally loaded
enquiry. Another option is to have the parents explain to the children
the reason for the consultation. The therapist then checks whether
they have understood this and their reactions to it.

Parents often express concern about talking openly in the presence
of their children lest they should criticize or humiliate them. The
parents' possible sense of shame or embarrassment may preclude them
from divulging feelings they harbour about problems facing the
family. From the outset the therapist takes care to encourage all family
members to communicate freely, both thoughts and feelings; he can
reassure them that they are invariably already acquainted with one
another's views. Kinston and Loader (1984, 1988) in their pragmatic
account of a standardized approach to the interview, describe several
possible tasks to promote family interaction.

In most cases, channels of communication open up by the end of the
initial session. The therapist takes a much more active role than is
customary in other psychotherapies in pursuing the chief goal at this
point, namely to involve the whole family. Of the many techniques
available to him those described by Minuchin (1974)—joining and
accommodation and tracking—are especially apposite. We also
consider the function of circular questioning (Palazzoli *et al.* 1980).

a) *Joining and accommodation*

The therapist forges links with each of the family members by clearly showing that he appreciates their unique positions and experiences. For example, in a family in which Peter has three older sisters the therapist may comment that it must be good being the only son and yet difficult as the youngest with so many older sibs. He can remark to the girls that it must be awkward at times having a younger brother and yet good that both sexes are represented in the family. He may note to the parents that despite the pleasures involved it must have been bewildering to accustom themselves to a son following three daughters. To accomplish such 'joining' the therapist 'accommodates' himself (or adjusts) to the family's particular style and patterns of communication, modifying his methods to facilitate their acceptance of him. An excellent manoeuvre is to relabel problem behaviours and connote them positively. For instance, in a family concerned about John's temper tantrums the therapist comments that John is 'good' at getting angry and 'wonders' which member is next best, and whether father or mother had this 'talent' when they were children.

(b) *Tracking*

Tracking is a suitable term to reflect the therapist's tasks in pursuing emergent themes; he keeps 'track' of what occurs in the session by asking the family to clarify or elaborate relevant aspects. Rather than challenging them he leads them by expressing interest in what he has heard, echoing their statements, and encouraging them to amplify. Although he may initiate communication his principal goal is to follow the family's lead (at the same time ensuring that all members participate).

(c) *Circular questioning*

This simple but most useful technique, introduced by the Milan group (Palazzoli *et al.* 1980), relies on the interconnectedness between and mutual influence of family members. The therapist, for example, may observe that one child has a particular skill in attracting his parents' attention by behaving provocatively, and does so when the parents are on the verge of arguing. The therapist pursues this by asking another child whether the pattern observed in the session is typical of family life. Following this inquiry, he may ask a parent what they make of the child's comments; the same child may then be invited to offer his view in turn of his parent's comments; and so the circular process can be extended boundlessly.

Exploring the presenting problem

The therapist encourages the family to describe the presenting problem in substantial detail in order that he may arrive at a diagnostic formulation and, as importantly, to demonstrate that he is 'actively' listening. When did the problem begin, who first noted it, what effect has it had on family members, who has benefited most from attention paid to the person with the problem, who conversely has been most distressed, who has done what to ameliorate the situation, with what results?

The therapist also elicits the family's own explanations of the problem, which helps him to understand maintaining factors (e.g. a family labelling a particular child as the source of everything bad). The therapist also observes directly ways in which problem behaviours manifest in the session: what provokes a child's angry outburst, what sets off an argument between siblings or between parents, what alliances exist, and so on. He may discreetly provoke characteristic ways of relating by directing group discussion, instructing the family to perform certain tasks like having a hyperactive child sit down before discussing a topic, or issuing a paradoxical injunction.

The therapist places the presenting problem/s in the context of the family's overall functioning. Pauline, for example, a 12-year-old girl experiencing school refusal, sat close to mother with father situated at the other end of the room. The therapist could have assumed from this arrangement that Pauline and mother had formed a collusive bond which excluded father. The therapist noted, however, that rather than looking to mother for reassurance when her problems were under scrutiny Pauline constantly sought eye contact with her father, reflecting a distinct affiliation. On probing, it emerged that father and daughter had an intense association which played a pivotal role in the school refusal.

Exploring the family life cycle and inter-generational issues

To appreciate why a family is troubled at a particular time, knowledge of their past history and development is invariably illuminating. In exploring their life cycle (see above) the therapist pursues a myriad of issues: for instance, what originally attracted the parents to each other;

ow did they feel about the birth and development of each child; how ave they responded to crises and significant family events over the ears? The children contribute to the picture provided by the parents; a rich fabric unfolds in time in which the presenting problems can be conveniently embedded.

As discussed earlier, the therapist also explores the parents' experiences as children in their own families, noting both the content and style of their accounts. Preparation of a family tree, sculpting, and other non-verbal techniques can enrich such an assessment (see p. 241).

Planning therapy

Before devising a plan of treatment the therapist formulates a hypothesis to explain the origins of the presenting problems and of those that have emerged during the assessment phase. Furthermore, he creates a list of goals by which he can evaluate outcome. In so doing it is helpful to see how presenting problems fit in with patterns of family functioning in the here and now, and with past handling of stress and change (Bentovim and Kinston 1991).

A wide range of hypotheses is needed to fit the diversity of dysfunction seen. For instance, a child's disturbance may reflect his anxiety about a fragile marital relationship; parents may be overwhelmed by the challenge of their adolescent daughter's development because they themselves experienced difficulties when negotiating this period; a family may encounter difficulties in coping with a major loss; a life crisis, such as financial loss, may dislodge a family's customary coping capacity; and many more.

A family map illustrating boundaries and relationship patterns can guide the therapist in setting treatment goals. These may need to be step-wise, that is, attempting to focus on one aspect of the family's dysfunction at a time. He may, for example, first deal with the anxiety of the children in the face of a deteriorating marital relationship. His next target may be the parents' difficulties. Later, focus may be on each parent's distinctive problems if it appears as if both mother and father require help in their own right.

The time interval between sessions and duration of treatment depend in large measure on the model adopted and the nature of the problems tackled. A structural family therapist who actively encourages the family to enact their problems in order to identify a solution for controlling a defiant child or assisting a clinging child to separate, needs to see the whole family at least weekly in the initial phase; this allows for sufficient intensity of work to be accomplished. Other models, particularly the Milan systems one, use a longer interval of three to four weeks between sessions to enable powerful interventions to be made; these often urge the family to be cautious about change.

Depending on his approach the family therapist has a choice of working solo or with a co-therapist, ideally of the opposite sex. Co-therapy is advantageous in that it provides all family members with a model of their gender, the two co-therapists can demonstrate effective ways of relating to each other which members can imitate, and in treating a group with so much happening, 'two pairs of eyes are better than one'. Family therapists generally favour working as part of a team whether with a co-therapist or consulting with colleagues behind a one-way screen. In another variation the team share their reflections with the family directly after observing the therapy session.

Duration of therapy lasts between a single session (in which it is obvious the problem is resolved or not appropriate for a family approach) or endures indefinitely, say in the case of a psycho-educational approach for a family with a chronically ill member, particularly schizophrenia.

CLINICAL ILLUSTRATION

A case history follows to illustrate the typical process of assessment and treatment.

Matthew, a 5-year-old with a much older brother aged 19, was referred because of disruptive behaviour which was jeopardizing his integration into school. He was fighting with other children to an extent that his mother worried lest he might injure a smaller child; he did not know his own strength.

A striking pattern emerged during the initial session: despite his parents sharing their intense concern about his behaviour, Mathew sat beside his mother singing in a nonchalant, even contemptuous manner. He ostensibly manifested complete indifference; there was not a hint of anxiety or pensiveness that one might expect in the circumstances.

The therapist noted that mother particularly both admired Mathew's 'clever' behaviour but at the same time was most anxious about how to cope with it, and fearful about what might happen if either she or father became angry with him. The therapist conjectured that both parents were anxious about violence and loss and therefore did not adequately control Matthew; he literally had to persist with his outrageous and contemptuous behaviour until somebody took notice of him.

The therapist experienced a quandary: should he advise the parents to assume control over Matthew or should he allow the pattern to continue in order to make further observations and thus gain a more comprehensive understanding of the family dynamics.

It was also abundantly clear during this session that the maternal grandmother, an important family member, was absent. She had always lived in the home, in fact occupying more room than the rest of the family combined. The therapist hypothesized that the parents hesitated to manage Matthew because there was so much resentment they could not express to the grandmother. It was learned that John, the older sibling, had been an anxious child and had had weight problems similar to Matthew. It became progressively clearer that the family were incapable of assuming control over their children or supporting them adequately.

Six family sessions followed. The main aim early on was to strengthen the bond between therapist and family so that patterns of behaviour could be openly explored, particularly the elucidation of the implicit rules that governed family interaction. As the history was elaborated, it emerged that both parents had experienced emotional deprivation as children and received little affection from the same-sex parent. The therapist's empathy with the parents' past distress enabled them to recall and share their own parents' hardships. The maternal grandmother who had been presented as a negative force, not allowing the family to have their space, was revealed more sympathetically. Instead of feeling aggrieved, the family, it could be seen, were caring for grandmother by not challenging her, thus trying to compensate for her past privations. It was also then noted that the parental difficulty to control the children over diet or behaviour reflected their concern about not depriving them in the way they themselves had felt deprived.

It then emerged that a strong tradition prevailed in both the parents' families of not expressing criticism or anger. Negative feelings had always had to be suppressed. Both parents were exceedingly anxious about the ventilation of any negative emotion lest it might harm the recipient. The therapist connoted the family's pattern and rules of not manifesting anger positively. Swallowing their feelings and sacrificing their own needs to care for others (grandparents and children) was interpreted as a dimension of parental caring.

In later sessions, the parents acknowledged the risks for Matthew of not supervising him adequately; if he ran on the roads or struck other children or he ate excessively. The parents were able to think the unthinkable—to take some measure of control. For instance, they reported their ability to be firmer with both grandmother and Matthew. The therapist also encouraged the parents to spend time in enjoyable pursuits as a reward for Matthew's compliance.

The family were again seen after a three-month break. The change in Matthew's behaviour was striking, but the parents showed considerable marital tension. It emerged that they were challenging other family inhibitions. In particular, both acknowledged breakdowns in their own parents' marriages; this confrontation with their past had sensitized them that angry expression might damage their relationship. The couple went on to explore their respective family legacies of losses and other painful events psychodynamically. Although a painful pursuit, the work involved proved beneficial to themselves, their relationship, and the family as a whole.

PROBLEMS ENCOUNTERED IN THE COURSE OF TREATMENT

Of the range of problems that may disrupt therapy only a few can be discussed here. Not all families improve even with well-planned intervention. Since the marriage is the axis around which the family revolves, a critical view of the parental relationship must be taken by the therapist when treatment seems to be 'stuck'. In some cases, a parent has a severe psychiatric problem in his or her own right and either individual treatment or more intensive family therapy is indicated. When family dysfunction has been present for several years and is well entrenched, it is not surprising that change does not occur readily.

Missed appointments should always be raised with the family through a telephone call or letter. The therapist may not appreciate how frightening treatment is for a family; they in turn may not reveal their distress when touching sensitive terrain. He therefore needs to monitor their reactions to particular sessions and be constantly alert to any cues of distress they emit. Absence of a member automatically requires family discussion as does his eventual return. Should a member not be able to attend the family is urged to inform him about what transpired. Premature drop-out is discussed below.

Poor progress may be attributable to the therapist. Thus, a vague, diffuse approach may provoke the family to wonder what they gain from attending. Therapy tends to wander, the outcome inevitably poor. This drift can be minimized if the therapist sets and maintains clear objectives and works assiduously towards them. Treatment can also be interfered with by the therapist unwittingly entering into an alliance with a member or a subgroup. He needs to check regularly that his interventions are objectively determined. Is the son with whom he feels sympathy in a similar position to the one he occupied in his own family? Is the husband on whose behalf he senses anger towards the wife paralleling his own marital experience or that of his parents? A therapist who feels blocked with a family may learn that they are grappling with a problem resembling one he experienced in his own family and which was never satisfactorily resolved. A female therapist encountering difficulty to divert a mother from scapegoating her son may learn that she, the therapist, unwittingly colluded with her own mother in undermining an elder brother.

Problems readily arise when a member violates the rules of openness by offering the therapist information but at the same time instructing him to withhold it from the rest of the family. The therapist, tempted to accept such communication, should desist vigorously, stressing that all information needs to be divulged to the whole family and that 'secrets' hinder even sabotage treatment. An exception are sexual problems in the parents which are best discussed with them alone. The children are then told that a separate meeting between parents and therapist has been planned to discuss matters of no direct concern to them. It is surprising, however, to what extent the parents' general relationship can be openly talked about in the family and how reassuring this can be to the children.

TERMINATION

If the therapist has negotiated a specific number of sessions with the family at the outset, termination is relatively straightforward. He will, however, need to remind them periodically about the schedule. Towards the end of the agreed programme a review of progress is helpful. Should problems remain the therapist can prepare a revised contract for additional sessions; indeed, two or three distinct phases of therapy each with their own goals are feasible.

Termination is usually smoother when the therapist is clear about objectives: delineating problems, setting goals (covering both amelioration of the presenting problem and improved family functioning), and formulating outcome criteria. A regular review of these goals guides the therapist further in planning the final phase. Some families, less ambitious in their goals, may terminate prematurely, either when their child's symptoms have waned or when they discover that the process of overall change is more demanding of them than they anticipated; keen clinical judgement is called for in responding to these circumstances.

TRAINING

The most difficult task for trainees is to make sense of the mass of information presented to them as they begin to work with families. They not only have to attend to the child with the presenting problem but also to each of the other members and to the family as a whole. To familiarize themselves with the ways families respond to therapy they need to observe them being treated by experienced practitioners through a one-way screen or on video-tape. Their own therapeutic efforts should be closely supervised. Here, again, the one-way screen and video-tape are invaluable teaching aids. The supervisor observes trainees' work with families and offers appropriate feedback; trainees have a parallel opportunity to note their own performance on tape. If members of supervision groups, they can benefit from the feedback of fellow trainees. There is a particular advantage in immediate feedback while issues are still fresh.

Therapists also gain from participating in a group of peers where, through techniques such as role-play and family sculpting, they study different patterns of adaptive and disturbed family functioning. Another rewarding method is for trainees to think back to their own significant family experiences. Constructing family trees is useful, even to the point of consulting directly with family members. In this way family 'secrets', buried for years, may be brought to light and their implications explored.

As we noted earlier there is a wide assortment of models of family therapy. Trainees need to experience and evaluate a few of them in order to select the one/s which best suits them. Observation of different therapists, their own efforts to practise various approaches, and a close reading of the literature facilitates this process. The Recommended reading contains sources providing detailed accounts of the main contemporary schools. For a useful account of training aspects, see Little (1991).

CONCLUSION

Family therapy has developed substantially since the 1950s.
Contemporary therapists function in an exciting but potentially
baffling field. Many different models compete for their attention and
important questions remain to be studied systematically (Gurman and
Kniskern 1981). Novices need to familiarize themselves with these
models and select one they can apply comfortably. Whatever their
choice they should not restrict themselves by setting up rigid
theoretical boundaries. As important as a coherent model is the
diligent formation of goals and a treatment plan for each family with
which they work.

REFERENCES

Ackerman, N. W. (1958). *The psychodynamics of family life*. Basic Books, New York.
Bateson, G., Jackson, D., Haley, J., and Weakland, J. (1956). Towards a theory of schizophrenia. *Behavioural Science*, **1**, 251–64.
Bentovim, A. and Kinston, W. (1991). Focal family therapy: joining systems theory with psychodynamic understanding. In *Handbook of family therapy*. Vol. 2, (ed. A. S. Gurman and D. P. Kniskern). Brunner/Mazel, New York.
Bentovim, A., Elton, A., Hildebrand, J., Vizard, E., and Tranter, M. (1988). *Sexual abuse within the family*. Wright, Bristol.
Bloch, S., Sharpe, M., and Allman, P. (1991). Systemic family therapy in adult psychiatry: A review of 50 families. *British Journal of Psychiatry*, **159**, 357–64.
Bloch, S., Hafner, J., Harari, E. and Szmukler, G. (1994). *The family in clinical psychiatry*. Oxford University Press, Oxford.
Bowen, M. (1966). The use of family theory in clinical practice. *Comprehensive Psychiatry*, **7**, 345–73.
Byng-Hall, J. (1973). Family myths used as defence in conjoint family therapy. *British Journal of Medical Psychology*, **46**, 239–50.
Byng-Hall, J. (1982). Dysfunction of feeling. Experiential life of the family. In *Family therapy: Complementary frameworks of theory and practice*, (ed. A. Bentovim, G. Gorell-Barnes, and A. Cooklin). Academic Press, New York.
Byng-Hall, J. (1986). Family scripts, the concept which can bridge child psychotherapy and family therapy thinking. *Journal of Child Psychotherapy*, **12**, 3–13.
Byng-Hall, J. (1991). The application of attachment theory to understanding and treatment in family therapy. In *Attachment across the life cycle*, (ed. C. M. Parkes, J. Stephenson-Hinde, and H. P. Marr), pp. 159–215. Routledge, London.
Carter, E. and McGoldrick, M. (eds) (1980). *The family life cycle: A framework for family therapy*. Gardner Press, New York.

De Shazer, S. *et al.* (1986). Brief therapy: focused solution development. *Family Process*, 25, 207–22.

Freud, S. (1977). *Case histories*, Vol. 1. Penguin, Harmondsworth. (Originally published 1909)

Gorell Barnes, G. (1994). Family Therapy. In *Child and adolescent psychiatry: modern approaches*, (ed. M. Rutter, E. Taylor, and L. Hersov), pp. 946–67.

Gurman, A. S. and Kniskern, D. P. (1981). Family therapy outcome: Research knowns and unknowns. In *Handbook of family therapy*, Vol. 1, (ed. A. S. Gurman and D. P. Kniskern). Brunner/Mazel, New York.

Gurman, A. S. and Kniskern, D. P. and Prusoff, B. (1986). Research on marital and family therapy—progress, perspective and prospects. In: *Handbook of psychotherapy and behaviour change: An empirical analysis* (3rd edn), (ed. S. L. Garfield and A. E. Bergin). Wiley, New York.

Haley, J. (1963). *Strategies of psychotherapy*. Grune and Stratton, New York.

Haley, J. (1971). *Changing families: a family therapy reader*. Grune & Stratton, New York.

Haley, J. (1977). *Problem solving therapy*. Jossey-Bass, San Francisco.

Hug-Hellmuth, H. (1921). On the technique of child analysis. *International Journal of Psychonalysis*, 2, 287–305.

Jackson, D. and Weakland, J. (1961). Conjoint family: some considerations on theory, technique and results. *Psychiatry*, 24, 30–45.

Kinston, W. and Loader, P. (1984). Eliciting whole family interaction with a standardized clinical interview. *Journal of Family Therapy*, 6, 347–63.

Kinston, W. and Loader, P. (1988). The family task interview: a tool for clinical research in family interaction. *Journal of Marital and Family Therapy*, 13, 67–88.

Klein, M. (1948). *Contributions to psychoanalysis 1921–1945*. Hogarth, London.

Lidz, T. (1973). *The origin and treatment of schizophrenic disorders*. Basic Books, New York.

Lieberman, S. (1980). *Intergenerational family therapy*. Croom Helm, London.

Little, H. A. (1991). Training and supervision in family therapy: A comprehensive and critical analysis. In *Handbook of family therapy*, Vol. 2. (ed. A. S. Gurman and D. P. Kniskern). Brunner/Mazel, New York.

Loader, P., Burck, C., Kinston, W., and Bentovim, A. (1981). A method for organising the clinical description of family interaction—the family interaction summary format. *Australian Journal of Family Therapy*, 2, 131–41.

McGoldrick, M., Pearce, J., and Giordano, J. (ed.) (1982). *Ethnicity in family therapy*. Guilford Press, New York.

Madanes, C. (1991). Strategic family therapy. In *Handbook of Family Therapy*, (ed. A. S. Gurman, and D. P. Kniskern) Vol. 2. Brunner/Mazel. New York.

Main, M., Kayman, N., and Cassidy, J. (1985). Security in infancy, childhood and adulthood : a move to the level of representation. In *Growing points in attachment theory in research* (ed. I. Bretherton and E. Waters). Monographs of the Society for Research in Child Development, 50, 66–104.

Minuchin, S. (1974). *Families and family therapy*. Tavistock, London.
Minuchin, S. and Fishman, H. C. (1981). *Family therapy techniques*. Harvard University Press, Cambridge, Mass.
Minuchin, S., Baker, L., Rosman, B. L., Liebman, R., Milman, L., and Todd, T. C. (1974). A conceptual model of psychosomatic illness in children. Family organisation and family therapy. *Archives of General Psychiatry*, **32**, 103–8.
Palazzoli, M. S., Boscolo, L., Cecchin, G., and Prata, G. (1978). *Paradox and counterparadox*. Aronson, New York.
Palazzoli, M. S., Boscolo, L., Cecchin, G., and Prata, G. (1980). Hypothesising–Circularity–Neutrality: Three guidelines for the conductor of the session. *Family Process*, **19**, 3–12.
Von Bertalanffy, L. (1962). General systems theory: a critical review. *General Systems*, **7**, 1–20.
Watzlawick, P., Beavin, J. H., and Jackson, D. D. (1967). *Pragmatics of human communication*. Norton, New York.
Watzlawick, P., Weakland, J., and Fish, R. (1974). *Change: principles of problem formation and problem resolution*. Norton, New York.
White, M. (1984). Pseudo-encopresis: from avalanche to victory, from vicious to virtuous cycle. *Family Systems Medicine*, **2**, 150–60.
White, M. (1986). Negative explanation, restraint and double description. A template for family therapy. *Family Process*, **25**, 169–84.
Zinner, J. and Shapiro, R. (1974). The family group as a single psychic entity, implications for acting out in adolescence. *International Review of Psychoanalysis*, **1**, 179–86.

RECOMMENDED READING

Bloch, D. A. (ed.) (1973). *Techniques of family therapy: a primer*. Grune & Stratton, New York. (An American text with useful contributions on home visits and action techniques.)
Bloch, S., Hafner, J., Harari, E., and Szmukler, G. (1994). *The family in clinical psychiatry*. Oxford University Press, Oxford. (A novel text which highlights family factors relevant to specific psychiatric states; contains an important chapter on assessment.)
Bentovim, A., Gorell-Barnes, G., and Cooklin, A., (ed.) (1989). *Family therapy: complementary frameworks of theory and practice*. Academic Press, New York. (A broad-based view, covering different approaches to theory and practice.)
Campbell, D. and Draper, R. (1985). *Applications of systemic family therapy: the Milan approach*. Grune & Stratton, New York. (A clear account of systems thinking; an updated chapter of their work can be found in *Handbook of family therapy*, Vol. 2 (ed. A. S. Gurman and D. P. Kniskern), pp. 325–62, Brunner/Mazel, New York.)

Glick, I. D., Kessler, D. R., and Sugarman, S. (1987). *Marital and family therapy* (3rd edn). Grune & Stratton, New York. (Probably the best American introductory text.)

Gurman, A. S. and Kniskern, D. P. (1981, 1991). *Handbook of family therapy*, Vols 1 and 2. Brunner/Mazel, New York. (These highly recommended volumes, complementary rather than the second replacing the first, include authoritive accounts of all the main models.)

Hoffman, L. (1983). *Foundations of family therapy*. Basic Books, New York. (An excellent historical perspective of different models.)

Satir, V. M. (1964). *Conjoint family therapy*. Science and Behaviour, Palo Alto, CA. (A classic text, particularly on communication.)

Skynner, A. C. R. (1976). *One flesh, separate persons. Principles of family and marital psychotherapy*. Constable, London. (An erudite account by a British pioneer of family therapy which attempts to integrate different approaches.)

11

Child psychotherapy

SULA WOLFF

In this chapter, Sula Wolff focuses on dynamic psychotherapy involving children as patients in their own right. This chapter is best read in conjunction with Chapter 10 on family therapy. In the first section she provides an account of the development of child psychotherapy and gives special attention to the contributions of Anna Freud, Melanie Klein, Virginia Axline, and Donald Winnicott. The main section of the chapter then follows—a description of practical aspects of therapy and the various therapeutic tasks involved; these include the role of the therapist, her relationship with the child's parents, the first interview, and termination. The indications and contra-indications for this type of treatment are also covered. Consideration is then given to research on outcome, and the chapter ends with an account of requirements for training.

When children are referred for psychiatric treatment, the approach is a dual one: to view the child in his own right and also as a member of a family, school, and community. Whatever the problem and intervention, the clinician is responsible to parents or other caregivers and, at times, especially if a teacher identifies the difficulty, to the school. But it is essential also to see children as developing individuals in their own right and, whatever their circumstances, to accept responsibility for their future. This may mean that, to ensure a child's best possible development, change must be brought about in the home or school environment. To this extent, the clinician becomes the child's ally and advocate, quite apart from any other therapeutic role.

The psychotherapies in child and adolescent psychiatry have multiplied over the years, and no single chapter can do justice to them all. This chapter will focus on individual child psychotherapy, including play therapy, based on psychodynamic principles. The reasons are twofold. First, individual child psychotherapy is still a common form of treatment in practice; and secondly, its principles inform all professional encounters with disturbed children.

Whenever a child is the referred patient and whatever the main treatment approach (whether behavioural psychotherapy, cognitive therapy, remedial education, family therapy, group or individual psychotherapy, or medication), communications with children should be such that: (1) they understand what is being conveyed to them; and (2) they benefit in the sense of feeling better and gaining developmentally. Such communications are based on the general principles of psychodynamic child psychotherapy which clearly have something to offer to all professionals who look after disturbed children, whether they be doctors, nurses, social workers, teachers, psychologists, or other therapists. And a psychodynamic framework, the foundation for therapeutic communications, continues to be indispensable in the formulation of children's psychological problems whatever the subsequent treatment (Shapiro and Esman 1992).

CHANGING CHILDHOOD ADVERSITIES AND TREATMENT METHODS

Major changes have taken place in the types of problems brought to therapeutic attention and in the range of professional services which provide treatment for young people. More and more children are identified as traumatized as a result of physical or sexual abuse, family breakdown, or major disasters. These may be family disasters as when one parent attacks or murders another, or public disasters resulting, for example, from fire, shipwreck, or war. And increasing numbers of children are referred to social, medical, and educational services with emotional and behavioural disorders due to neglect or deprivation of adequate parental care (Callias *et al.* 1992).

A second striking change has been the development over the past 40 years of multiple treatment methods in child and adolescent psychiatry (Shapiro and Esman 1992). In the early years of the child guidance movement efforts were largely limited to once-weekly individual therapy for the child using methods derived from psychoanalysis and from client-centred (Rogerian), non-directive, therapy, together with social casework for parents. Analytic, non-directive, and activity-based methods of group psychotherapy for children (e.g. Foulkes and Anthony 1957), and at times for parents, were an occasional later addition, and are currently often used for children and adolescents with shared traumatic experiences such as sexual abuse. Behaviour modification techniques began to play an increasing part from the 1950s onwards (Herbert 1994) and the family therapies, originating at around the same time, flowered in the 1970s (Gorell Barnes 1994) and remain popular with therapists. Family approaches, including those using behavioural methods, are described in Chapter 10.

Much effort has always been invested in treating parents with the expectation that children benefit indirectly. Parent training has been imaginatively developed, for example, in helping parents to apply behavioural principles to cope with their children's conduct disorders (Bank *et al.* 1991; Callias 1994); and to teach parents to control their toddlers less coercively and more effectively, using a one-way screen and immediate therapist feedback and encouragement.

In the 1980s, cognitive therapy began to be used both for adults and children (Petti 1991) and cognitive therapies, individually tailored to the child's inner preoccupations, are now effectively applied in childhood depression and anxiety states (Kendall and Lochman 1994).

'Consultation work' with other professionals, an increasing commitment of most clinicians in child psychiatry, is based on the idea that other people caring for children, such as teachers, nurses, and child-care staff can, with help, increase their understanding of disturbed children and their parents, and improve their own treatment skills.

It must be said, however, that the scientific basis for these dramatic shifts remains insecure. We shall see that of the many different interventions used, only behavioural and cognitive methods have been adequately evaluated.

Although analytic, non-directive, and cognitive psychotherapies take note, explicitly or implicitly, of the child's inner life, of emotional and cognitive developmental levels, and of the underlying causes for a disorder, this is not so in the case of behavioural approaches. The principles underlying these treatments are precisely the same for children as for adults. In practice, behaviour therapy with children is often, and to excellent effect, undertaken by parents or teachers. It is important to stress that, as Heinicke and Strassmann (1975) point out, behaviour therapy constitutes a profound change in a child's environment. Family therapy also needs to be looked at from the viewpoint of its impact on the individual child.

The dynamic and non-directive psychotherapies involving children as patients by themselves, with which this chapter is concerned, are not in conflict with behavioural, family, or other approaches. On the contrary, different treatments are often helpfully combined either sequentially or concurrently, although different therapists may need to be involved. Despite the multiplicity of treatments for children and their families, considerable uniformity in approach prevails in different clinical centres.

THE IMPORTANCE OF ASSESSMENT

At a time when reorganization of services in many countries has made it difficult to maintain multidisciplinary teams, and disturbed children are often seen in settings without any child psychiatric involvement, the importance of assessment and diagnosis, that is, of correctly identifying the nature of a child's difficulties and their multiple and interacting causes, cannot be stressed enough. Cross referral between agencies and psychiatric liaison are essential. For example, children with early childhood autism, Asperger's syndrome, schizoid personality, severe developmental problems, and attention deficit disorders should not be treated with any 'all-purpose' psychotherapeutic or family approach. Specific interventions, beyond the scope of this chapter, are indicated. In particular, children with depression, easily overlooked, require diagnosis and specific treatment.

MODELS OF CHILD PSYCHOTHERAPY

Individual psychotherapy offered to children is usually weekly and short term (three to six months). Brief interventions are often helpful (Kolvin *et al.* 1981), especially when patients are prepared for this in advance (Frank 1974; Holmes and Urie 1975), and families are unable to commit themselves to a more intensive and open-ended contract.

The schisms between clinicians for whom the contribution of psychoanalysis to the theory and practice of psychotherapy is indispensable and those, family and behavioural therapists among them, who derogate the teachings of psychoanalysts on account of their unproven efficacy or lack of scientific foundation, remain wide. Yet it seems, especially in the practice of family therapy, that the hypotheses set up to understand family systems, the intervention strategies devised, and their apparent 'common sense', succeed because the really skilled practitioners, in fact, developed their new methods on the basis of a thorough grounding in psychodynamically oriented psychotherapy (see Will and Wrate 1985).

Newcomers are disadvantaged unless they bring to their understanding of maladaptive behaviour and of the reactive emotional and behavioural disorders of childhood, a clear grasp of their origins at different stages of life, and of defence mechanisms (A. Freud 1946*a*, 1965); of the structure of the self; of transference phenomena; and, most of all, of both cognitive and psychoanalytic findings and theories about child development (Erikson 1968; Piaget and Inhelder 1969). (For a summary of cognitive and psychosocial development in childhood see Wolff 1989.)

These topics lie beyond our remit, yet psychotherapy with children repeatedly provides powerful and poignant experiences for clinicians of the validity of both psychoanalytic and cognitive developmental theories. In particular, many children openly manifest defence mechanisms which, in adults, are totally outside conscious awareness and the animistic, pre-rational world of the under-sevens is often dramatically revealed.

The founders of child psychoanalysis: Melanie Klein and Anna Freud

Following Sigmund Freud's analysis of 'Little Hans', with the child's father as therapist and only a single encounter with the phobic 6-year-old in his father's presence (S. Freud 1909/1959), Anna Freud in Vienna, and later in London, and Melanie Klein in London developed theories and techniques for the direct psychoanalysis of children. Both believed that many child psychiatric disorders develop on the basis of unconscious neurotic conflicts and that they improve as a consequence of self-observation, self-awareness, and insight, aided by commentary of the therapist which facilitates maturation of the ego. Both held that insight does not occur without a process of 'working through'. Both also believed that in interaction with the therapist, in play and/or words, the child repeatedly displays his basic conflicts and that the interpretation of feelings, thoughts, and motives underlying such conflicts enables the child to master them and, in the process, to mature.

Klein (1961, 1963) was the first to equip a play-room with small, non-mechanical toys, representing people, animals, cars, and trains, etc., drawing and cutting-out materials, water and sand. She took everything the child did in the sessions as a significant transference communication and saw the analyst's prime tasks as understanding and interpreting the symbolic content, or meaning of the child's play on the basis of a coherent framework of theory (both of child development and of the genesis of symptoms). At the same time, she held that the analyst must be aware of the unique life situation and idiosyncratic experiences of each child patient, while also alert to recurrent dominant anxieties, emotions, and object relations which find their symbolic expression in play. The repeated re-enactment of the child's anxiety-laden life experiences and the therapist's continuing commentary on their underlying meaning constitutes the helpful 'work' of analysis.

Anna Freud (1946*b*) took issue with Klein's view of the transference in child analysis. She saw the therapist not only as a recipient of projections but also as a real person, even an educator, for the child. Non-transference aspects of the relationship are especially important for severely deprived children and for children with 'ego-deficits', that is, children whose functioning is impaired by constitutional factors (including borderline or schizoid children). For these, the therapist assumes the role of an auxiliary ego. For all children, however, quite apart from his interpretative functions, the therapist inevitably becomes a model for identification, a provider of real gratification, and takes on the role of mediator between the child and the parents, the school, and sometimes the courts. Fatherless children, for example, may best be helped by a male therapist. Anna Freud thought that the part played by toys in therapy was overrated stressing that:

Analysis is neither abreaction, which would be associated with lay therapy nor 'corrective emotional experience' . . . It is rather the changing of the inner balance or focus to bring about that widening of consciousness which is insight into motivation. These are three different concepts of the therapeutic process. Insight does not occur without a working through process' (Sandler *et al.* 1980, p. 70).

She did not regard the psychoanalytic process as unique: ordinary, good methods of upbringing also foster children's self-observations and insight into motivation and feeling, their own, and those of their parents.

Psychoanalytically oriented psychotherapy, as we shall see, adopts basic principles and techniques derived from psychoanalysis but the experience is less intense and less protracted, and the aims are more circumscribed.

Non-directive play therapy: Virginia Axline

Axline's two volumes (1967, 1971), eloquent accounts of Carl Roger's non-directive psychotherapy applied to children, are written for teachers and other non-medical professionals as well as for psychiatrists. Axline's play therapy can be practised by teachers, social workers, and other care staff in children's homes as well as in psychiatric clinics. Children are treated individually or in groups and, an unusual feature, they can bring their friends!

Her writings are examined here because, although not new, they provide vivid examples of good practice. Her basic notion that each individual has the potential for self-realization leads to the aim in play therapy to release curative forces. Even without treating parents play therapy helps children through self-understanding to become better able to withstand adverse conditions.

While her theories of personality development and of psychopathology are anti-Freudian and relatively unclear, Axline conveys a way of interacting with children and parents which serves as a model. Her books are filled with practical examples of how to deal with common problems like the reluctant child in the waiting room, the child who wants to take toys home, physical attack by one child on another, and how to interact with disabled children.

Axline's eight principles for therapists are:

(1) the rapid creation of a warm and friendly relationship;

(2) total acceptance of the child as she is;

(3) establishing permissiveness so that the child is free to express feelings openly within the relationship;

(4) alertness to feelings expressed by the child and reflecting these back so that she gains insight;

(5) a deep respect for the child's capacity to solve her own problems if given the opportunity, and leaving the child with the responsibility for choices and for initiating change;

(6) no attempt to direct the child's behaviour or conversation—where the child leads the therapist follows;

(7) no attempt to rush treatment;

(8) setting limits only to the extent of anchoring treatment in reality and making the child aware of her responsibility.

Axline does not see regard for transference as essential and is opposed to fostering dependence or removing responsibilities from the child. Her play-room contains both small, representational toys and material for artistic creativity, and also large toys such as rockers and punchball, puppets, and dressing-up clothes. Her approach is especially commended for beginners working with disturbed children

Although entirely unself-critical and at times quixotic, Axline's writings have withstood the passage of time. But specialist therapists need to add more focused interventions to her recipe if psychiatrically-disturbed children are to be helped within a reasonable time.

Winnicott's contribution

Donald Winnicott, a psychoanalyst and paediatrician, developed his own quite original and imaginatively effective method for helping children with neurotic conflicts and their parents in the setting of a busy out-patient practice. He would ask parents to tell him about the problem, its development, and background. He would have a single, lengthy interview with the child, using his now famous 'squiggle' game as the main mode of communication. Taking turns, he and the child would draw a squiggle on a sheet of paper, get the other one to complete the picture and comment on what it might represent.

Because of his exceptional combination of gifts (together with his own original concepts): acute empathic understanding of children, serious concern, and the capacity to allow his own childhood self to participate playfully in the encounter, he often achieved more in one session than others could during prolonged treatment. Follow-up was often by telephone with the parents. Whether other less intuitive therapists can use his methods as effectively remains in doubt. While giving us ample illustrations of his approach, Winnicott (1971), himself influenced by Klein, did not establish a 'school' or training programme of his own. Yet his legacy of concepts, such as 'good enough' parenting, the facilitating environment, and the transitional object, has been very fruitful. In particular, his ideas about the child's capacity to experience an internal world, an external reality, and also an 'intermediate area of experience', that is, an area of play containing transitional objects in which the child can soothe himself and come to terms with the other two realms of experience, has been illuminating for play therapists (Coppolillo 1991).

ohn Bowlby's contribution: attachment theory

Bowlby's monumental work on attachment, separation and loss (e.g. Bowlby 1979; Holmes 1993; and for a summary see Wolff 1989) constitutes a major contribution to knowledge about child development and has had enormous impact on child-care practices and on hospital procedures. Attachment theory has also influenced treatment approaches to mothers of young children (Fonagy *et al.* 1994; Murray and Cooper 1994). Its effect on child psychotherapy has been to shift attention away from concerns with children's possible Oedipal conflicts to concerns with their primary attachments. The quality and security of these often provide a more relevant basis for understanding developmental difficulties and symptoms, especially of deprived and traumatized children, and for knowing how to intervene helpfully.

THE PROCESS OF THERAPY

Every point made in the introductory chapter applies also to children.

Qualities of the therapist: personal characteristics

Although Kolvin and his colleagues (1981), in a major research enterprise, found extraversion, assertiveness, and openness in therapists rather than empathy and warmth related to good outcome, we must remember that this finding derives from a study of group psychotherpay for children. There has been no other challenge to the three qualities deemed to be essential in psychotherapists—respect, empathy, and non-possessive warmth (Truax and Carkhuff 1967), to which Reisman (1973) added the wish to be of help. These qualities are integral to all civilized relationships between adults but are less universally cultivated by grown-ups in their approach to children. Therapists inevitably bring to their encounters with children memories of how they themselves were treated in youth. Lewis (1991) stresses the 'regressive pull' and the frequent occurrence of 'rescue fantasies' evoked by children in the counter-transference. Unless child therapists are among the fortunate few with clear early memories and unguarded about their own childhood selves, special efforts are needed not to be patronizing and educative but seriously attentive to child patients and, just as in psychotherapy with adults, to be tactful (Lewis 1991) and scrupulously to avoid value judgements. When a child shares one of his school

successes, a morale-boosting 'You must have been pleased wit'
yourself' is preferable to 'That's very good'. If the following term end
less happily, it will help the child to see the therapist invested not in hi
actual success but rather in his capacity to cope, even with set-backs

Lewis (1991) suggests that what appears to help most is a rea'
affectionate relationship with the therapist in which the child feel
understood and optimism is conveyed. Children can then 'borrow' th'
therapist's qualities to help them cope with their lives.

Qualities of the therapist: the special knowledge base for work with children

Because children are less able to describe their thoughts and feelings
accurate empathy is possible only if one can make informed guesses
about how the child at his particular stage is likely to have experience(
certain events and circumstances. This requires a working knowledg(
of cognitive, social, and emotional development in childhood (Wolf'
1989). The under-sevens, for example, tend to personalize thei'
experiences so that when a father leaves home after repeated violen'
quarrels with his wife, they often believe the quarrels must have beer
about them or that, if only their father had loved them more, he would
have stayed. If a 4-year-old is admitted to hospital after an accident,
she is likely to interpret this as punishment for some misdeed. Logica'
relationships are hard to grasp in these early years and children find i'
difficult to reason on the basis of observations. An intelligent, adopted
half-Chinese boy of seven, for example, was unhappy with his face and
disliked other children calling him 'chinky'. He knew his adoptive
parents were not his first parents. He longed for the people he had
heard so much about, who had looked after him (as foster parents)
during his first year of life. Although he could see from photographs
that they were not Chinese, he clung to his belief that *they* must have
been his 'real' parents.

We also have to be aware that timing of events and circumstances
affects both how children are likely to think and reason about their
experiences and what the emotional impact of these will be. Exposure
to prolonged group care, for example, can expand the horizons of a
12-year-old, but seriously impair a child's capacity for emotional
responsiveness if it occurs during the first three years of life. And the
accidental loss of a finger tip, for example, stressful at any age, may
have a quite disproportionate emotional impact if it occurs between
three and six years when, symbolically, the injury can represent a

etaliatory punishment for excessive competitive assertiveness or sexual experimentation.

Moreover, young children cannot give clear accounts of their life histories. It is essential to get these from their parents in order to understand the meaning and significance of what children tell one. The sudden tears of a 10-year-old recounting how his mother took his rather too destructive kitten to the vet to be put down, conveyed their full meaning only when one knew that he was the one remaining child his single, schizotypal mother now looked after. Long before his birth she had abandoned three other children, and quite recently had given up a further baby for adoption.

The first interview

Children are brought for treatment, usually by their parents, sometimes at the request of teachers, social workers, or the courts. It is adults who identify the problem. One of the therapist's initial tasks is to clarify with the child why he has come, what the problem is, and what the therapist can do to help. The first interview provides many opportunities to demonstrate a therapeutic attitude.

The therapist conveys interest in the child's own view of the encounter and makes clear her own readiness to be frank. When children are referred for stealing or soiling, for example, symptoms usually evoking angry concern in parents and teachers and shame and guilt in the child, it is helpful after an initial discussion of more neutral topics, for the therapist frankly to declare her knowledge: 'Your mother is very worried about your stealing. That must be a big worry for you too.' In a non-judgemental way the therapist conveys that she sees (i.e. quite deliberately 'reads') the aberrant behaviour as a symptom the child himself would wish not to have; that this symptom gives rise to anxiety; and has a meaning the child may not know of himself. Because the therapist is careful not to put direct questions, the child is likely to respond not with defensive denial but with a more open revelation of his feelings. If this is not possible in the first interview, the therapist can helpfully acknowledge that it may be 'too difficult' to talk about that just now.

From the start, children should be clear that the purpose of treatment is to help them understand better what may be troubling them, and that play is an important part of treatment (see also Wolff 1992).

The role of the therapist

The most distinctive features of child psychotherapy are th relationship between therapist and child and the modes o communication between them. These features spring from the child' immaturity and actual dependence on adults. Anna Freud (Sandler *e al.* 1980) thought children were more difficult to analyse because o their intolerance of anxiety and frustration, their preference for actio over words, their inability to engage in 'free association', and th 'inavoidable intrusion of parents'!

(1) *Transference*

Although Klein (1963, 1961) held that the transference in chil psychoanalysis was equivalent to that of adult patients, Anna Freuc (1946*b*) stressed two clear distinctions (Sandler *et al.* 1980). These ar important also for psychotherapy. First, when children interact with their therapist as they would with their parents, projecting feelings on to the therapist and expecting specific responses in turn, the parents are in the present and not the past. The patient is not interacting with others 'as if' he were under the control of powerful parents; he is actually still a child. While in treatment children certainly have the experience that other adults can be different from their parents; they cannot, as adult patients can, put their parents behind them. Secondly, the therapist, however neutral, is always a real adult person in the life of the child and to that extent both nurturing and educative. He becomes both an auxiliary ego, helping the child to cope and to mature, as well as an alternative role model.

(2) *Setting limits*

It is an error to think that children benefit from releasing aggression as if there were a certain amount which had to be let out. In fact when this happens children often become very anxious, terrified of their own power and its possible dangers. As in adult therapy, children are encouraged to reveal their feelings (in words and in play) with no limits on content and form. The intervention is to help children understand, tolerate, and master their feelings, not to enact them in reality. But, when occasionally children do become wild and possibly destructive, the therapist scrupulously avoids the common adult to child prohibition: 'Don't do that', a response most likely to result in non-compliance with loss of face for both child and therapist. Instead, while welcoming the child's expression of feelings and wishes, the therapist assumes full responsibility for the maintenance of safety without conveying that more self-control is expected than the child can manage. The message is 'I won't let you hurt yourself or me, or damage the room . . . If you feel so angry that you can't control yourself, I will help to make sure no harm is done.' Often simple comments on the child's feelings and acknowledging their validity is enough to prevent their enactment. Sometimes, the therapist has to step in more actively, even holding a child on her lap, until control has been regained. This is anxiety-reducing: it relieves the child of responsibility and guilt without inducing shame. It also presents a model of non-hostile control.

(3) The therapist's relationship with the parents

Therapists are accountable both to the children they treat and to parents. Moreover, the child's attendance depends on the parents' willingness to come as much as (sometimes more than) on the child's. Therapists are also dependent on parents for essential information. And, finally, if the child is to change, the parents must be able to tolerate this. If we help an inhibited, phobic girl to become more openly assertive, negativistic, and questioning, we must be sure that her parents can put up with such behaviour. It can be helpful, in the child's presence, to ask the parents whether their daughter can ever get angry with them; to suggest, if this never occurs, that the symptom may be an expression of 'bottled-up' feelings; and that an important stage in the treatment is for the child to become more awkward and oppositional with her mother and father. Many parents declare themselves willing to accept this, while a few are adamant that they could never tolerate 'cheek'. Whatever the response, the parents' real attitudes can then be acknowledged by child and therapist in treatment. Most parents require support and many quite active treatment while their child is in therapy. Often, especially when the presenting problem indicates open conflict and mutual hostility between parents and child, a period of psychotherapy for child and parents separately and with different therapists can helpfully precede family interviews.

The emotional and behavioural difficulties of children often, but by no means always, arise from family conflict and parental personality disturbance, and they fulfil a function within the network of family transactions. A constipated 3-year-old boy, for example, ate poorly and woke up each night crying for his mother. She, grossly overweight,

would regularly rise to make a midnight feast of 'hot chocolate' for
herself and him. She always went to bed early in anticipation of her
toddler's demands, frustrating her husband's needs for sex and
affection. She justified this pattern to herself in terms of not wanting
to wake her hard-working husband. But she was also clear that
although she wished it were otherwise, ever since her son's birth she
had been unable to face having intercourse. Her husband resented his
son but passively accepted the situation, remembering the violence he
had witnessed between his own parents as a child, which he wanted at
all costs to avoid in his own family.

A fine judgement is always needed about the most appropriate
treatment method and, in particular, whether the initial approach
should involve the family as a whole or whether, if the child's
intrapsychic disturbance and his needs require this, the parents can
tolerate and support a period of individual psychotherapy for the
child. Ornstein (1994) advocates 'child-centred family treatment'
consisting of three stages: a diagnostic family interview; individual
assessment, including psychotherapeutic assessment of the child; and
'integrative' family sessions in which the meaning underlying the
child's manifest behaviour is 'translated' for the family.

(4) *Frankness and confidentiality*

In general, as with adults, the therapist approaches children with
genuineness and frankness, demonstrating that important matters
affecting them can be talked about without fear. But one must always
remember the child's cognitive level and what aspects of an event are
likely to make the biggest impact. The aim is not to have children
understand the details of a life event but to declare the topic open and
to help them express their own thoughts and feelings about the
experience. This is especially important when there is a possible family
secret surrounding, for example, a child's adoption, the loss and
replacement of a mother in early childhood, or a father's
imprisonment. Children are often aware of these events but dare not
reveal their knowledge for fear of upsetting their parents. The
therapist must be absolutely clear about what the parents have told
the child, and he may need to help parents towards greater frankness.
Some parents are adamant that secrecy must prevail and this does not
close the door to treatment. But, once children reveal what they know
in the course of treatment and are helped to convey this to their
parents, parental attitudes are likely to change.

Yet the requirement of frankness is less than absolute. When a mother reveals in private that she is the only one who knows that her 12-year old boy is not her husband's son, is it necessarily helpful to press her now, as a prerequisite of treatment, to face her unsuspecting family with this shattering news? When the alcoholic father of a backward 8-year-old in foster care kills his alcoholic wife and is imprisoned for murder, does it help to present the facts to the boy against the wishes of the foster parents, except in terms of an 'accident' caused by drink, in which his mother died and for which his father was held responsible, although he tried (as indeed he did too late) to get help?

A major difficulty in maintaining confidentiality has arisen with increasing recognition of child sexual abuse and pressure to apply criminal as well as child care law. Glaser (1991), in her review of treatment in sexual abuse, stresses the contribution of individual psychotherapy for affected children but suggests that full confidentiality can rarely be maintained. Affected children need help to understand from the start that the therapist cannot guarantee privacy and that their disclosures may be revealed in a court of law.

Apart from legal constraints and the rare and shocking circumstances referred to above, a quality of frankness between therapist and child should be preserved.

As in adults, therapy with the child is private. The products of play remain in the room which parents or other concerned people, such as the child's social worker, should not as a matter of course, enter. Nor are the child's communications revealed to others, except when the child demands this or the therapist thinks it will be helpful and the child agrees. Evidence of battle scenes in the sand-tray and of paint on hands and paper remain part of the evanescent fantasy shared by child and therapist, clearly separated from the outside world.

Returning the child to the family

In contrast to the treatment of adults, child therapy ends by returning the child not to his own care alone but to that of the parents. The therapist aims not only to have children look at themselves more squarely but to promote a more courageously open relationship between children and parents which can better meet their emotional needs as they grow up. Parents must thus come to understand their child better. Indeed, many bring their child for treatment for this purpose. When the parents' personalities are essentially healthy, the therapist can often, after a period of treatment with the child, act as a mediator enabling the child to have his say in joint interviews with parents. Such encounters should occur only with the child's agreement and when the therapist is confident the parents can tolerate the communications.

THE TASKS OF DYNAMIC CHILD PSYCHOTHERAPY

The following publications contain good advice for the novice: Axline (1967, 1971), Reisman (1973), Adams (1982), Lewis (1991), Coppolillo (1991), Jennings (1993), and Schaefer and Cangelosi (1993).

General principles and aims

Basic to child as to adult dynamic psychotherapy is the idea that repetitive maladaptive behaviour and psychogenic symptoms are expressions of thoughts and emotions outside the patient's awareness. Because the experiences are in conflict either with the child's conscience or aspirations (super-ego or ego-ideal) or with real demands of parents, they are repressed (i.e. kept out of conscious awareness) by a range of defence mechanisms.

A primary aim is to create a relationship in which the child will feel so secure that defensive manoeuvres can be abandoned and inner thoughts and feelings faced squarely, however dangerous or foolish they may seem. It is the therapist's job to help children like themselves and their inner lives better. The validation of the child's thoughts and feelings through the idea that any child of his age, who has had those particular experiences, would have reacted similarly, will help children to feel better. Self-esteem is raised and anxiety lessened. Many repressed thoughts and feelings stem, even in childhood, from the past when the child was cognitively less mature than now. And to recognize this also brings relief. Whether the crucial feature of child psychotherapy is the therapeutic relationship or the therapeutic transaction remains an open question (Rosenfeld *et al.* 1994).

The importance of the child's actual environment

It is increasingly recognized that clear-cut childhood neuroses are rare and that many children suffer as a consequence of neglect, physical or sexual abuse, inadequate opportunities for development, and unavailable or inconsistent parenting. Interpretations alone do not help such children. They need developmental help in the form of both interpretation and support (Alvarez 1991*a*). For such children the therapeutic experience is 'corrective' of past misperceptions and misinterpretations, and also represents an 'oasis' in their lives, with temporary relief and distance from their real, external world of turmoil and conflict (Lewis 1991). Often it is also necessary, with the help of colleagues in social work or education, to modify the child's circumstances.

Elizabeth Newson (1992) has made a case for avoiding interpretations altogether in the treatment of very deprived children, making no demands, and giving them instead an experience of mastery and of being in control; such children should have their therapist's total attention during regular, predictable sessions.

When children experience real conflict, because of excessive parental demands or because parents are intolerant of normal child-like modes of being, the therapist must strive, with his colleagues to promote change in parents. When constitutionally healthy parents are themselves under excessive pressure or suffer from psychiatric disorders, such as depression or personality difficulties, which interfere with the upbringing of their children, practical help or psychiatric interventions focusing on their own needs can lead to a shift in their reactions to their children. Often, interventions for parents using behavioural, cognitive, or family therapy techniques, outside the scope of this chapter, are helpful.

When parents are absent or unable to change (e.g. if they are psychotic, brain-damaged, or have schizoid, schizotypal, borderline, or antisocial personality disorders), auxiliary parental care, such as a residential school, may have to be sought for the child.

Four basic tasks

The therapist's tasks are to:

— facilitate the creation of a non-critical and secure relationship with children;

— help them express freely their inner thoughts and feelings;

— understand the underlying meaning of their communications; and

— reflect this meaning back to the children.

Care is needed in implementing the last, important task when children lack real security in their lives. An 8-year-old who has lost two parents

and whose temporary foster placement is about to break down wil
benefit from reflecting back to him feelings he expresses. However, h
may not be able to face his repressed fury and underlying grief unti
new parent figures have made a permanent commitment. He needs al
the defences he can muster even if, to preserve a cheery front, he has to
soil or steal. Once new security has been found, interpretativ
treatment can begin.

(1) *Creating a therapeutic relationship*

The principles of non-critical acceptance and a friendly but non
intrusive approach apply as in adult psychotherapy. But with childrer
one has to explain more and question less, aware of children':
disadvantage in relation to adults: they know less in general terms
their understanding is different and they are socially less skilled.

Questions demand answers and children may not know or ma}
think they do not know what to say. It is better to turn a question into
a statement. The child is then free to take or leave it (e.g. 'I was
wondering if your mother knew how you felt' or 'That must have beer
quite upsetting for you'). If the child is too anxious to reply, the
ensuing silence is not a mark of either failure or non-compliance.

Children should never be 'put on the spot' by questioning them
about matters the therapist already knows about, especially if they are
likely to react defensively, for example, about stealing. The therapist
should frankly say what he knows in such a way that the child need
feel no shame (e.g. 'Stealing is a very common problem in childhood. I
know it has been a problem for you too.') Children should always be
helped to avoid lying in treatment.

Adams (1982, p. 107) is clear about the need to explain to children
the purpose, aims, and process of treatment. '. . . a general or
permanent stance of non-direction . . . will turn off most children',
who interpret it as meanness. The therapist should feel free to share all
information he has had from parents with the child, but tell them
nothing about the child except with his knowledge and agreement, and
preferably in his presence. This has the additional advantage of
modelling for parents how children can be helped to say what is on
their minds.

As a symbolic expression of the therapist's wish to understand the
child seriously at her level, she always sits at the same height. Even
small children, if busy at a table or participating in a family meeting,
sit on adult chairs, while the therapist sits on a small chair when the
child, sitting or standing, is at the sand-tray.

Although child therapists should be more communicative and more giving, even, for example, sending postcards during holidays or after the end of treatment, they should, at least until treatment has been completed and just as in psychotherapy with adults, guard against revelations about their personal lives. Of course, if asked one can explain that one does not actually sleep in the clinic. But it does not help to reveal facts about one's family. All too readily this becomes a standard for hurtful comparisons with the child's family. Children should be free to imagine the therapist's family in any way they chose, and such communications should be treated strictly as transference phenomena.

(2) *Helping children express their thoughts and feelings*

This requires opportunities for children to communicate through play with small representational toys and creative activities (drawing, painting, modelling, puppet play). Enquiries about their earliest memories, their three magic wishes if anything could be granted to them, what they want to be when grown up, and what their dreams are about, all encourage children to convey their fantasy lives. They are also helped when their therapists try to determined what thoughts and feelings their drawing or play conveys to him and what might be on their minds.

For example: 7-year-old John was brought to the clinic because of aggressive attacks on his mother. She had a mild schizophrenic defect state and he recalled vividly her delusions, involving him, when he was 3 years old. He was repeatedly asking her for money to buy sweets and ice cream, and at night his hard-working and worried father was always angry with him.

In the first session John drew a 'fight' between a large and confident looking 'woodpecker' and a small, misshapen dog. When asked who would win, he paused and said: 'the woodpecker, because it's bigger'. When asked who he thought should win, John replied 'the dog'. His therapist then commented that she guessed he really wanted his mother to win over him and that he probably felt quite bad when she did not. John explained at length how he always asked his mother for money and how she always gave it to him. When asked what she *should* do, he replied: 'Not give it to me.' 'My ma's going to buy me a piano', he went on to say, and this seemed to make him uneasy.

Different techniques are needed for children of different ages. Toddlers often feel most at home, at least initially, with a sand-tray equipped with animals and 'people' of different kinds, and with water.

Children in middle childhood express themselves well with crayons, paint, and plasticine and through more structured make-believe play (e.g. a doll's house). Even at this stage children often need to regress to more infantile play in order to express less differentiated thoughts and feelings; play and paperwork are also helpful in mediating therapeutic conversations. Older children and adolescents may prefer to talk merely using clay, plasticine, or drawing as accompanying activities. Patient and therapist going for a stroll can also be of help for older inhibited children.

Jigsaws and board or card games are less helpful, except for extremely inhibited youngsters. They permit little expression of fantasy and, because interesting in themselves, they often divert patient and therapist from their tasks.

(c) *Understanding the underlying meaning of children's communication*

Comments on the underlying meaning of children's communications encourage further communication so that these two processes are intimately linked. When John, for instance, referred to the piano his therapist thought this meant that his mother would give him anything he asked for, however big, rather than that a real piano was about to be purchased.

Guesses about certain universal connections in childhood are often appropriate, for example, that fear of the destructive effect of one's impulses leads one to be more rather than less aggressive in an attempt to reassure oneself that nothing really bad can happen; or that phobic anxiety when parents go out—in case an accident should befall them—often stands for feelings of anger towards those very parents which the child, usually for good reason, is too fearful to face.

(d) *Interpretations*

The reflections to John of the underlying meaning of his communication went beyond a commentary on how he felt. It was already a form of interpretation.

In contrast to classical psychoanalysis, it is important in psychoanalytically oriented, brief psychotherapy that interpretations should be framed in such a way that they enhance children's positive feelings about themselves (their self-esteem) and are ego-building but, at the same time, just as in psychoanalysis, they foster insight and the giving up of inhibiting defences. When an 11-year-old with anorexia nervosa reports that she dreamt it was kinder to eat vegetables rather than people, it is inappropriate to point out her cannibalistic impulses.

t is more helpful to focus on her defence of reaction formation: to tress her wish to be kind, her discomfort when she is angry, and her preference to eat nothing at all rather than risk hurting anyone. When, n time, she reveals her frustration at her mother's restrictiveness, a comment indicating that such feelings are universal in children of her age is likely both to give relief and to encourage further expressions of previously suppressed or repressed emotions.

Interpretations are now thought by some practitioners to be more helpful when they focus on the here and now than on the past (Lewis 991; Alvarez 1991*a*). In contrast to the impression gained by the naïve reader of much of the psychoanalytic literature, interpretations should be a comforting 'corrective experience' and not an 'unmasking' device (Adams 1982). Alvarez (1991*a*) also stresses the need to avoid reductionist interpretations of fantasies in terms of defences against the pain of loss or absence, especially in the case of deprived, abused, or depressed children. Instead, she advocates the positive evaluation even of boastful fantasies and lies, in terms of their expressions of hope for the future. She suggests that therapists focus not only on the present and the past but help children in their search for new views of their future.

Two feelings central to unconscious conflicts in adults and children with neurotic disorders are anger and sexual longing. In child psychotherapy Adams (1982) helpfully suggested focusing first on anger. Adult sexual preoccupations can confuse and seduce children and foster excessive dependency, misplaced when treatment is time-limited. This does not mean that one should disregard children's unsatisfied sexual curiosities. Therapists can often be helpful mediators, enabling parents to enlighten their children. This increases intimacy between child and parents and often promotes the child's status with other children.

Interpretations of the transference play an important part. A comment to a silent child that it is difficult to talk to a person one barely knows, opens up the relationship between child and therapist as a topic for discussion. Once familiar with the treatment setting, aggressive pre-school and early school-aged children often become extremely hostile towards their therapist. They may project on to her feelings for an impulsive and physically punitive parent and their fears of their own destructiveness. The therapist repeatedly provides a corrective experience by taking full responsibility for kindly and non-threatening control, by relating the child's present behaviour to his experiences outside the treatment setting, and by focusing on feelings of affection as well as on anger and disappointment. Even a father violent in drink usually loves his children and does not intend to cause harm. Much aggression in childhood is a means of testing the strength of parental affection: how bad can one be without being rejected?

At termination, an awareness of the meaning to the child of the end of the relationship, in the light of his experiences of the loss of other important people, can help to end therapy positively. Disguised disappointment and anger have to be acknowledged. A consolation is that there will be mutual remembrance: people do not disappear from one's mind. And follow-up postcards are allowed.

Perhaps the most important goal of interpretations is to reduce anxiety by fostering a more mature view of the world. Neurotic symptoms, even in adults, tend to have their origins in those stages of childhood when thinking is still pre-causal and animistic (Piaget and Inhelder 1969) and when, unless care is taken to explain things to children in a child-centred way they can understand (Donaldson 1978), anxiety-inducing misperceptions and misconceptions are rampant. In particular, the distinction between thoughts and wishes on the one hand and actions and consequences on the other is often blurred. Child therapists need to stress repeatedly that murder and bloodshed in the sandpit have no consequences in real life and that thoughts and words, however bad, carry no risk.

In treating adolescents, Swift and Wonderlich (1990) suggest prompt interpretation of negative transference reactions but wariness about commenting on positive transference, so as to avoid idealization of the therapist. Conscious links should be made before unconscious ones, and no interpretation should be longer than seven words!

Interpretations are never made with certitude, as if the therapist knows best, but rather as tentative offerings. It is up to the child to see whether they fit.

Matching therapeutic resources to the child's needs: duration of treatment

Much individual child psychotherapy is once-weekly except when children are so ill or disturbed that they need to be treated in hospital. Short-term treatment can be sustained more easily by parents, is more economical, has on the whole proved effective (see Kolvin *et al.* 1981), and can be carried out without change of therapist by trainees of different disciplines under supervision. This is the most common form of child psychotherapy despite the fact that more frequent and more long-term treatment may be more effective (Heinicke and Strassman 1975; Wright et al. 1976).

(1) Brief, dynamic psychotherapy is focused

All brief treatments have a focus, based on a full assessment, including aetiology and underlying psychopathology, and the psychiatric status of the parents. The emergent formulation of the child's conflicts is open to revision in the light of subsequent information, but it helps to keep the primary aims of treatment in mind throughout. These aims may be to reduce the anxiety of a sleepless toddler about the possible destructive effects of his angry impulses on the parents; or to counteract the self-doubts of an over-compliant 6-year-old who steals from her step-mother for fear of being openly assertive, in case she is once more rejected; or to help a 12-year-old girl with school phobia to see that her angry, oppositional impulses could not possibly have caused her widowed mother's depression.

Psychotherapists are now less ambitious in their goals (Shapiro and Esman 1992), prepared, especially with adolescents, to accept more limited results. This is in the knowledge that symptomatic improvement can be growth-enhancing by evoking more positive responses from others which in turn reinforce self-esteem.

(2) The role of long-term supportive psychotherapy

When children have physical or educational disabilities, or a constitutional impairment, as in the case of hyperkinetic or schizoid/Asperger disorders, they are likely to experience chronic stress. A more long-term, if less frequent, contact with a clinician (unlikely to move on) can be helpful both for child and parents. Older children burdened by deficiencies within their own families, for example, having a psychotic mother or being the only child in a one-parent family, are greatly helped in their development by knowing that their therapist identifies with their needs and future plans, and will be available long term. This is so even when, following a short intensive period of treatment, sessions occur only a few times a year.

Indications

Amid the wealth of treatments available and in the absence of research-based knowledge about which treatment works best for which conditions under what circumstances, choice of treatment may seem arbitrary.

There is agreement, however, that psychodynamic psychotherapy is suitable for reactive rather than constitutionally based disorders. If emotional or behavioural symptoms are likely to respond to environmental change alone, such as a shift in family interaction or in teachers' approaches, then family therapy or teacher consultation may be the intervention of choice.

If the disorder is more deep-seated, the result of past traumatic experience and has led to maladaptive use of defences and developmental arrest, especially when the picture is that of a neurosis, individual psychotherapy is indicated, quite apart from other treatment (e.g. family therapy, parent or teacher counselling, behaviour modification, antidepressants) that may also be necessary.

Contra-indications to exploratory psychotherapy: approaches to children with 'ego-deficits' or schizoid/Asperger disorders, and autism

Psychoanalysts regularly treat children with 'borderline' states whose defensive structure is abnormal. Such children have also been described as having Asperger's syndrome or schizoid or schizotypal personality disorders (Wolff 1991). Psychoanalysts previously held that in the treatment of these children defences needed strengthening rather than to be interpreted in order to avoid fantasy and anxiety from escalating uncontrollably (see, for example, Rosenfeld and Sprince 1965). Many child analysts no longer believe this, and use easily comprehensible interpretations for such patients (Alvarez 1991*b*). But this occurs within the setting of frequent sessions, even daily, continued for years.

Psychotherapists need to be absolutely clear about diagnosis before embarking on short-term dynamic psychotherapy. The latter helps many children who are constitutionally healthy, have normal defences and suffer from neurotic, emotional, or conduct disorders. It can be harmful for those with schizoid/Asperger disorders and for some brain-damaged children. Interpretations can further impair already limited capacities to distinguish fantasy from reality, increase a propensity for paranoid projection, and lead to frightening and explosive losses of impulse control.

This approach is ineffective for autistic children, as well as inappropriate, because expectations will be aroused in parents that cannot be fulfilled. Autistic children and their families need a different approach (see Howlin and Rutter 1987).

Constitutionally impaired children respond better to supportive, non-intrusive methods which take the chronicity of their condition into account. Greater tolerance by the school and family can help such children towards better social and educational adjustment. Parents are enlisted as allies in treatment and informed clearly that they are in no way responsible for their child's difficulties; thus, the burden of having a difficult child is not compounded by misplaced guilt.

Psychotherapy for severely deprived children

Psychoanalysts used to believe that children without a permanent home, (i.e. those lacking basic security), should not be exposed to interpretative therapy. However, foster parents and child-care workers often seek treatment for the seriously deprived in their care because they worry about these children's level of aggression, withdrawn behaviour, or unusual sexual activity.

Attempts to help traumatized children in care cope better in whatever homes they have, or to prepare them for a permanent new home by means of intensive and long-term analytic psychotherapy have been described (Boston and Szur 1982). These authors help the reader to grasp the extreme difficulties faced by such children and their therapists, but there has been no attempt to evaluate outcome. It is clear, however, that only experienced therapists, able to treat the child for several years, should attempt such interventions (see also Newson 1992, for an alternative approach to such children).

OUTCOME

Kolvin *et al.* (1981) in their evaluative study of psychological treatments for disturbed children, dispel the gloom induced by previous research (Levitt 1963) that outcome is no different from no treatment at all. Many of the apparently treated children in these early studies had received psychiatric care but not psychotherapy, and the baseline of success derived from untreated children, many of whom had developmental disorders where the spontaneous improvement rate was much higher than that of other clinic attenders.

However, reviews make clear that the good results of most acceptable outcome studies, including Kolvin's own, cannot be generalized to ordinary clinical practice. It may come as a surprise that most good outcome studies (see Kazdin *et al.* 1990; Weisz and Weiss 1993), perhaps because of ethical difficulties in random allocation to treatment and non-treatment or waiting list control groups, recruited for study non-referred disturbed children from within schools. Treatment tended to be group-based rather than individual; relied more on behavioural and cognitive methods than on the psychodynamic, eclectic, and family-oriented approaches most often used in practice; was brief (8–10 weeks) rather than extended (27–55 weeks); de-emphasized parent and family involvement, and also consultation with teachers. Moreover, therapists often were specially trained and supervised to carry out the treatment being evaluated, under conditions quite unlike those of a busy clinic.

Kazdin *et al.* (1990) in their review of over 200 studies found that behavioural and cognitive methods were effective, improvement continuing beyond the end of treatment. Efficacy of other commonly used methods has been much less adequately studied. Barrnett *et al.* (1991) reviewed 43 studies of non-behavioural psychotherapy, in which treated children were compared with a control group. Since these studies were all methodologically flawed, the writers conclude that past notions of ineffectiveness are invalid but equally, there is no clear evidence that non-behavioural treatment works. Weisz and Weiss (1993) too, in their summary of meta-analyses, conclude that cognitive and behavioural treatments are effective because they have been adequately studied. Up to now, psychodynamic psychotherapy, family therapy, and eclectic methods have been rarely and inadequately researched. In an interesting meta-analysis of the efficacy of non-behavioural psychotherapy (Weisz *et al.* 1987), better outcomes correlated with better research methodology (Shirk and Russell 1992), suggesting that child psychotherapy may yet prove to be effective.

There are exceptions to the dearth of good outcome studies in non-behavioural child psychotherapy. Fonagy and his colleagues have analysed the records of the Anna Freud Centre in London to arrive at predictors for the efficacy of child psychoanalysis (Fonagy and Target 1994; Target and Fonagy 1994). Their findings are, perhaps not surprisingly, that improvement rates were higher for children with emotional rather than disruptive disorders; and for younger rather than older children, especially when given intensive (i.e. four or five times weekly) treatment. Moran *et al.* (1991), in a well-controlled study showed that a brief psychoanalytic approach, together with parent counselling, helped significantly to stabilize the control of children's 'brittle', that is, poorly controlled, diabetes. Remarkably in this study, as in the controlled trial of family therapy for asthmatic children (Lask and Matthes 1979), objective indices of physical status were applied as outcome measures.

The field of child psychotherapy is clearly wide open for imaginative, well-controlled outcome studies.

TRAINING

As for other forms of psychotherapy, training in dynamic child psychotherapy has three components: (1) acquiring a knowledge base—and about this no more will be said here; (2) supervised clinical practice; and (3) a personal therapeutic experience.

In the past only specialized institutes offered intensive postgraduate courses as well as case supervision for trainees in child psychotherapy, while they simultaneously underwent a personal analysis. Other institutions, including universities, have began to provide such experiences. Fully trained child psychotherapists are few in number and usually work in psychiatric settings within a health service or in special residential schools and other child-care agencies (Callias *et al.* 1992). Here they apply their skills not only in direct treatment but as consultants to other professionals responsible for the treatment, care, or education of disturbed children.

Most therapists acquire skills during their training in departments of child and adolescent psychiatry. In fact, many trainees in adult psychiatry value these attachments because of the available training in methods of psychological treatment for children, parents, and families. Some departments, however, are so committed to family therapy that children are rarely seen individually, even for an initial interview, or so keen to apply cognitive or behavioural methods, that trainees have little chance to acquire skills in individual dynamic psychotherapy. This robs newcomers of the opportunity to learn how to communicate therapeutically with children; and without this skill, their efficacy even as family or cognitive therapists is likely to be impaired. All child psychiatry clinics and departments, whatever their orientation, should ensure that trainees from relevant disciplines (psychiatrists, social workers, psychologists, nurses, and occupational therapists) obtain experience of how to assess and treat children individually.

Supervision may take place in three settings: in regular meetings of trainee and supervisor (often the consultant, sometimes a trained child psychotherapist); in weekly or twice-weekly multidisciplinary meetings; and in special child psychotherapy groups or workshops.

During regular, preferably weekly, *individual sessions* the consultant orients the trainee to the work and plans his experience in the light of training needs. Opportunities exist for regular, detailed discussion of the treatment of only a few patients but this helps trainees in treating other children too, whose progress and management is attended to more briefly. The merit of individual supervision is that, without in any way encroaching on the trainee's privacy, revelations can be made that are salient for the treatment of children and which are rarely possible in a team or workshop. One trainee, for example, a single mother, was able to discuss her initial hesitancy during the first interview with a boy who was the only child of an unmarried mother. Another trainee, himself deprived of mothering in childhood, was able to see this not as a disadvantage (as it might be in relation to his colleagues), but as helping him to understand similarly deprived children better.

During *multidisciplinary team meetings* the focus on individual child psychotherapy depends on the team itself: whether its composition is stable and whether concerns exist other than the care of patients, relating, for example, to interprofessional collaboration or to work overload. Management decisions inevitably take priority and difficult cases inordinate time. But it is enjoyable and makes for cohesion if individual psychotherapy with children can feature regularly. Most important, it is more illuminating to discuss a child's psychotherapy in a meeting attended by both the child's and the parents' therapists, so that a complete picture is drawn.

Group workshops provide a forum for discussion between members from different disciplines but with the advantage of less pressure than in team meetings from urgent management, personal, or team problems. The workshop can focus on the therapeutic process at a more leisurely pace. If the group is cohesive and stable, personal revelations relevant to treatment enhance interest, enjoyment, and mutual understanding. Workshops also offer opportunities for reading and discussion of the literature, and for formal case or topic presentations.

It is extremely helpful through video- and audio-recording to note other therapists at work, and salutary to hear or view oneself. The benefit of objectifying performance must be set against time taken and on the encroachment on free-floating discussion.

CONCLUSION

The principles of psychotherapy for children are the same as for adults. But the framework differs because of the centrality of personality development in childhood and because children are dependent on their parents and on a network of other adults responsible for their education and care. The rewards are exceptional. Although the notion that early intervention prevents later mental ill health or delinquency is still open to proof, opportunities to reduce severity and duration of childrens' distress are considerable, as is the chance to exert a benign influence on their lives and those of their families.

REFERENCES

Adams, P. L. (1982). *A primer of child psychotherapy*, (2nd edn). Little, Brown, Boston.

Alvarez, A. (1991*a*). Wildest dreams: aspiration, identification and symbol-formation in depressed children. *Psychoanalytic Psychotherapy*, **5**, 177–89.

Alvarez, A. (1991*b*). Workshop—the psychotherapist and the borderline and psychotic child: a developmental view of defence. In Occasional Papers No. 6, *Psychotherapy—Pure and applied*, (ed. S. Ramsden), pp. 18–19. Association for Child Psychology and Psychiatry, London.

Axline, V. M. (1969). *Play therapy*, pp. 73–7. Ballantine, New York.

Axline, V. M. (1971). *Dibs in search of self*. Penguin, London.

Bank, L., Marlowe, J. H., Reid, J. B., Patterson, G. R., and Weinrott, M. R. (1991). A comparative evaluation of parent-training interventions for families of chronic delinquents. *Journal of Abnormal Child Psychology*, **19**, 15–33.

Barrnett, R. J., Docherty, J. P., and Frommelt, G. M. (1991). A review of child psychotherapy research since 1963. *Journal of the American Academy of Child and Adolescent Psychiatry*, **30**, 1–14.

Boston, M. and Szur, R. (ed.) (1983). *Psychotherapy with severely deprived children*. Routledge, London.

Bowlby, J. (1979). *The making and breaking of affectional bonds*. Tavistock, London.

Callias, M. (1994). Parent training. In *Child and adolescent psychiatry: modern approaches* (3rd edn), (ed. M. Rutter, E. Taylor, and L. Hersov), pp. 918–35. Blackwell, Oxford.

Callias, M., Miller, A., Lane, D. A., and Llanyado, M. (1992). Child and adolescent therapy: a changing agenda. In *Child and adolescent therapy: a handbook*, (ed. D. A. Lane and A. Miller), pp. 3–38. Open University Press, Milton Keynes.

290 *Child psychotherapy*

Coppolillo, H. P. (1991). The use of play in psychodynamic psychotherapy. In *Child and adolescent psychiatry: a comprehensive textbook*, (ed. M. Lewis), pp. 805–11. Williams & Wilkins, Baltimore.

Donaldson, M. (1978). *Children's minds*. Fontana, Glasgow.

Erikson, E. H. (1968). *Identity and the life-cycle*. Faber, London.

Fonagy, P. and Target, M. (1994). The efficacy of psychoanalysis for children with disruptive disorders. *Journal of the Academy of Child and Adolescent Psychiatry*, 33, 45–55.

Fonagy, P., Steele, M., Steele, H., Higgitt, A., and Target, M. (1994). The Emanuel Miller Memorial Lecture 1992: The theory and practice of resilience. *Journal of Child Psychology and Psychiatry*, 35, 231–57.

Foulkes, S. H. and Anthony, E. J. (1957). *Group therapy: the psychoanalytic approach*, pp. 169–88. Penguin, London.

Frank, J. D. (1974). Therapeutic components of psychotherapy: a 25-year progress report on research. *Journal of Nervous and Mental Diseases*, 159, 325–42.

Freud, A. (1946a). *The ego and the mechanisms of defence*. Hogarth, London.

Freud, A. (1946b). *The psycho-analytical treatment of children*. Imago, London.

Freud, A. (1965). *Normality and pathology in childhood: assessment of development*. Hogarth, London.

Freud, S. (1959). Analysis of a phobia in a five-year-old boy. In *Standard edition*, Vol. 3. Hogarth, London. (Originally published 1909.)

Glaser, D. (1991). Treatment issues in child sexual abuse. *British Journal of Psychiatry*, 159, 769–82.

Gorell Barnes, G. (1994). Family therapy. In *Child and adolescent psychiatry: modern approaches*, (3rd edn), (ed. M. Rutter, E. Taylor, and L. Hersov), pp. 946–67. Blackwell, Oxford.

Heinicke, C. M. and Strassmann, L. M. (1975). Toward more effective research on child psychotherapy. *Journal of the American Academy of Child Psychiatry*, 14, 561–88.

Herbert, M. (1994). Behavioural methods. In *Child and adolescent psychiatry: modern approaches*, (3rd edn), (ed. M. Rutter, E. Taylor, and L. Hersov), pp. 858–79. Blackwell, Oxford.

Holmes, D. S. and Urie, R. S. (1975). Effects of preparing children for psychotherapy. *Journal of Consulting and Clinical Psychology*, 43, 311–18.

Holmes, J. (1993). *John Bowlby and Attachment Theory*. Routledge, London.

Howlin, P. and Rutter, M. (1987). *Treatment of autistic children*. Wiley, Chichester.

Kazdin, A. E., Bass, D., Ayers, W. A., and Rodgers, A. (1990). Empirical and clinical focus of child and adolescent psychotherapy research. *Journal of Consulting and Clinical Psychology*, 58, 729–40.

Jennings, S. (1993). *Play therapy with children: a practitioner's guide*. Blackwell, Oxford.

Kendall, P. C. and Lochman, J. (1994). Cognitive-behavioural therapies. In *Child and adolescent psychiatry: modern approaches*, (3rd edn), (ed M. Rutter, E. Taylor, and L. Hersov), pp. 844–57. Blackwell, Oxford.

Klein, M. (1961). *Narrative of a child analysis*. Hogarth Press for the Institute of Psychoanalysis, London.

Klein, M. (1963). *The psychoanalysis of children*. Hogarth, London.

Kolvin, I., Garside, R. F., Nicol, A. R., Macmillan, A., Wolstenholme, F., and Leitch, I. (1981). *Help starts here: the maladjusted child in the ordinary school*. Tavistock, London.

Lask, B. and Matthews, D. (1979). Childhood asthma: a controlled trial of family therapy. *Archives of Disease in Childhood*, **54**, 116–19.

Levitt, E. E. (1963). Psychotherapy with children: a further evaluation. *Behaviour Research and Therapy*, **1**, 45–51.

Lewis, M. (1991). Intensive individual psychodynamic psychotherapy: the therapeutic relationship and the technique of interpretation. In *Child and adolescent psychiatry: a comprehensive textbook*, (ed. M. Lewis), pp. 796–805. Williams and Wilkins, Baltimore.

Moran, G., Fonagy, P., Kurtz, A., Bolton, A. and Brook, C. (1991). A controlled study of the psychoanalytic treatment of brittle diabetes. *Journal of the American Academy of Child and Adolescent Psychiatry*, **30**, 926–35.

Murray, L. and Cooper, P. J. (1994). Clinical applications of attachment theory and research: change in infant attachment with brief psychotherapy. In *The clinical application of ethology and attachment theory*, (ed. J. Richer), pp. 15–24. Association for Child Psychology and Psychiatry, Occasional Paper No. 9.

Newson, E. (1992). The bare foot play therapist: adapting skills for a time of need. In *Child and adolescent therapy: a handbook*, (ed. D. A. Lane and A. Miller), pp. 89–107. Open University Press, Milton Keynes.

Ornstein, A. (1994). Resolved: the therapist–patient relationship is the crucial factor to change in child psychotherapy: affirmative. *Journal of the American Academy of Child and Adolescent Psychiatry*, **33**, 1050–2.

Petti, T. A. (1991). Cognitive therapies. In *Child and adolescent psychiatry: a comprehensive textbook*, (ed. M. Lewis), pp. 831–41. Williams and Wilkins, Baltimore.

Piaget, J. and Inhelder, B. (1969). *The psychology of the child*. Routledge & Kegan Paul, London.

Reisman, J. M. (1973). *Principles of psychotherapy with children*. Wiley, New York.

Rosenfeld, S. and Sprince, M.P. (1965). Some thoughts on the technical handling of borderline children. *Psychoanalytic Study of the Child*, **20**, 495–517.

Rosenfeld, A. A., Onesti, S. J., Ornstein, A., and Esman, A. H. (1994). Resolved: the therapist–patient relationship is the crucial factor to change in child psychotherapy, *Journal of the American Academy of Child and Adolescent Psychiatry*, **33**, 1047–54.

Sandler, J., Kennedy, H., and Tyson, R. L. (1980). *The technique of psychoanalysis: discussions with Anna Freud*. Hogarth, London.

Schaefer, C. E. and Cangelosi, D. M. (ed.) (1993). *Play therapy techniques*. Aronson, Northvale, NJ.

Shirk, S. R. and Russell, R. L. (1992). A reevaluation of estimates of child psychotherapy effectiveness. *Journal of the American Academy of Child and Adolescent Psychiatry*, **31**, 703–10.

Shapiro, T. and Esman, A. (1992). Psychoanalysis and child and adolescent psychiatry. *Journal of the American Academy of Child and Adolescent Psychiatry*, **31**, 6–13.

Swift, W. J. and Wonderlich, S. A. (1990). Interpretation of transference in the psychotherapy of adolescents and young adults. *Journal of the American Association of Child and Adolescent Psychiatry*, **29**, 929–35.

Target, M. and Fonagy, P. (1994). The efficacy of psychoanalysis for children: prediction of outcome in a developmental context. *Journal of the American Academy of Child and Adolescent Psychiatry*, **33**, 1134–44.

Truax, C. B. and Carkhuff, R. R. (1967). *Toward effective counselling and psychotherapy: training and practice.* Aldine, Chicago.

Weisz, J. R. and Weiss, B. (1993). *Effects of psychotherapy with children and adolescents.* Sage, London.

Weisz, J. R., Weiss, B., Alicke, M. D., and Klotz, M. L. (1987). Effectiveness of psychotherapy with children and adolescents: A meta-analysis for clinicians. *Journal of Consulting and Clinical Psychology*, **55**, 542–9.

Will, D. and Wrate, R. (1985). *Integrated family therapy: a problem-centred psychodynamic approach.* Tavistock, London.

Winnicott, D. W. (1971). *Therapeutic consultations in child psychiatry.* Basic Books, New York.

Wolff, S. (1989). *Childhood and human nature: the development of personality.* Routledge, London.

Wolff, S. (1991). 'Schizoid' personality in childhood and adult life: the vagaries of diagnostic labelling. *British Journal of Psychiatry*, **159**, 615–20.

Wolff, S. (1992). Aspects of child psychotherapy. *Current Opinion in Psychiatry*, **5**, 361–4.

Wright, D. M., Moelis, I., and Pollack, L. L. (1976). The outcome of individual psychotherapy: increments at follow-up. *Journal of Child Psychology and Psychiatry*, **17**, 175–85.

RECOMMENDED READING

General

Adams, P. L. (1982). *A primer of child psychotherapy* (2nd edn). Little, Brown, Boston. (A helpful introduction to child psychotherapy.)

Lewis, M. (1991). Intensive, individual psychodynamic psychotherapy: the therapeutic relationship and the technique of interpretation. In *Child and adolescent psychiatry: a comprehensive textbook*, (ed. M. Lewis), pp. 796–804. Williams & Wilkins, Baltimore. (An outstanding brief overview of the field.)

Coppolillo, H. P. (1991). The use of play in psychodynamic psychotherapy. In *Child and adolescent psychiatry: a comprehensive textbook* (ed. M. Lewis), pp. 805–11. Williams and Wilkins, Baltimore. (Techniques and principles of play therapy are reviewed with special emphasis on Winnicott's contribution.)

Models of child psychotherapy and psychoanalysis

Axline, V. M. (1969). *Play therapy*. Ballantine, New York. (A helpful, practical guide for the novice.)

Freud, A. (1946). *The psycho-analytical treatment of children*. Imago, London. (A brief glimpse of Anna Freud's style.)

Klein, M. (1963). *The psychoanalysis of children*. Hogarth, London. (A more ponderous work conveying Klein's theories and techniques.)

Winnicott, D. W. (1964). *The child, the family and the outside world*. Penguin, London. (Essays for the general reader, providing examples of Winnicott's ideas and style.)

Child development

Bowlby, J. (1979). *The making and breaking of affectional bonds*. Tavistock, London. (A series of essays conveying Bowlby's ideas as they evolved.)

Donaldson, M. (1978). *Children's minds*. Fontana, London. (A critique of Piaget, in the light of more recent experimental work on cognitive development.)

Erikson, E. H. (1971). *Identity, youth and crisis*. Faber, London. (An outline of Erikson's views of personality development. An overview of constitutional, psychodynamic, cognitive and social aspects of personality development, and their relevance in clinical practice.)

Wolff, S. (1989). *Childhood and human nature: the development of personality*. Routledge, London.

12

Supportive psychotherapy

SIDNEY BLOCH

Supportive psychotherapy continues to have several connotations, but in this chapter refers to a form of treatment used for the chronically impaired psychiatric patient. After attempting to define the term, Sidney Bloch considers the aims of treatment and its indications. A typical patient is briefly described. A section follows on the nature of the therapuetic relationship in, and the components of, supportive therapy. With practical issues in treatment discussed, a model whose central concept is that of an 'institutional alliance' is recommended. The problem of dependency is then examined and the chapter ends with brief accounts on research and training.

The term 'supportive psychotherapy' has many different meanings. In this chapter, it will be used to refer to a form of psychological treatment given to patients with chronic and disabling psychiatric conditions for whom fundamental change is not a realistic goal. Applying the term thus, it is likely that supportive therapy is one of the most commonly practised types of psychotherapy. Apart from its widespread use in psychiatry, the therapy is also applied by, among others, general practitioners and social workers, and, less formally, by other professionals like the clergy and teachers.

At the time of the second edition of this book scanty attention had been paid to supportive therapy in the literature or by researchers. This state of affairs was not surprising: supportive therapy was perhaps the most nebulous of all psychotherapies and tended to be recommended only when no specific form of treatment was available. Commonly, it was also regarded as an inferior form of treatment for use only in patients for whose problems we lacked effective techniques.

Fortunately, the picture has changed since the mid 1980s with a growing interest in the pivotal role supportive therapy can play in the care of the chronically ill and in those with severe personality disorders (e.g. see Hartland 1991; Rockland 1989*a*, 1995; Novalis *et al.* 1993).

Review articles by Rockland (1993) and Winston *et al.* (1986) are noteworthy contributions well worth reading. Further reference to some of this material is made in the sections that follow. We now turn to a defintion of supportive therapy and consider its aims, indications, therapeutic components, and the problems that may arise in the course of treatment. I shall also discuss a model which has particular utility and provide a clinical case illustration.

DEFINITION

The definition of supportive therapy has always proved elusive (Novalis *et al.* 1993; Pinsker 1994; Holmes 1988). First, we must emphasize that we are dealing with a form of treatment in which therapist support is a core component. All therapies obviously entail an element of support but this is only one of several therapeutic factors used, and not the main one underlying treatment.

The derivation of the word 'support' helps to clarify the type of therapy we are considering: Supportare: Sup = Sub + portare—to carry (*Oxford English Dictionary*, Oxford University Press, Oxford, 1978). The therapist 'carries' the patient; he helps to sustain him, to bolster him. The implication is that certain patients are so impaired by their psychiatric condition or severe limiations of personality that they depend on a form of professionally derived psychological aid in order to 'survive'.

With the above in mind and for our purposes, supportive therapy can be defined as a form of psychological treatment provided to a patient over an extended period, often years, in order to sustain him psychologically, because he is unable to manage his life adequately without this long-term help. An alternative definition by Gilbert and Ugelstad (1994) stresses 'supporting and strengthening the potential for better and more mature ego functioning in both adaptational and developmental tasks'.

The inability to cope may be transient or enduring. If temporary, the person typically experiences a stressful life event such as bereavement, divorce, or loss of job which leads to a degree of emotional upheaval not matched by his own integrative resources. Additional help from elsewhere is called for. The person is in crisis and the treatment necessary is crisis intervention; this is dealt with in Chapter 5 and will not be discussed further here.

Enduring incapacity to manage autonomously is seen in patients disabled by their chronic psychotic or neurotic state, or by the limitations of their personality. They may require supportive therap~ indefinitely. We are concerned with this type of patient and with hi~ need for long-term help. We limit ourselves to supportive therapy a~ practised in the community although the points to be made pertain t~ patients living in hospitals, hostels, or half-way houses.

A clear distinction between supportive and exploratory (synonym~ are interpretive, insight-oriented, dynamic, expressive) implied in th~ above account is subject to debate. Kernberg (1984), for example refers to a spectrum with supportive and expressive at the two end~ and some admixture and movement possible dependent on the degre~ of patient impairment and clinical progress. Pine (1986), again from a~ psychoanalytic perspective, advances the notion of how interpretation is given in specific ways for the psychologically vulnerable, that is, the therapist minimizes the vulnerability through a number of supportive strategies, thus making interpretive interventions possible.

Pinsker's (1994) contribution on the issue of theory in supportive therapy illuminates further the complexity of arriving at a uniform definition. He concludes that since supportive therapy is 'not based~ upon a theory of mind or personality or psychopathology, it should not be thought of as a unique modality of treatment but rather as a body of techniques or tactics that function with various theoretical orientation . . .'

This chapter is written with the same observation in mind but with a crucial proviso: various theoretical principles derived from several schools—systems, psychoanalytic, behavioural, cognitive, self-psychology, attachment, and object-relations among them—are applicable to the practice of supportive therapy. They can be usefully incorporated in varying ways and measure according to clinical circumstance.

Thus, Dewald (1994), in a clear description of relevant principles, utilizes psychoanalytic terminology but is careful to avoid equating supportive therapy with a modified form of psychoanalysis exclusively.

Buckley's (1994) position interestingly applies concepts from several schools which he argues are useful for understanding both the techniques and potential efficacy of supportive therapy. For example, Kohut's emphasis on an empathic stance is a means to foster and maintain a positive transference and yet enable the patient to appreciate that 'the idealized object is unavailable or imperfect'. Winnicott's 'holding environment' is another instance of creating the appropriate framework for therapy; the patient feels secure enough to feel real rather than merely existing and to relate to others as oneself.

BACKGROUND

Supportive therapy has a long tradition. For centuries, designated members of society have helped those who were psychologically disabled. Religious orders particularly played, and continue to play, a part as 'therapist'. In addition, in relatively cohesive societies, relatives and friends have served as providers of long-term support to those in need of it. With the advent of 'professional' psychotherapy, psychiatrists turned their interest to the application of psychological measures for their patients, but confined themselves to the neuroses, and later to certain personality disorders. Chronically ill patients, however, were relegated to the back-wards of mental hospitals, and there limited to custodial care.

The discovery of antipsychotic drugs in the 1950s, and the adoption of community based treatment soon after, paved the way for large numbers of patients with chronic psychiatric conditions to be cared for outside the mental hospital. One corollary has been the increasingly relevant role of supportive therapy. The changes have also brought many problems in their wake; a salient question today is how mental health professionals can care effectively for people with severe, long-term difficulties who live outside of institutions, often isolated and with minimal or no natural supports.

AIMS OF TREATMENT

The aims of supportive therapy will be influenced to a great extent by characteristics in the patient—age, diagnosis, prognosis, social circumstances, personal resources, and the like—but common objectives can be summarized as follows:

(a) To promote the patient's best possible psychological and social adaptation by restoring and reinforcing his abilities to cope with the vicissitudes and challenges of life.

(b) To bolster his self-esteem and self-confidence as much as possible by highlighting assets and achievements.

(c) To make him aware of the reality of his life situation e.g. of his own limitations and those of treatment—of what can and cannot be achieved.

(d) To forestall a relapse of his clinical condition and thus try to prevent deterioration or re-hospitalization.

(e) To enable the patient to require only that degree of professiona
    support which will result in his best possible adaptation, and sc
    prevent undue dependency.

(f) To transfer the source of support (not necessarily all of it) from
    professionals to relatives or friends, provided the latter are
    available and in a position, psychologically and materially, to
    assume the role of caregiver.

INDICATIONS

Supportive psychotherapy is indicated in psychiatric patients who are
severely impaired both emotionally and in their interpersonal
relationships and in whom there is no prospect of basic
improvement. Werman (1984) sums it up this way: '. . . supportive
psychotherapy assumes that the patient's psychological equipment is
fundamentally inadequate.' Because of their condition they simply
cannot live their lives without some form of external help. They are
relatively intolerant of life's stresses, on occasion even of trivial
demands. Commonly, they encounter difficulty in seeking help,
whether from professionals or others, in an adaptive way or in
applying help that is offered. Life changes often disrupt their
equilibrium, leading to symptom formation or increased dependency
on others. Relatives and friends who might be a source of support are
often absent, or unable to respond satisfactorily to the patients' needs.
The severity of their conditions and associated vulnerability preclude
the application of forms of psychotherapy that involve the acquisition
of insight as a central therapeutic factor and aim for so-called
'structural' change.

Dewald (1994) captures the gist of the criteria for supportive
therapy:

Supportive therapy is usually indicated for people who have difficult, unstable,
or limited interpersonal relationships; for those who are not introspective or
curious about themselves and their psychological functioning; for patients
whose reality resources preclude the necessary frequency or expense of
intensive psychotherapy; or for those whose interest is predominantly in
symptomatic change and whose capacity for self-initiating behaviour is
limited.

In terms of conventional diagnosis patients who may benefit from a
supportive approach come from the following groups:

a) chronic schizophrenia and related psychoses including delusional and schizo-affective disorders (Kates and Rockland 1994);

b) recurrent or chronic affective disorders including unipolar, bipolar, cyclothymia, and dysthymia;

c) long-standing neurotic and somatoform disorders including phobic and anxiety states, adjustment disorders, somatization, and hypochondriasis (Kellner 1982; Karasu 1986);

d) severe personality disorders including dependent, paranoid, schizoid, borderline, narcissistic, and histrionic types (Kernberg 1984; Rockland 1992; Paris 1993).

Clearly, not all patients within these clinical categories are impaired, and many may progress satisfactorily with insight-oriented psychotherapies and medication. We are here concerned with those who are severely and enduringly impaired. As a consequence, their needs have to be considered in terms of how they might be best assisted to accomplish *their* best possible adjustment and its maintenance.

Determining whether a patient of the type outlined is suitable or not for supportive therapy does not usually pose a problem. Conversely, the treatment has no place in those in whom there is evidence of personal resources and strengths, sufficient for independent coping with life's demands. As noted in Chapter 5, it can be used as part of 'intensive care', that is, in crisis intervention when a person with normal coping ability is overwhelmed by major stress, necessitating the therapist assuming responsibility temporarily.

A TYPICAL PATIENT IN SUPPORTIVE THERAPY

Sally was born into a professional family, the oldest of three children. Her father, an eminent lawyer, and her mother, a highly committed school teacher, were emotionally unavailable as the children grew up. Moreover, father was persistently irascible and critical of all three children when they failed to meet his expectations. Sally had little to do with her two brothers, four and seven years her junior. Indeed, each child seemed to retreat into a world of their own. Growing up in this family was a lonely, distressing experience for Sally. She did not find much solace elsewhere. Although she acquitted herself reasonably at school, she could not sustain any friendships. The result was an isolated teenager prone to ultra-sensitivity and exquisite vulnerability to even the mildest challenge or pressure.

Much the same pattern prevailed at university. By dint of hard slogging, Sally graduated in her early twenties with an arts degree; her achievement brought her little joy and nothing in the way of family congratulation. She could not land a suitable job, not for want of trying, and wandered from one temporary or part-time post to another. Still threatened by closeness in relationships, she remained isolated and lonely. Casual sexual relationships ensued, apparently a desperate means to make human contact. On becoming pregnant through one of these encounters, she became determined to have the child despite the partner's disinterest and her parents' marked ambivalence. She was supported materially by the latter for the first two years of David's life but mounting conflict culminated in a breakdown of the arrangments. Sally was now truly on her own—a mother, long-term unemployed, friendless and receiving a single parent benefit—at the age of 32.

Sally's psychiatric 'career' began with her self-referral, aged 27. Buffeted by feelings of rejection, loneliness, and low self-regard, she stressed her need for 'emotional support'—she could no longer cope with what she saw as her family's rejection and an uncaring, harsh society. Although no explicit psychotic phenomena were identified, Sally's paranoid-like stance was noted, as was her incapacity to trust the ward staff. A comprehensive assessment pointed to severe personality difficulties, with schizoid and avoidant features to the fore. The recommendation was for a trial of exploratory psychotherapy with the caveat that her fragile sense of self and tendency to use primitive defences might well preclude the development of an effective therapeutic relationship and the application of psychodynamic techniques, especially the interpretation of unconscious conflict, defences, transference, and resistance.

It required only a matter of weeks to confirm that the caveat had been justified. Sally become severely distressed in the course of the early sessions, to the point of growing suspicious about the therapist's intentions. The latter for her part, fearing an impending psychotic break, consulted with a senior colleague. They agreed readily that Sally was certainly, at this point, not a suitable candidate for an exploratory approach. Rather, her vulnerability and fragility pointed to the appropriateness of supportive therapy. This was launched by the same therapist following a careful description of the new, substitute approach and its rationale. Sally welcomed the change, ostensibly relieved that support was to be a foremost ingredient.

The clinical judgement proved correct. Sally has continued to be seen in the clinic, although the original therapist had to be replaced following her depature for a new job. The frequency of sessions has varied from weekly to monthly dependent on Sally's clinicial state and life situation. For example, she was seen weekly during the last trimester of her pregnancy and puerperium, and for the duration of a conflict-laden episode with her parents. Apart from the centrality of the therapeutic alliance, an assortment of strategies has been deployed according to clinical necessity (see below). Attempts have also been made to promote more effective coping in Sally as a mother by arranging for her membership of a new mothers' club. Minimal family intervention was attempted—the aims modest given the entrenched history of conflict and alienation—in order to ameliorate the continuing tensions and to promote links between the grandparents and their sole grandchild. Sally has also been persistently encouraged to exploit her own assets. For example, she has participated in a local social club's activities and has done voluntary teaching in a literacy programme.

The likelihood of Sally requiring indefinite supportive therapy is high, in as much as her capacity to live autonomously is distinctly limited. Yet, a monthly frequency of sessions appears adequate and admission to a psychiatric hospital unlikely (unless a major crisis supervenes).

For two further case illustrations, most vividly portrayed, see Holmes (1988).

THE THERAPIST–PATIENT RELATIONSHIP

The typical patient for whom supportive therapy is indicated experiences difficulty in maintaining relationships with others, both intimate and general. An intense relationship entailing closeness and trust poses a threat. This must be borne in mind in considering the nature of the link between patient and therapist in supportive therapy (Rada *et al.* 1969). This is well illustrated in a classical study by Balint *et al.* (1970). Patients who requested repeat prescriptions (mainly of psychotropic drugs) from their general practitioners made frequent contact with them but always indirectly. They were isolated with long-standing maladaptive traits who 'tolerate badly any proximity or intimacy with their partners'. They maintained a safe distance from their doctors chiefly by 'offering them bodily complaints' and receiving repeat prescriptions from them; the drug represented the 'something' they needed badly. These patients were incapable of making use of a warm alliance, the basis of almost all psychotherapy.

Thus, the relationship between patient and therapist in supportive therapy is of a particular kind: the therapist assumes a helping role, attends sensitively to the patient's needs through various strategies (to be discussed below), but promotes only a modest level of closeness (Crown 1988).

Another reason for this type of relationship is more pragmatic: patients receiving supportive therapy have chronic conditions requiring help for extended periods, often for life. The same therapist will usually be unavailable for such a long-term commitment as he moves from one clinical service to another or to a new position elsewhere. Fostering too intense a relationship only paves the way for a greater sense of loss in the patient and the risk of deterioration when the therapist departs. An obvious alternative is for the patient to 'relate' to the 'institution'; we return to this later when considering potential models of providing supportive therapy.

Apart from the issue of closeness, the other feature that typifies the therapist–patient relationship is the directive role the therapist plays. He assumes a measure of responsibility—not seen in other forms of psychotherapy—on the premise that the patient is chronically impaired and vulnerable, unable to live autonomously. To an extent the bond resembles that between parent and child, that is, the therapist creates and maintains a link through which she offers the security and care the patient needs (Winnicott 1965; Meyer 1993). The therapist also uses the relationship as a vehicle to implement a number of specific therapeutic strategies.

COMPONENTS OF SUPPORTIVE THERAPY

What are the components of supportive therapy? In this section we discuss each of them separately, although in practice they are not at all discrete. Teasing them out, however, will make their specific application more obvious. We should also note that they are not considered in any order; any of them may be applied at any time and in varying combinations.

1) Reassurance

The therapist reassures patients in at least two ways: by removing doubts and misconceptions, and by pointing to their assets. Patients commonly harbour thoughts or sentiments about themselves which are ill-founded and lead to considerable distress. For example, a middle-aged married man who believed he was losing his sanity was much relieved at the therapist's reassurance that he was definitely not destined for such a fate and that his feelings of jealousy were an exaggeration of a normal emotion and perfectly understandable in the light of his deprived upbringing. Reassurance can be used to good effect to relieve fears in the patient that he is crazy or becoming so, that he will be permanently detained in a hospital, that he has a serious physical illness, or that his symptoms are unique to him alone, etc.

The chronic psychiatric patient has invariably also lost self-confidence; on assessing his life, he can see nothing but failure and missed opportunities. Although this may well be true in part, he tends to omit from his self-appraisal any assets and abilities. The therapist can bolster his patient's esteem by pointing these out. A caveat is indicated—reassurance must, to be effective, be realistic. To promote hope unreasonably through reassurance that is groundless may be effective in the short term, but is bound to backfire later. The therapist therefore aims to create a climate of hope and positive expectation, but without deceit and disingenuousness.

(2) Explanation

This strategy is used quite differently in supportive therapy compared to psychotherapy in which the chief goal is to promote insight (see Chapter 2). We should stress that, in the former, explanation (or to use the customary term, interpretation) of such phenomena as transference, resistance, defences, and unconscious determinants of behaviour, is inappropriate and best avoided. Instead, explanation focuses on day-to-day practical questions, on the current and external reality with which the patient contends. The goal is not to promote self-understanding of a psychodynamic kind but to enhance the ability to cope by clarifying the nature of the problems and challenges the patient faces and how he can best deal with them.

This reality testing is pivotal for the chronically impaired patient. He has to become aware of the nature of his condition and of any unrealistic fantasies he may nurture. He must also appreciate the limits of the therapist and of his techniques (i.e. 'I cannot expect a magic cure from my therapist'). Following appropriate explanation, he is better equipped to accept that he must live in spite of his chronic difficulties in the best way possible. He should acknowledge: 'I have to live with this for a long time to come, perhaps life-long; what can I do in collaboration with the therapist to face the future?'.

The therapist may clarify a broad array of issues among which are the nature of the symptoms (e.g. 'Your headaches are due to your scalp muscles tightening up when you feel tense and not to a brain tumour'); the reason for taking medication (e.g. 'These tablets will make you more relaxed and this in turn will help to prevent your breaking down again'); the reason for relapse (e.g. 'It's not surprising you are feeling distressed given the pressure you have been under since your husband became ill'); and so forth. Note that all the examples are in straightforward, everyday language. Explanations in technical language or peppered with jargon may impress the patient but exert no impact since they are beyond his comprehension.

(3) Guidance

Supportive therapy usually entails guiding the patient in a range of situations, mainly through direct advice. As with explanation, the stress is on practical issues, including the most fundamental—budgeting, personal hygiene, nutrition, and sleep. Advice may be necessary in respect of work (e.g. how to apply for a particular position, whether to change jobs, how to approach a boss to make a reasonable request); or about family (e.g. how best to relate to an aged parent, what to do about a rebellious adolescent son); or about leisure (e.g. how to join a social club, how to pursue a hobby).

The therapist's goal is not merely to assist the patient to deal with a particular issue but also to teach him requisite skills for coping with other similar problems. Ideally, he is shown how to assess common pressures and identify appropriate measures to deal with them; in this way he becomes better placed to handle stress and to tackle decisions on his own. Particularly pertinent here is teaching the patient how and when to seek help appropriately. Many patients have been unable to do this throughout their lives, often calling for aid when the situation is dire, or conversely frustrating their caregivers, professional or natural, by insatiable or pervasive demands. Moreover, they may have expressed their difficulties exclusively in terms of bodily symptoms, or made impulsive suicide attempts, or delayed consultation until they vere either excessively distressed or functioning very poorly. In ummary, the therapist tries both to enhance the patient's coping kills and to teach him how to ask for help when this is clearly iecessary.

Occasionally, advice proves inadequate; *persuasion* is then another herapeutic option. The therapist moves from a gently directive stance o a more controlling one as he tries to convince the patient to think or ict in a particular way. This may relate, for example, to an decision the)atient is obviously obliged to make or to a specific programme of iction the therapist senses the patient should pursue. The therapist nust feel confident of his ground before resorting to this strategy and)referably use other means like advice and explanation beforehand. Fhe danger always lurks that persuasion will reflect the therapist's own)ersonal attitudes and beliefs rather than be more objectively ¿rounded.

(4) Suggestion

In this strategy, similar to guidance, the patient is offered less choice in considering whether to comply. The therapist aims to induce change by influencing him implicitly or explicitly. An example of implicit influence is the therapist manifesting approval of desirable behaviour: 'The way you stood up for yourself was terrific', with the obvious implication that the patient ought to replicate the behaviour. As was the case with persuasion, guidance and explanation in which the patient plays a more collaborative role are preferable to suggestion and should be attempted first.

(5) Encouragement

To encourage a patient is such common sense that we are apt to take it for granted. The most effective use of encouragement is made, however, when the therapist is keenly aware what he is trying to achieve. Patients with long-standing difficulties need 'injections of courage' repeatedly, but this is best done in relation to particular circumstances in their lives or therapy. Thus, rather than encourage in vague general terms, the therapist does so in specific contexts. These vary considerably from patient to patient. What remains consistent are its objectives: to combat feelings of inferiority, to promote self-esteem,

and to urge the patient to adopt courses of action or behaviours o
which he is hesitant or anxious (Lamb 1981).

The therapist encourages in myriad ways according to need an
circumstance. For example, he can use the full force of he
authoritative, benevolent role by commenting: 'From my lon
experience of dealing with the sort of problem you describe, I an
fully confident you will be able to master it.' She may also demonstrat
her sense of confidence non-verbally through a display of eagernes
and optimism. As with reassurance, the therapist exploits past o
current progress by positive reinforcement, explicit or tacit. He may
comment: 'Last year you proved how effectively you could discus
your work schedule with your boss—I'm certain you have it in you t
do it this time too.'

Caution is necessary regarding encouragement; its use may be no
only futile but also counter-therapeutic if given inappropriately. To
encourage a patient unrealistically, towards a goal hopelessly out o
his reach, may well have a contrary result to that intended: he become
dispirited as he battles to attain what the therapist hopes for but which
he himself finds too demanding. The limitations imposed by the
patient's condition and resources must be respected. In any event, he
should be encouraged to take small steps so that the chance of
negotiating them successfully is increased. Each mastery experience
then promotes self-confidence and serves as a source of encouragement
for subsequent initiatives (see Chapter 1).

(6) Effecting changes in the patient's environment

Patients with a chronic psychiatric condition are markedly influenced
by social forces, both human and institutional, that impinge on them.
The deleterious effects on the schizophrenic patient of a family
atmosphere typified by high 'emotional expressiveness' is a good
illustration. In supportive therapy a cardinal consideration is the
patient in his social context; the goals of removing or altering
detrimental elements and conversely, of maximizing potentially
beneficial ones. The therapist therefore regularly asks herself:
'How can I help to modify my patient's social environment to best
advantage?'

Stressful factors need to be carefully assessed so that they can be
suitably modified. The range is infinite, the following common: the
patient's job has become too demanding and outstretched his
psychological resources; the family atmosphere is tense; the housing

situation is poor; he is socially isolated; he is under financial pressures, etc. Environmental changes of a more positive kind (i.e. adding to the patient's world), are as important as the removal of stress. Thus, encouraging the patient to participate in social activities like those found in Elderly Citizens' Clubs, the church, and community centres, or helping him to launch or resume hobbies and pastimes, can be of considerable value. Social contact is enhanced but in a protective setting, and the patient derives pleasure from intrinsically worthwhile pursuits.

There are two dimensions to this strategy: (1) working directly with the patient by helping him, for example, to obtain a suitable job or to approach the appropriate authorities for sickness or other benefits, or putting him in touch with social clubs and the like (social workers are most helpful with these aspects); and (2) working with people who are important to the patient, particularly relatives. Here, straightforward counselling often helps both relatives, and, indirectly, the patient. If we recall that one aim of supportive therapy is the transfer of some of the source of support from professional to family or friends (assuming, of course, they exist) it follows that the more skilled and prepared they are for the task, the more likely they are to succeed. The job is no easy matter. Caring for a chronically ill patient calls for perseverance and discretion (Bloch *et al.* 1995). The therapist assisting relatives or friends can use many of the strategies we have already discussed including guidance, encouragement, and reassurance.

Failure of the supportive therapy of the chronically ill patient may well be due to the therapist's neglect of the family's needs. He may have overlooked or underestimated the marked positive effects on the patient's welfare that can result when optimizing the family's role as ally. The family's successful incorporation, however, requires they be fully informed and counselled, and then instructed as to what to do and how to do it. In addition, family members need help in their own right to care for their relative as the process can be burdensome and frustrating.

In long-term care, the need occasionally arises to alter the patient's environment radically because his condition has deteriorated or he has become exposed to a particularly noxious situation. Options include admission to a psychiatric ward, attendance at a day hospital, or participation in a sheltered workshop or occupational therapy programme. Such a development need not be construed by either therapist or patient as a failure if both appreciate that the patient's resources will periodically be outstretched by circumstances.

(7) Permission for catharsis

The relative security typifying the therapeutic relationship permits the patient to share with a sense of relief pent-up feelings like fear, grief, sorrow, concern, frustration, and envy. The clinic is commonly the sole place where the patient can feel sufficiently safe to do this. The therapist, by showing that he is a sympathetic, active listener who accepts the patient unconditionally, grants him permission to share his 'secrets', whatever they are and however painful or embarrassing they may be. Although sharing of emotionally charged material is not necessarily effective in itself (Yalom *et al.* 1977), the process leads to a sense of relief and serves as a vehicle for other strategies.

ASSOCIATED COMPONENTS OF THERAPY

Apart from the specific type of relationship and the above therapeutic strategies, other methods can be added to a programme of supportive therapy when appropriate. Drug treatment may well have a place (e.g. maintenance antipsychotics in chronic schizophrenia or lithium to prevent recurrent mood swings). The role of benzodiazepines, still used far too widely in general practice, is dubious and any potential positive effects outweighed by the physical or psychological dependence that may develop. Although the 'tablet' has symbolic value and serves as a tangible reflection of the therapist's interest such grounds for prescribing are entirely unsound; the therapist should clarify the precise place for psychotropic medication in a particular patient and only use it when solid clinical criteria are met.

Other methods usefully adjunctive to supportive therapy include relaxation training, social skills training, attendance at a social club, and occupational therapy. Treating the patient together with spouse or family may be indicated but the approach adopted is primarily supportive rather than dissecting the nature of intra-familial relationships. The therapist uses the strategies discussed above to help the family cope more effectively as a group.

SUPPORTIVE PSYCHOTHERAPY IN PRACTICE

More often than not, trainees are assigned to patients for long-term supportive therapy. Typically, the therapist 'slides' into the work rather than mapping out clear objectives or devising a comprehensive plan. Therapy tends, as a result, to be unfocused, even haphazard.

Supervision is commonly limited as if supportive therapy were straightforward. This state of affairs is regrettable given that the work, in fact, demands as sophisticated and critical a set of skills as for insight-oriented therapies.

In launching supportive therapy, it is helpful to pose a series of interlocking questions (Greenberg 1986). How often will I see the patient? How long will each session be? How long will therapy continue for? Is it likely that I will refer this patient to his general practitioner in the foreseeable future? Will he require long-term care from a mental health professional? At what point will I review the effectiveness of therapy? Should anyone else be involved in treatment, for example, spouse, other relative? Should I draw upon community resources such as a support organization, (e.g. Schizophrenia Fellowship)? Is medication necessary? If yes, under what circumstances?

These are but some of the questions the therapist needs to ask. Accompanying the inquiry is the preparation of a problem list: an attempt to clarify in what specific areas help is necessary. The use of a problem-oriented approach not only guides the therapist in setting realistic goals but also enables him to assess the value of his interventions. Much of this preparatory work should be shared with the patient in a collaborative spirit.

Anticipating hurdles that may hamper therapy is useful from the outset. In particular, what is the risk of the patient becoming overly dependent on me? How likely is he to co-operate with my recommendations? Will it be necessary to set any limits? What arrangements should I make regarding sessions requested between appointments, the patient's use of emergency services, and my availability on the telephone? Do I need to set conditions to obviate problems?

Periodic review is an inherent feature of a long-term treatment like supportive therapy. As mentioned earlier the problem list will be valuable for this purpose. In addition, certain questions need to be asked: Is my original plan working? Am I making the patient worse in any way? Is he becoming unduly dependent? Have any new problems arisen? Should I modify goals set previously? Am I still the most appropriate person to provide help? If not, who is best suited—the general practitioner, the family?

Careful thought to these points facilitates more efficient and effective treatment. However, the question arises whether an optimum model is available in applying supportive therapy?

A MODEL OF SUPPORTIVE THERAPY
IN A MENTAL HEALTH SERVICE

In this section, we consider a model which appears to be eminently suitable. Although first reported in the early 1960s, its recommendations are as sensible today as then, and no apology need be offered for citing it. In 1962, MacLeod and Middleman described their 'Wednesday Afternoon Clinic' (WAC), a pattern of supportive care for chronically ill psychiatric patients. Other similar clinics sprang up thereafter, particularly in the United States (see, for example, Sassano and Stone 1975; Masnik *et al.* 1980; Rada *et al.* 1969; Brandwin *et al.* 1976). Their structure and function warrant close examination. The clinic is held regularly, on the same day of the week at the same time. Patients assessed as suitable attend at intervals ranging from weekly to twice monthly. Although they are seen by appointment they do have free access, especially in seeking an earlier meeting.

Staffing arrangements call for two constant figures: a receptionist and a co-ordinator. The receptionist, rarely given enough credit in mental health services, is important in providing continuity. The co-ordinator is most conveniently a psychiatrist, since prescribing drugs applies in many cases. The remaining staff, among them psychiatrists, psychologists, social workers, occupational therapists, and psychiatric nurses, work in the clinic as permanent members or for a period of several months, usually as part of training.

Let us follow the 'career' of a typical patient (who has been deemed suitable). On arrival he is greeted by the receptionist and ushered to the waiting room where he can avail himself of light refreshments. There he meets other patients whom he gets to know over time. This informal prelude to the actual therapy session is of inestimable value in itself in that the clinic is perceived as homely and welcoming. The receptionist plays a cardinal role in this respect, fostering the climate necessary to reduce anxiety and a sense of isolation. The 'coffee atmosphere' also allows the patient to appreciate that he is not unique. He is seen by a therapist, either the same or a different one, for about 20 to 30 minutes. During that time therapeutic strategies discussed earlier come into play.

At the end of the clinic, staff meet to review progress of patients seen and to discuss any problems in treatment that have been encountered. This meeting enables the staff to become familiar with the treatment of all patients which in turn: (a) facilitates a consistent approach; and (b) promotes continuity of care despite any staff changes. The results of the discussion are recorded in the file of each patient including suggestions for future treatment. In addition, any trainees present learn about the principles and practice of supportive therapy while the entire staff support one another for what can be demanding work.

A key rationale behind this model is the notion of an 'institutional alliance', that is, the patient forms a relationship with the 'clinic' rather than with a single therapist (Daniels *et al.* 1968). As discussed on p. 301, the patient we are considering is threatened by too intimate a relationship. The fact that he is treated by different therapists but in the secure framework of the clinic suits his needs well. A pragmatic issue is also pertinent—the patient is likely to require indefinite care. Because of their training obligations and job movements, staff will generally not be available for such a long-term commitment. Problems of loss would then arise for the patient. In contrast, the clinic meets regularly—without exception, always dependable; there is no threat of the patient being abandoned by it.

In summary, the model incorporates the institution as the everpresent, constant, and accessible source of help. The waiting room, refreshments, receptionist, and rotating staff together comprise the agency of support. Personal attention is given but at a level which can be tolerated by the patient; moreover, losing a particular therapist is not a catastrophe.

A MODEL FOR SUPPORTIVE THERAPY IN GENERAL PRACTICE

To set up this type of clinic is not always feasible. In any event some patients do not require psychiatric assistance *per se* and can be given long-term supportive therapy by their general practitioner. Indeed, this is common practice. A reasonable approach here is for the GP to negotiate an agreement with the patient as follows: he will be seen regularly, once a month on average, for a specified period, usually for about 15 to 20 minutes. The time allocated 'belongs' to the patient and the appointments guaranteed. When the programme is so utterly predictable the patient feels secure while the GP is spared anguished telephone calls or maladaptive requests for additional sessions. Clinical experience suggests that the patient adheres to the agreement, probably because he feels confident that his 'lifeline' will remain intact.

During the session, the GP is an active listener, displaying interest in the patient. As in the WAC, he applies the strategies discussed previously. Particularly relevant in general practice is the approach to somatization. Since the patient commonly expresses his psychic distress through the body and seeks relief from physical symptoms, the GP gently encourages him to 'express his feelings with his mouth rather than with his body' (Wahl 1963). At the same time it is made clear that the doctor does not regard the physical symptoms as imaginary. On the contrary, he explains how emotional states can produce pain and other physical symptoms.

Since the model allows for continuing contact, there is no pressure to accomplish a set amount in any one session. After all there will be opportunity to talk further the following month, and thereafter.

PROBLEMS IN THE COURSE OF TREATMENT

A principal risk in practising supportive therapy, no matter the model used, is fostering dependency to a degree that the patient relinquishes any sense of responsibility for himself and comes to rely entirely on his therapist. As Kolb (1973) cautions: 'In employing supportive therapy, the physician should bear in mind the dangers that he may thereby encourage dependence and a regressive passivity in the patient.' Whatever the nature of the patient's clinical state the 'prospect exists that dependency (intrinsic to treatment) will escalate and persist in a way that is not necessarily in the patient's long-term interests' (Bloch 1977). Dependency in some measure is inevitable in every therapist–patient relationship but even more so in supportive therapy where the patient is actually permitted to 'lean on' the therapist. The thorny question arises as to how much leaning is appropriate? The condition of the patient will often dictate the answer but in general the therapist's goal is to promote self-sufficiency to the maximum degree possible and to transfer some of the source of support to family and other intimates.

One could argue that dependence on the therapist in the chronically impaired is of no consequence. A parallel is prescribing narcotic drugs in the terminally ill—concern about drug addiction is not relevant since palliative care is paramount. The drawbacks with the patient in supportive therapy, however, are that he is robbed of any opportunity to act independently and that, should the therapist depart, for whatever reason, the patient will rapidly crumble unless he finds a substitute source of support.

Neki (1976), in an excellent review of dependency in psychotherapy, highlights the resistance that Western therapists harbour to the patient's yearning for dependency on them; they work assiduously to promote self-reliance and full autonomy. Such efforts are perfectly applicable to those psychotherapies which aim towards personality change but quite unsuitable in the case of supportive therapy where the therapist has to accept his role as a principal source of support, albeit taking care not to nurture undue passivity and dependency. Not uncommonly, the therapist assumes the supportive role initially but later encounters difficulty in grappling with the patient's entrenched dependent stance and his own discomfort in trying to reduce the level of support offered. He may resort to setting limits or 'withdraw'. The relationship inevitably is strained and therapy thrown into disarray. The patient clings all the harder as the therapist, angry and frustrated, endeavours to keep him at bay.

A therapist may instil dependency unwittingly out of a need to prove to himself and others that, first, he exerts a pivotal role in helping patients, and secondly, even in chronic cases he can be useful. In many of the conditions he deals with there is only equivocal evidence that his efforts are beneficial. He may well deflect unconsciously the uncertainty of his helpfulness by relying on the concept of support. Since supportive therapy by definition denotes an active role for the therapist he can derive comfort that he is a benevolent figure.

Supportive therapy is not regarded by many therapists as satisfying as intensive psychotherapy where one participates in a journey of discovery with goals specified and often accomplished. For the chronic patient there is no chance of 'cure' and the therapy tends to be less engaging, to some even dull. Moreover, therapists often find supportive therapy arduous and frustrating. They are repeatedly confronted with their relative ineffectiveness in the face of a range of conditions—fertile ground for the growth of demoralization.

In addition, as we saw earlier, the patient typically cannot tolerate the close relationship that ideally (and gratifyingly to the therapist) obtains in the relationship of the intensive psychotherapies; this is a potential further source of frustration (Kahn 1984).

The WAC model becomes all the more relevant in the light of these pressures. The clinic shoulders the major task and no one therapist is over-burdened. Furthermore, the staff provide support to one another (Sassano and Stone 1975). The general practitioner obviously lacks this opportunity although he may, if in a group practice, use his colleagues as a source of support. He also has recourse to refer complicated patients to a specialist clinic.

Supportive therapy practised in an appropriate setting can, despite what we have noted, satisfy and challenge. A patient achieving a goal, no matter how limited, can be rewarding for him and his therapist (Daniels *et al.* 1968). The positive experience for the latter is more likely to occur if she remembers to '. . . content herself with settling for what is possible' (Lamb 1981).

RESEARCH

The effectiveness of supportive psychotherapy is extremely difficult to assess (Conte and Plutchick 1986; Conte 1994; Rockland 1993). Criteria of outcome have to be tailored to patients who are enduringly impaired. Moreover, we are dealing with a diagnostically heterogeneous group. Obviously, we would have to tease out these groups to test efficacy adequately. We would also need to note other treatments being given (e.g. medication, non-professional support like social clubs, and so on). Forming a control group against which to test effectiveness would be clinically and ethically problematic.

With regard to the problem of outcome assessment, suitable criteria might include: the pattern of clinic attendance (e.g. failure to keep appointments, dropping out of treatment, excessive use of the clinic); incidence of psychiatric hospitalisation; use of emergency facilities; the overall pattern of help-seeking; quality of relationships with family and others; work performance and ability to cope with everyday tasks.

Given these methodological hurdles it is no surprise that outcome studies continue to be rare. The WAC model has been examined although only impressionistically. MacLeod and Middleman (1962) compared the outcome of patients in treatment at their WAC clinic with similar types of patients attending a conventional out-patient clinic and found 'considerably more indications of improvement' in the former. Brandwin *et al.* (1976) in assessing their 'continuing-care clinic' used hospitalization as a criterion and compared the rate for a period before the patients began their clinic attendance and for a period thereafter. The proportion of patients admitted, frequency of admissions, and total number of in-patient days were all substantially reduced while attending the continuing-care clinic.

Another study supports these findings. Masnik *et al.* (1980) followed up patients who had attended a supportive, 'coffee' group for an average five years. According to therapists' ratings, patients improved symptomatically and in their ability to cope, albeit modestly. Re-hospitalization rates also diminished. Improvement correlated only with attendance, suggesting that the group served as a support system with peer identification and encouragement as notable therapeutic elements.

In summary, supportive therapy as practised in a clinic designed for the chronically ill appears to achieve better results than conventional out-patient approaches but further systematic research needs to be done to confirm these trends.

TRAINING

Training programmes have, until the 1990s, tended to emphasize the hospital treatment of the chronically ill. Following their discharge into the community, trainees are often left to their own devices as to how to continue care. Their training has also lagged behind the development of the community mental health movement over the past two decades (Rockland 1989).

What are the requisite ingredients of training? Instruction on theory has been seen as less pertinent than in other therapies because no theoretical model has stood out as more relevant than others. Indeed, no psychotherapy school has adopted the chronic patient under its wing, although the picture has changed since the 1980s as psychodynamically-oriented theorists like Kernberg (1984) and Rockland (1989, 1993) have begun to commit themselves. Alongside this movement has been the participation of behaviourally focused practitioners. Treatment remains more empirical than theoretical and consists of a number of related procedures that experience has shown to be beneficial. As important as theoretical knowledge is the trainee's familiarity with the nature of chronic illnesses—clinical course, aetiology, prognosis—for which supportive therapy is indicated. He will then be more aware of the needs and problems these patients present.

Practising supportive therapy under supervision is undoubtedly the main aspect of training. By working with various types of patients over at least a year the trainee accomplishes several tasks. His attitudes to their care becomes more realistic and positive. Instead of regarding them nihilistically as 'incurables' the trainee appreciates that a specific approach is necessary, where goals are limited (Daniels *et al.* 1968). To the novice, these goals are frustratingly minuscule, but later he can understand that for the patient their achievement may be immensely

Supportive psychotherapy

rewarding. The therapist thus learns that he can be helpful. Another attitude to modify is the commonly held one that supportive therapy is merely 'brief, commonsensical chats . . . which consist of little more than sympathetic listening and more-or-less considered advice' (Smail 1978). The trainee realizes that treatment involves much more, with specific skills being of the essence.

Teaching should relate closely to patient care. The WAC model is most appropriate. As mentioned earlier a group of trainees assembles together to discuss the cases seen. Each therapist compares his encounters with those of his peers as well as receiving suggestions from an experienced clinician who serves as supervisor. A useful spin-off is that trainees from different professions—psychiatry, clinical psychology, social work, nursing and occupational therapy—participate in the same programme with the advantage of interdisciplinary exchange and sharing of different perspectives in the care of the chronic patient. If a WAC-type clinic is unavailable clinical experience under supervision remains the core of training.

CONCLUSION

Supportive therapy with the chronically impaired psychiatric patient has the main aim of promoting his best possible adjustment. To achieve this the therapist enters into a particular type of relationship with the patient and uses a range of specific strategies such as explanation, reassurance, and guidance. Undue dependency is without doubt the most important problem facing the therapist; its prevention requires careful skill. A useful model of treatment which revolves around the concept of an 'institutional alliance' can help to minimize the problem of dependence as well as provide suitable care. The effectiveness of this model, however, and of supportive therapy in general, still remains to be tested.

REFERENCES

Balint, M., Hunt, J., Joyce, D., Marinker, M., and Woodcock, J. (1970). *Treatment or diagnosis. A study of repeat prescriptions in general practice.* Tavistock, London.

Bloch, S. (1976). Supportive psychotherapy. *British Journal of Hospital Medicine*, **18**, 63–7.

Bloch, S., Szmukler, G. I., Herrman, H., Benson, A., and Colussa, S. (1995). Counselling caregivers of relatives with schizophrenia: themes, interventions and caveats. *Family Process* (in press).

Brandwin, M. A., van Houten, W. H., and Neal, D. L. (1976). The continuing care clinic: outpatient treatment of the chronically ill. *Psychiatry*, **39**, 103–17.

Buckley, P. (1994). Self psychology, object relations theory and supportive psychotherapy. *American Journal of Psychotherapy*, **48**, 519–29.

Conte, H. (1994). Review of research in supportive psychotherapy: An update. *American Journal of Psychotherapy*, **48**, 494–504.

Conte, H. and Plutchik, R. (1986). Controlled research in supportive psychotherapy. *Psychiatric Annals*, **16**, 530–3.

Crown, S. (1988). Supportive psychotherapy: A contradiction in terms? *British Journal of Psychiatry*, **152**, 266–9.

Daniels, R., Draper, E., and Rada, R. (1968). Training in the adaptive psychotherapies. *Comprehensive Psychiatry*, **9**, 383–91.

Dewald, P. A. (1994). Principles of supportive psychotherapy. *American Journal of Psychotherapy*, **48**, 505–18.

Gilbert, S. and Ugelstad, E. (1994). Patients' own contributions to long-term supportive psychotherapy in schizophrenic disorders. *British Journal of Psychiatry*, **164**(Suppl. 23), 84–8.

Greenberg, S. (1986). The supportive approach to therapy. *Clinical Social Work Journal*, **14**, 6–13.

Hartland, S. (1991). Supportive psychotherapy. In *Textbook of psychotherapy in psychiatric practice*, (ed. J. Holmes). Chuchill Livingstone, Edinburgh.

Holmes, J. (1988). Supportive analytical psychotherapy. *British Journal of Psychotherapy*, **152**, 824–9.

Kahn, E. M. (1984). Psychotherapy with chronic schizophrenics. *Journal of Psychosocial Nursing*, **22**, 20–5.

Karasu, T. (1986). Supportive psychotherapy. Psychosomatic medicine and psychotherapy. *Psychiatric Annals*, **16**, 522–5.

Kates, J. and Rockland, L. H. (1994). Supportive psychotherapy of the schizophrenic patient. *American Journal of Psychotherapy*, **48**, 543–61.

Kellner, R. (1985). Functional somatic symptoms and hypochondriasis. *Archives of General Psychiatry*, **42**, 821–33.

Kernberg, O. (1984). Supportive psychotherapy. In *Severe personality disorders*. Yale University Press, New Haven, CT.

Kolb, L. C. (1973). *Modern clinical psychiatry*. Saunders, Philadelphia.

Lamb, H. R. (1981). Individual psychotherapy. In *The chronically mentally ill*, (ed. J. A. Talbot). Human Sciences Press, New York.

MacLeod, J. and Middleman, F. (1962). Wednesday afternoon clinic: a supportive care program. *Archives of General Psychiatry*, **6**, 56–65.

Masnik, R., Olarte, S., and Rosen, A. (1980). 'Coffee groups': a nine-year follow-up study. *American Journal of Psychiatry*, **137**, 91–3.

Meyer, W. (1993). In defense of long-term treatment: on the vanishing holding environment. *Social Work*, **38**, 571–8.

Neki, J. S. (1976). An examination of the cultural relativism of dependence as a dynamic of social and therapeutic relationships. *British Journal of Medical Psychology*, **49**, 11–22.

Novalis, P. N., Rojcewicz, S. J., and Peele, R. (1993). *Clinical manual of supportive psychotherapy*. American Psychiatric Press, Washington, DC.

Paris, J. (1993). The treatment of borderline personality disorder in light of the research on its longterm outcome. *Canadian Journal of Psychiatry*, 38(Suppl. 1), 28–34.

Pine, F. (1986). Supportive therapy: A psychoanalytic perspective. *Psychiatric Annals*, 16, 526–9.

Pinsker, H. (1994). The role of theory in teaching supportive psychotherapy. *American Journal of Psychotherapy*, 48, 530–42.

Rada, R. T., Daniels, R. S., and Draper, E. (1969). An out-patient setting for treating chronically ill psychiatric patients. *American Journal of Psychiatry*, 126, 789–95.

Rockland, L. H. (1989). Psychoanalytically-oriented supportive therapy: Literature review on techiques. *Journal of the American Academy of Psychoanalysis*, 17, 451–62.

Rockland, L. H. (1989a). *Supportive therapy: A psychodynamic approach*. Basic Books, New York.

Rockland, L. H. (1992). *Supportive psychotherapy for borderline patients: A psychodynamic approach*. Guilford Press, New York.

Rockland, L. H. (1993). A review of supportive psychotherapy, 1986–1992. *Hospital and Community Psychiatry*, 44, 1053–60.

Rockland, L. H. (1995). Advances in supportive psychotherapy. *Current Opinion in Psychiatry*, 8, 150–3.

Sassano, M. P. and Stone, C. L. (1975). Supportive psychotherapy: Thursday afternoon clinic. In *Psychiatric treatment: crisis, clinic, consultation* (ed. C. P. Rosenbaum and J. E. Beebe). McGraw-Hill, New York.

Smail, D. J. (1978). *Psychotherapy: a personal approach*. Dent, London.

Wahl, C. W. (1963). Unconscious factors in the psychoanalysis of the hypochondriacal patient. *Psychosomatics*, 4, 9–14.

Werman, D. S. (1984). *The practice of supportive psychotherapy*. Brunner/Mazel, New York.

Winnicott, D. W. (1965). *The maturational process and the facilitating environment*. International Universities Press, New York.

Winston, A., Pinsker, H., and McCullough, L. (1986). A review of supportive psychotherapy. *Hospital and Community Psychiatry*, 37, 1105–14.

Yalom, I. D., Bond, G., Bloch, S., and Zimmerman, E. (1977). The impact of a weekend group experience on individual therapy. *Archives of General Psychiatry*, 34, 399–415.

RECOMMENDED READING

Kernberg, O. (1984). Supportive psychotherapy. In *Severe personality disorders*. Yale University Press, New Haven, CT. (A thought provoking chapter by one of the 'masters' of the therapy of the severely disorderd personality.)

Novalis, P. N., Rojcewicz, S. J., and Peele, R. (1993). *Clinical manual of supportive psychotherapy*. American Psychiatric Press, Washington, DC. (As the title suggests, a 'how-to book, concentrating on principles and detailed clinical applications.)

Rockland, L. H. (1989). *Supportive therapy: A psychodynamic approach*. Basic Books, New York. (A clinical account of supportive therapy applied within a psychoanalytic framework.)

Rockland, L. H. (1992). *Supportive therapy for borderline patients*. Guilford Press, New York. (A psychodynamically oriented model of supportive therapy directed towards the special needs of the borderline patient.)

Rockland, L. H. (1993). A review of supportive psychotherapy 1986–1992. *Hospital and Community Psychiatry*, **44**, 1053–60. (Useful review of the literature which suggests a growing consensus about the aims and methods of supportive therapy.)

Werman, D. (1984). *The practice of supportive psychotherapy*. Brunner/Mazel, New York. (Application of psychoanalytic principles with an attempt to differentiate between supportive and insight-oriented psychotherapy; contains many illuminating clinical vignettes.)

13

Ethical issues in psychotherapy practice

T. BYRAM KARASU

Some new as well as old and enduring ethical issues in the conduct of psychotherapy are discussed, with emphasis on contemporary socio-economic concerns about health care reform and accountability. These include the general areas of the scientific validity, goals, and values of treatment, and of the special nature of the therapeutic relationship between clinician and patient. More specific subjects are confidentiality and privileged communication, and sexual boundary violations and exploitation, such as sexual contact, sexism, and of most recent controversy, suggestion in sexual abuse. T. Byram Karasu makes recommendations for the promotion of proper ethical practices of psychotherapists during training and treatment.

Basic standards of conduct have been set down for all physicians since antiquity (Castiglione. 1947). The Hippocratic Oath of the fourth century BC forms the enduring foundation for contemporary codes of doctors as well as other helping professions (e.g. American Psychological Association 1981; American Psychiatric Association 1985). Special ethical problems, however, affect psychotherapeutic practice that differ in shade and degree from those in the physical branches of medicine. The unusual emotional bond that develops between therapist and patients lies at the root of these differences. It has been compared to that of parent and child and is unlike other professional or contractual relationships, such as teacher to student, clergy to parishioner, or lawyer to client (Gabbard 1989). It is distinct, not only in the intimacies of personal life that are revealed but due to deep-seated dependency, attraction and affection, including sexual feelings, that are often aroused.

Some new as well as old and enduring ethical dilemmas in the practice of psychotherapy derive from this unique relationship. An overriding issue involves the social and personal values or ideologies—often implicit—that are transmitted, even by the presumably neutral therapist. Two specific subject areas of major moral and legal importance are those of confidentiality and privileged communication, and therapist–patient sexual behaviours and boundaries.

VALUES IN PSYCHOTHERAPY

The values of psychotherapy are expressed in the overall nature of its belief systems, methods, and goals. Major ethical concerns include: (1) controversy over how 'value-free' the psychotherapist is, or ought to be; (2) unproven validity or efficacy, and possible negative effects of treatment; and (3) of contemporary consideration, the financial/ethical interface between aims and costs. All of these impact on therapeutic responsibilities, plans, and practices of the moral therapist.

The 'value-free' fallacy

A neutral and accepting stance by the therapist is often believed to be the backbone of the therapeutic endeavour. The clinician suspends judgement by attentively listening and being objective towards the patient and nature of his problems. Theoretically at least, this means that practitioners are expected to exercise professional restraint and are admonished against imposing their personal views or values. In reality, however, the idyllic notion of psychotherapy as 'value-free' is considered a fallacy (Strupp 1974).

The current understanding is that all therapists embody particular social standards, value orientations, or personal preferences—unconsciously, if not consciously. Therapists and other helping professionals are 'secular moral agents' who implicitly represent certain 'good' values, like beneficence, fidelity, and responsibility to others (Thompson 1990). Their expertise also gives them licence to apply some of the basic tenets of their professional belief systems. At bottom, they must inevitably decide what constitutes health or adaptation and the difference between normality and psychopathology. Even diagnoses can represent a form of value judgement (Torrey 1974).

Some even question whether opting for 'cure' of presumed psychopathology violates personal freedom to decide what change one wishes to make. Should the therapist help the patient to rebel against a repressive or abusive environment, adapt to a particular cultural norm, or to adjust to his current condition? This issue has recently arisen in relation to psychiatry's traditional definition and treatment of homosexual patients. On a diagnostic level, the earlier nomenclature of homosexuality as a perversion or sexual deviation has been challenged and changed. The newer view of such behaviours as a sexual orientation preference (rather than psychiatric disorder) reflects greater acceptance of alternative life styles, and is less stigmatizing to the patient by removing this phenomenon from psychiatric nomenclature.

On a practical level, the therapist may still be obliged to take a stand with regard to his *own* view of the patient's clinical status and purpose of treatment: Does the clinician foster heterosexuality as an ultimate goal, or rather, help these individuals to maximize the quality of their *homo*sexual life (Schwartz and Masters 1984)? Other social, cultural, and religious values are expounded whenever the clinician, directly or indirectly, encourages the unwed woman to get an abortion, the married man to cease having affairs, the troubled couple to divorce, the failing student to remain in school, the traumatized child to leave home, or the sexually abused daughter to take legal action against her father. Is it always unethical to take one or another position? Can the moral therapist be expected to withhold good advice or renounce sound standards in the name of neutrality?

Unexpressed values

The greatest fear is that prejudiced clinicians may hide their beliefs or biases behind professional claims of neutrality. It is well known that practitioners typically have an implicit predilection for their own schools or methods. This is not unethical *per se*; it serves as part of their professional identity and offers consensual support for, confidence in, and commitment to their work. Accompanying this, however, is often a reluctance to acknowledge, utilize, or inform patients of alternative forms and goals of treatment. For example, the dynamic psychotherapist traditionally tends not to prescribe medication for mild to moderate insomnia, anxiety or depression. The presumed justification is that the patient's discomfort and suffering have a motivating function for psychological exploration.

A landmark malpractice suit occurred when a patient (also a physician), having made a remarkable recovery with antidepressant medication, sued a prior psychiatric facility for having treated him with psychodynamic psychotherapy alone—to which he had shown no improvement. The judge ruled in his favour. A 'respectable minority rule' (i.e. following a course of treatment that is practised by a recognized segment of the profession) has been generally accepted in legally establishing whether there is negligence in the standard of care. Thus, recent knowledge of the useful integration of psychotherapy and pharmacotherapy may make it increasingly necessary for psychotherapists to educate patients about other options, such as the availability of medication. But just how much does the ethical therapist need to tell the patient?

The goals of psychotherapy are varied and complex: they can be short-term (alleviation of acute anxiety or depressive symptoms) or long-term (resolution of unresolved conflicts, personality change), non-specific (i.e. inner peace, greater insight) or specific (removal of a phobia). Long-term treatment holds the ethical danger of keeping patients beyond necessity, whereas brief therapies can be abortive. For example, the behavioural psychotherapist generally believes that the symptom *is* the neurosis, so that he is perfectly justified, therapeutically and ethically, in aiming solely at symptomatic relief or removal. But, if others in the profession recognize that they may merely be providing superficial or temporary relief for a deeper disturbance, are these clinicians deceiving themselves—and their patients—by failing to recommend alternative approaches? As utilization of multiple modalities and combined treatment regimens become more commonplace, can the use of a single strategy or school be construed as a form of negligence?

Unproven validity and efficacy

A cardinal principle in contemporary ethics states that a health professional should practise a method of healing founded on a scientific basis. He should neither lend endorsement nor refer patients to persons, groups, or treatment programmes with which he is not familiar, especially if their work is based only on dogma and authority and not on scientific validation and replication. He is also admonished against voluntarily associating professionally with anyone who violates this principle. A basic ethical issue is the extent to which such dictums are—or more aptly, can be—carried out in actual practice.

There are a host of unresolved research problems in psychotherapy. They include the anecdotal nature of individual case reports, the elusiveness of many basic concepts (e.g. repression, transference, defence mechanisms, insight), and the complexity of therapist, patient, and relationship variables that are involved (APA Commission on Psychotherapies 1982). It is especially difficult to equate the respective outcomes, processes, and diverse methods espoused by different schools from 'talking' cures (psychoanalysis) to 'screaming' cures (primal therapy) or 'reasoning' cures (cognitive therapy), from behaviour modification to hypnotherapy, group marathons, or sex therapy. One must question the extent to which each of these approaches are valid and effective (including negative or side-effects), and therefore morally defensible. Despite specific claims and counter-claims in behalf of one or another modality, classic research suggests that 'all' psychotherapeutic approaches may be equally efficacious. This is largely attributed to *non*-specific factors, or 'common elements', that therapeutic methods of all types share: a healing setting, a mutual belief system between therapist and patient, offering hope for help, a trusting relationship, and enhancement of a sense of mastery (Frank and Frank 1991).

Even if different therapies are scientifically proven essentially equal in their positive effects, this does not necessarily mean that are equally ethical in their respective practices. Some believe that techniques utilizing direct manipulation (behaviour modification) or subliminal suggestion (hypnotherapy) are more susceptible to misuse than those designed to expand self-awareness (dynamic psychotherapy). Others maintain that therapeutic influence cannot be easily exerted against a patient's will. The answer to the ethical issue of involuntary influence may be a relative one, that is, the *degree* of control, suggestion, or persuasion that is imposed, from which no therapies or therapists are completely exempt.

Unrealistic goals and compromised values

A survey of practitioners and researchers in the field has found that a major factor in negative effects of psychotherapy was the specific issue of undertaking unrealistic tasks or goals (Hadley and Strupp 1976). Frequently, the patient over-endows the clinician's powers as part of his psychopathology. This may perpetuate irrational demands and excessive expectations which sustain the erroneous impression that therapy and therapist can solve everything. Such distortions can be compounded by the therapist's failure to discuss, describe, or even acknowledge goals before and during treatment. It should be pointed out that fostering optimism—and dependency—is an appropriate function of the clinician's attempt to secure and sustain motivation. But it can also become inappropriate: the clinician may unconsciously create or change goals, prolonging treatment out of his own counter-transferential wishes (e.g. narcissistic need to sustain an exalted position, not wanting to be abandoned by the patient, fear of financial strain). Greenson (1967) has warned that any aspect of therapy that makes the patient an addict to treatment is undesirable.

The other side of this ethical coin is arising as economic pressures are favouring short-term policies. Today it is probably much less likely that the patient is at risk of becoming an addict to treatment; rather, he is in greater danger of being subject to insufficient or superficial treatment. Pharmacotherapy, behavioural and cognitive therapies, brief dynamic psychotherapy, and group approaches are all in the direction of cost-efficiency, so that they will increasingly become the preferred modalities of the future. What may become compromised in the process is the reduced availability to deal with individual themes and enduring problems, the trading in of long-term goals for short-term ones, and making professional decisions based not on what is best therapeutically, but what will be most expedient financially.

For example, trying to curb the rising cost of treating workers for mental illness and substance abuse, a growing number of businesses are turning to a new way of measuring treatment—by computers (Freudenheim 1994). It gives therapists the ability to compare the symptoms of their patients with a large database of presumably similar cases, upon which to tailor treatment. This reduces expenses but also attempts to bring a degree of precision to practice that it does not possess. Does the therapist let his own professional judgement prevail, or does he succumb to financial pressure?

Similarly, there is the issue of the clinician's commitment to a multidisciplinary orientation that utilizes alternative approaches and resources versus personal threat from other disciplines (e.g. psychology, social work, pastoral counselling), that overlap with the roles and responsibilities of the therapist. From an increasing cost-effective perspective, how does the practitioner morally deal with referrals, the blurring of professional boundaries, and the competitive effects on his own practice? In the best interests of the patient, is there an ethical line that lies between purpose and price?

THE THERAPEUTIC RELATIONSHIP

The pivot of psychotherapy is the therapeutic relationship, which differs from all other professional or fiduciary relationships (Gabbard 1989). A *fiduciary* relationship is defined by a designated circumstance in which a person places trust and confidence in another, usually of special training or expertise, to act in his best interests. Possible ethical conflicts in this type of relationship are generally the result of the concept of authority on which they rest: in its purist sense, it refers to credit or acceptance that is entitled to the person by virtue of one's professional position; but it also can refer to power that requires submission due to the status difference between the parties involved.

The interpersonal relationship takes on an additional element in psychotherapy because of the development of strong *transference*, in which an early parent–child bond is unconsciously re-established and re-enacted by the patient towards the therapist. The nature of this interaction constitutes a strength of psychotherapy because it is through this vehicle that the clinician learns about the patient. However, it also represents psychotherapy's greatest ethical weakness in that it implicitly places the therapist in an idealized position of power and persuasion as parental surrogate.

Different types of therapist–patient bond

It has long been believed that faith in the healer is a necessary element in cure and that therapeutic leverage would be weakened by viewing such a person in too prosaic a light (Burling *et al.* 1956). In addition, dependency is one of the most common features of all patients and allows for the early establishment of the helper–helpee bond. Different types of relationship are formed in different therapies (Karasu 1977), and at different times within the same therapy (Karasu 1980). For example, the typical *transference* relationship, which offers the therapist a unique vehicle for exercising enormous (idealized and often irrational) influence over the patient, can be balanced by a *therapeutic alliance*, which conducts the tasks of therapy as a mutual and rational exploration. Taken further, a *therapeutic partnership* (Goldberg 1977) establishes an explicit and agreed upon treatment plan: this can consist not only of agreed goals, but means for attaining them, ongoing evaluation of therapy and methods of addressing dissatisfactions.

Not all therapists agree about the nature of the therapeutic relationship. Some suggest that an authoritarian fiduciary model gradually has been replaced by an egalitarian contractual model (Redlich and Mollica 1976); but others more recently observe the beginnings of a trend in the reverse direction: a dissolution of the dyad and a re-medicalization of the bond that increases distance between doctor and patient (Schultz-Ross *et al.* 1992). The perpetuation of the 'sick role' is a social value issue, and the encouragement of patient dependency is a technical issue. But the question remains, how does the therapist deal with their ethical implications?

SPECIFIC ISSUES: CONFIDENTIALITY

The protection of privacy: confidentiality and privilege

The general notion of privacy refers to the state of being separate from the physical company or observation of others; more specifically, it refers to freedom from unauthorized intrusion (*Webster's dictionary* 1989). In psychotherapy, the issue of privacy becomes particularly pertinent, not simply in regard to one's person (as in a physical examination) and/or with reference to specific illness-related information, discussion, or decision-making that naturally occurs in any doctor's office. The scope of its contents are not circumscribed to strictly medical matters and may go beyond the sensitivity and stigma associated with many physical ailments. Psychological problems pertain to some of the most secret and troubling thoughts and feelings about one's private life. Its revelations are frequently fraught with fear, shame, or guilt about socially unacceptable and undesirable events and behaviour. The special sanctity of psychotherapy is therefore crucial because of the inherently intimate nature of patient communications, which can include innermost confessions about self—and others. In fact, many countries grant the privacy between psychiatrist and patient the same absolute protection as that accorded to husband and wife, or lawyer and client (Dubey 1974).

Two related stipulations are designed to safeguard information shared with the psychotherapist: *confidentiality* and *privilege*. Confidentiality is concerned with the protection of patients' disclosures in a therapeutic setting; *privilege* extends that protection to decisions about specific material to be potentially released, usually for judicial or quasi-judicial purposes. Confidentiality has a long ethical history in the medical field (Castigione 1947); privilege is of relatively recent legal origin (Schwitzgebel and Schwitzgebel 1980).

Confidentiality thus constitutes a major patient expectation and right, its protection a professional duty, and its violation an ethical transgression. This stipulation means utmost care and impeccable therapist judgement regarding all formal and informal verbal exchanges as well as written reports and case records. This ideal can be compromised in relation to the requirements of treatment, training, or administrative responsibilities. For example, potential ethical dilemmas for the psychotherapist can arise in contact with family members, in therapeutic consultation with other professionals or social agencies, in bureaucratic accessibility to clinical notes and hospital records, in training use of patient presentations and teaching aids (including the utilization of case material for one's own professional writings), and even, in the more insidious instance of 'gossip' among colleagues, personal friends, or acquaintances.

At the same time, privilege (or privileged communication) is another established patient right, recognized only by legal statute, whereby a patient may bar his therapist from testifying about that person's treatment. It is a decision that has been ultimately placed in the hands of the patient, not the therapist. A Supreme Court ruling in the United States more specifically expresses the regulations and limitations of therapist–patient privilege regarding admissible evidence:

A patient has a privilege to refuse to disclose and to prevent any other person from disclosing confidential communications, made for the purpose of diagnosis or treatment of his mental or emotional condition, including drug addiction, among himself, his psychotherapists, or persons who are participating in the diagnosis or treatment under the direction of the psychotherapist, including members of the immediate family.

Exceptions to confidentiality: waiving patients' rights

The legitimate (and sometimes, not so legitimate) needs of third parties create constraints to the principle of confidentiality. Two famous cases are those of US vice-presidential candidate Thomas Eagleton, whose publicized psychiatric records resulted in his withdrawal from candidacy, and the 'Watergate' burglary of the unreleased office records of Daniel Ellsberg's psychiatrist by the US Government, for their presumed use in a pending treason trial. The increasing subpoena of patient records in court cases have made it imperative to set finer guidelines for waiving of confidentiality. It also behoves the therapist to devise record-keeping practices so that privacy can be protected (e.g. use of coding systems). Stricter standards of writing style and content also avoid dangers of informal, vague, idiosyncratic, or overly technical notes that create misunderstanding and distortion. It is also imperative that the clinician properly inform the patient of the realistic limits to the protection of confidentiality.

There are two major circumstances under which the patient's right to confidentiality is waived: when the patient chooses to do so (i.e. the patient–litigant exception to testimonial privilege) and when the therapist must do so (i.e. protection of public peril).

Patient–litigant exception to testimonial privilege

Despite patients' general wish for, expectation of, and right to confidentiality, a major exception is often made in instances of legal action, as when the patient wants information released because he is a plaintiff in an emotional damages lawsuit. An ethical dilemma often arises here, not between clinician and court, prosecuted party, or a third party (e.g. workman's compensation board), but between therapist and patient. This is due to the therapist's contention or erroneous belief that he should have the last word on the nature of privilege. Rather, patient consent is always needed (alone, or only if the patient desires, with professional help). The psychotherapist has no choice; he must release case records or provide professional testimony as legally mandated.

Nonetheless, at least three situations constrain this patient right. There is no privilege if: (1) the psychotherapist in the course of diagnosis or treatment has determined that the patient is in need of hospitalization; (2) the court orders an examination of the physical, mental, or emotional state of the patient; and/or (3) a communication regarding the patient's condition is essential to a legal claim or defence. Release of information to a professional third party, such as a supervisor, may also be a recognized exception in so far as it would impede the 'quality control' of care (Slovenko 1975).

Protection of public peril: the Tarasoff decision

The primary exception to the therapist's protection of patient confidentiality, which occurs irrespective of the patient's wishes, arises in the context of prospective danger to others. The famous Tarasoff decision enunciates the maxim that: 'Protective privilege ends where public peril begins.' It refers to the requirement that therapists warn authorities and potential victims of possible endangerment expressed to them by their patients (*Tarasoff* v. *Regents of the University of California* 1974). The ground-breaking case involved the confidential disclosure by a young male out-patient of his plan to kill his former girlfriend. Faced with an ethical dilemma, the therapist made a professional decision to waive patient confidentiality in two ways: he sought help by consulting two colleagues and he notified the police. The patient, who had been legally detained on disclosure of this information, was released from custody shortly thereafter, on denial of violent intent. In addition, he retaliated the therapist's breach of confidence by breaking off treatment. Two months later, when the patient actually committed the planned murder, both therapist and supervisor were sued by the victim's parents for failure to inform their daughter of the impending peril. The legal result was the clinician's 'duty to warn' the endangered person.

This case highlights the complex dilemma of weighing the right of confidentiality of individuals versus protection of society from danger. It is often a delicate balance on both conceptual and practical levels; it presumes that the psychotherapist is an expert in predicting violent behaviour (can perhaps even prevent it). It also compromises patient confidentiality as well as treatment by lowering the threshold of privacy. The clinician is morally and legally placed in an extremely difficult position. He is liable not only for failing to warn the prospective endangered party, but for invasion of privacy, and even defamation of character, if the potential danger fails to materialize. At the same time, the fidelity of the treatment process is at risk; the therapist may lose the betrayed patient at a time when therapy is most needed.

In addressing protective privilege versus public peril, there is concern about the social control function that is defined and reinforced by such rulings (Gurevitz 1977). This goes beyond therapists' expected duties and expertise; it requires them to perform a function that is not ordinarily mandated to their profession. In the light of these criticisms, Roth and Meisel (1977) have made a series of recommendations that allow for the utmost protection of confidentiality: (1) educating their patients beforehand of its limitations; (2) applying various social and environmental manoeuvres to reduce peril, including continued management

pecifically addressed to the dangerous situation, and if that fails,
ossible involuntary hospitalization; (3) informing police; and (4)
nforming the endangered person and other third parties.

rotection of private peril: danger to self

n addition to ethical issues around the objective danger to others is
he subjective danger to self—suicidal acts. A complicated conceptual
onflict pertains to one's philosophical or religious sentiments
egarding to the taking of one's own life. It is considered not only a
iagnostic issue (Is suicide an illness?) and functional problem that
nay require intervention (emergency or therapeutic care), but an
xistential one that questions the very value of human life (Heyd and
Bloch 1991).

In dealing with the suicidal patient, an ethical dilemma pivots on the
question of whether (and when) to intervene. One extreme example,
the so-called 'rational' suicide, occurs when a patient holds some
'objective' reasons for wanting to take his own life such as terminal
illness or the spectre of progressive disability. It raises diagnostic,
therapeutic, as well as spiritual questions with ethical implications. Are
all suicide attempts to be considered pathological, and must all lives be
saved? If so, are they therefore subject to immediate psychiatric
intervention, including involuntary hospitalization? Must the moral
clinician actively discourage such life-threatening behaviours
regardless of the specific circumstances? Or may he assist the
'rational' suicidal patient to make peace with an irreversible and at
best difficult decision?

In addition, some of the same questions and dilemmas arise as in
danger to others, such as: how responsible is the therapist in
predicting—and preventing—danger to self? At what point must
confidentiality be compromised by informing other professionals (e.g.
hospital staff) or more problematically, the family of the prospective
suicide? (Do suicidal ideation and wishes suffice? Is there a line
between threats and actual attempts where confidentiality may be
breached?)

Confidentiality and the future

In recent years, the protection of confidentiality of the traditional
therapist–patient relationship has been under unprecedented pressure,
as third-party insurance and peer-review organizations require

specified information about treatment. Three forces have been identified in the escalating conflict between the right to secrecy and the right to information: (1) increasing involvement of the government in areas that were previously considered as private, such as business regulation, product control—and health care; (2) the technological revolution in data collection, storage and retrieval (e.g. wire-tapping computerized records, video-tapes); and (3) in the light of the individual's greater threat of invasion of privacy, increased awareness of consumer rights.

On the basis of the above, major questions concerning confidentiality in psychotherapy are: Whose agent is the psychotherapist—the patient, the family, society, the law? What are the goals or motives of sharing a confidence—better evaluation and treatment, professional support and validation, counter-transferential need (e.g. self-aggrandisement, personal titillation)? And what are the risks and ramifications of divulging such information—jeopardy of patient trust, termination of treatment, a possible lawsuit?

SPECIFIC ISSUES: SEXUAL RELATIONS AND BOUNDARIES

All major mental health professions have explicit sanctions against sexual intimacy within the therapeutic situation. It reflects the unanimous belief in the damaging effects of such behaviour.

Understanding therapist–patient intimacy

The structure of therapy sets the stage for potential sexual transgression. It issues from the special nature of the relationship, especially the expected establishment of transference 'love' for an idealized father figure and the reciprocal counter-transferential response that it may arouse in the therapist. Specifically, the intensity of their bond can activate sexual feelings and fantasies, while potentially weakening objectivity needed to retain ethical boundaries. Graphic sexual content, which has traditionally been explored in dynamic psychotherapy, may also reinforce such thoughts and emotions. At the same time, the patient may be implicitly modelling his behaviour on that of the therapist by identification or by receiving covert permission to ease super-ego standards as part of the therapeutic process.

It is of utmost importance that both the mental health and legal profession understand the psychodynamics of therapist–patient sex and the circumstances under which it is most likely to occur. Such knowledge helps to assess the validity of the charges made, the extent of damage done, and the nature of punitive action to be taken. It also facilitates *post facto* treatment of the victim and rehabilitation of the perpetrator. Education should help the therapist to comprehend the gravity of violating sexual prohibitions, to recognize clinically patient patterns in those who have had sex with other therapists in the past and, it can be hoped, to prevent such actions from being repeated by identifying the signs of susceptibility of both parties in the present.

Several common themes of the therapist increase the likelihood of sexual involvement with the patient. They include: (1) confusion of one's own need to be loved with those of the patient, especially where the therapist is vulnerable due to personal problems; (2) the fantasy that love in and of itself may be curative; (3) the therapist's proneness to collude unconsciously with the patient in re-enacting past incestuous involvement; (4) the close link between therapeutic zeal and sexual prowess; and (5) the tendency of some therapists to act out their hostility toward their mentors or the profession in general by exploiting the relationship, particularly through sexual violation (Gabbard 1991).

Certain features of the the sexually victimized patient have also been observed. The term 'therapist–patient sex syndrome' has recently been coined to depict a distinct clinical entity having acute, chronic, and/or delayed elements; they may be evident before exploitation occurs or reveal later (Pope 1989): (1) an irrational attachment with marked ambivalence, in which the patient experiences intense love and gratitude as well as hate and fear of the therapist, and in which he may feel exploited, but trapped; (2) guilt in which the patient feels responsible for the sexual feelings or acts that occur during treatment; (3) emptiness and isolation whereby the patient feels empty or unreal unless replenished through sexual involvement; (4) sexual confusion in which an insecure or dependent patient is easily convinced that even non-sexual problems of inhibition or lack of motivation can be solved through intimacy; (5) impaired ability to trust, in which blind trust can turn to exaggerated mistrust of others after transgression with the therapist has occurred; (6) reversal of roles and identity, in which the therapist's needs are brought into treatment as if he were the patient; (7) emotional lability or dyscontrol, in which there is a chaotic surge of conflicting emotions; (8) suppressed rage, in which positive feelings for the therapist is a cover for anger and disappointment; (9) cognitive dysfunction, whereby attention and concentration are disturbed; and (10) increased suicidal risk, in which self-hate and recriminations are acted out against oneself.

Typically, therapists' libidinal or promiscuous behaviours represent a counter-transferential by-product of the therapeutic process, a form of lovesickness. (A US survey revealed that nearly three-quarters of those therapists sexually involved with their patients insisted they were in love at the time; Gartrell *et al.* 1986). Under these vulnerable circumstances, sexual transgression is not a new problem in psychotherapy. It is known that sexual contact (i.e. a range of erotic activities, including sexual intercourse) has occurred since the dawn of psychoanalysis, even though it was never sanctioned. More recent reports confirm these findings and suggest that all levels of the profession are implicated, from trainees to highly experienced professionals.

Society's value system has influenced the way in which sexual activities are viewed, and in turn, how one should deal with such transgressions within the therapeutic context. For example, during the 1960s and 1970s there was increasing acceptance of sexual permissiveness, including the endorsement of touching and presumably 'non-erotic' physical behaviours, especially by members of the 'human potential movement'. The 1990s are seeing a reversal of this trend. In psychotherapy, there is less theoretical emphasis on sexuality as the major motivating force, but more stress on actual sexual misconduct and abuse (Schultz-Ross *et al.* 1992).

Ethical and legal options in sexual transgression

Currently, therapists who violate sexual boundaries may face censure, possible dismissal from professional organizations through the action of their ethics committees, the risk of malpractice litigation, and in some US states, criminal prosecution (Gabbard 1991). The recommendation by some experts, such as Masters and Johnson (1976), that the therapist be charged with criminal or statutory rape, has yet to be accepted.

There are several unanswered questions about the criminalization of therapist–patient sex, which need to be explored if this is going to be a form of therapist censure. The controversy over criminal sanction may be viewed from several standpoints, including philosophical, clinical, legal, and empirical (Deaton *et al.* 1992):

(1) Philosophically, the definition of consent (versus coercion) is at the center of the criminal charge. We need to know what constitutes mutual consent within the therapeutic relationship—how much is genuine, rational, and autonomous as opposed to pathological, irrational, and coercive? In the light of the fiduciary relationship and unconscious forces that are acted upon, is the patient always a non-consenting party and the therapist always the perpetrator?

(2) The clinical standpoint directly issues from the above: what is the nature of the therapeutic alliance and how does it differ from other professional and personal relationships? Definite differences have been found both theoretically and in practice, especially with regard to its time parameters—when is it over? The therapeutic relationship is never over; transference distortions remain unresolved long after therapy has terminated (Gabbard and Pope 1989).

(3) From a legal perspective, the right to privacy interfaces with the nature of consent, as mutual consent has been used as a defence in these cases. It has even be suggested that it was the therapist who had not consented.

(4) Finally, from an empirical perspective, there is the question of the effects of such criminal actions—are they really a deterrent? And if the therapist is deemed a criminal, should patient victims be compensated?

Recent cases

(1) A female psychiatrist was sued by the family of a male medical student who had committed suicide while under her care. During the patient's ninth hospitalization for psychotic depression shortly before his death, he had instructed his sister to look for the source of his troubles in his apartment. She found elaborate clinical materials including tapes, articles, handwritten letters, flash-cards, and children's stories that contained explicit erotic fantasies as well as 'behavioural' directives by the therapist. The patient claimed that she read sexual fantasies to him, masturbated in his presence, and engaged him in 'kinky' sex. The clinician counter-claimed that these materials were explicitly prepared to assist the patient in viewing her as a loving and caring maternal figure.

Although the therapist denied and was exonerated of all charges of misconduct and of responsibility for the patient's suicide, she had, however, admitted to 'unconventional' treatment. It was specifically designed to deal with a virtually untreatable case, someone who was a chronically suicidal, highly volatile drug addict, and victim of horrendous child abuse. (For a long period, she even treated him free of charge.) The therapy included a variety of regressive techniques such as flash-card suggestion (while inviting him to bring stuffed animals to sessions). During these episodes, she recorded in vivid detail his highly primitive, oral, erotic fantasies about her—as well as her own, equally intense, erotic reactions to him.

On investigation by the relevant medical board, there was insufficient evidence that she had actually had sex with the patient; nor could she be legally blamed for his suicide. But the entirety of their therapeutic encounter was exposed, the quality of her treatment was found professionally unacceptable, and with a ravaged reputation, she ultimately resigned (Cotts 1992). The questions arise: are all unconventional therapies unethical? When the therapist did consult her colleagues, was she remiss in not revealing her own fantasies? Was the confidentiality she protected not the patient's, but her own?

(2) A male psychiatrist, one of several who had treated the renowned poet Anne Sexton, agreed to release taped sessions to a publisher for the posthumous publication of a biography of her life. Two issues arose, one of confidentiality, the other of sexual misconduct. The former referred to the fact that the psychiatrist claimed, after Ms Sexton's death by suicide, that the release of such records would be in keeping with her wishes: she had agreed to have sessions recorded and she was a famous public figure who wanted the world to share the knowledge of her artistic life. The uncensored material revealed many intimate details in her tumultuous and tragic story amidst a highly productive career (e.g. manic-depressive illness, violent and suicidal episodes, child abuse, alcoholism, drug addiction, promiscuity, lesbianism, marital discord, separation, and adultery). It also included multiple affairs both outside of—and within—the therapeutic situation. And she named names, particularly that of a former psychiatrist. Had the current psychiatrist acted improperly with regard to confidentiality? At the same time, could his behaviour be defended by the profession with regard to therapist sexual violation? Although the psychiatrist claimed no financial remuneration for the release of her records, was he nonetheless acting in his own interests of personal acclaim? As a dual dilemma, should confidentiality be waived to redress sexual transgression?

Sexism

Sexual relations can theoretically occur with male or female patients (and even between same-sexed therapist and patient); yet its most frequent and pervasive expression is in the male therapist–female patient dyad. Person (1985) has observed that in women treated by men, the erotic transference is more often overt, consciously experienced, intense, long-lived, and directed toward the therapist. In contrast, in men treated by women, it is muted, relatively short-lived, appears more in dreams than in conscious experience, and is frequently transposed to a female figure outside the therapeutic relationship. This phenomenon may be attributed to differences in male-female psychological development as well as to socio-cultural influences, in which women are more prone to define themselves through love relationships than through work achievement. It also places them in greater danger of exploitation when psychotherapy reiterates this fundamental leitmotif.

Sexual intimacy with female patients may be simply the tip of the iceberg of the more pervasive practice of sexism in psychotherapy (Seiden 1976). Sex-role stereotypes are expressed in different standards of psychopathology for each gender, including unchallenged assumptions that dependency and passivity are normal for women whereas assertiveness and independence are normal for men (Broverman *et al.* 1970); unhappiness of females in traditional roles has usually been considered neurotic by male therapists (Rice and Rice 1973). Research on the psychology of women at home, work, and in psychotherapy also reveals that they have long been the targets of a 'blame-the-mother' tradition in mental health, which looks upon them as a major cause of psychosis in their children (i.e. 'schizophrenogenic'). Such sex biases are reinforced by the finding that female therapists are much less likely to have had supervisors of their own gender as role models during training (Seiden *et al.* 1974).

Perhaps the most insidious aspect of sexism is the power differential, or 'one-down' position, in which women are typically placed in psychotherapy, as in life. Both psychopathology and treatment of the female patient are thus re-enactments of the overall feminine fantasy that an idealized relationship with a powerful male is the most desirable—and acceptable—solution to one's problems. Another damaging effect is that the erotic transference as played out in psychotherapy can also mask other important conflicts of women (Person 1985).

Sexual biases may gradually be corrected with a more balanced ratio of female to male therapists and supervisors, and as women are encouraged to assert themselves against chauvinistic values and behaviours. More important is the ethical need for a conscious recognition by 'both sexes of the silent assumptions that penetrate psychotherapy theory and practice.

Suggestion in childhood sexual abuse

Sexual abuse in childhood has become a subject of increasing attention and alarm in both the clinical literature and popular press. Early memories of sexual molestation are often reported during psychotherapy, as they have been since the dawn of psychoanalysis. They were the basis for Freud's original 'seduction theory'; he believed that his patients (frequently female) had been seduced by their fathers in early childhood. This thesis was initially proposed to explain hysterical symptoms and then extended to other neuroses. However, on further observation, it was repudiated and replaced by the notion of erotic incestuous desires as a universal phenomenon. The recollection of these experiences were believed to reflect the emergence of unconscious repressed fantasies, not facts.

The earlier conceptual stance has recently re-emerged with new fervour (Masson 1985). This has manifested as greater emphasis on, belief in, and evidence for the occurrence of actual early sexual violation. Major victims include young children who present with sexual abuse as their chief complaint (as discovered and referred by a teacher, school counsellor, or paediatrician), as well as adolescents and adults who come to therapy as rape victims, incest survivors, or battered wives. Others seek treatment for a range of less obvious abuse-related symptoms, including sexual dysfunction, chronic insomnia, anorexia, depression, low self-esteem, or borderline personality problems, which are eventually traced to early incestuous relations.

From an ethical perspective, this clinical and potentially criminal scenario places the psychotherapist in a pivotal position with respect to the truth or falsehood of such allegations. It poses a dilemma in terms of the extent to which the clinician supports and validates the reported experiences, and presents a legal quandary regarding prospective legal action against presumed perpetrators. This has direct implications for the treatment of the sexual victim, past or present, and for alleged abusive parents, or other significant surrogate figures in the formative years, such as family relatives, school teachers, or members of the clergy. The situation is particularly pressing due to recent changes in legislation in the United States that enormously extends the statute of limitations in damage suits. In fact, the concept of repressed memory made criminal history in 1991 when a father was convicted of murder, based on his daughter's *post facto* recollections 22 years after the event.

It is now possible for a person to sue for sexual misconduct anytime within three years—not of the event itself, but from the first time it is recovered from memory (Washington 1989; *Peterson* vs. *Bruen* 1990). This legal statute is a variation of the 'delayed discovery doctrine' that is used in the rest of medical malpractice. Analogous to the patient who only discovers upon X-ray examination years afterwards that his current condition is the result of a surgeon's much earlier mistake, so the psychiatric patient's memories were hidden from view until the process of psychotherapy exposed them (and the perpetrator) many years later. The above enactment has resulted in a deluge of claims 20, 30, and even 40 years after the abusive events, especially as details of long-lost recollections are retrieved from memory and brought into awareness within the therapeutic situation.

The 'repressed memory controversy'

Both children and adults are remembering and admitting their early traumas with unprecedented frequency. It has raised to a legal level of inquiry the crucial question of the authenticity and validity of repression. Ethically, it has put the psychotherapist at the centre of an unexpected conflict, the so-called 'repressed memory controversy' (Loftus 1993). Are all repressed memories real? And if so, to what extent may the earnest therapist have inadvertently aided and abetted in their recovery? Since the accuracy of buried memories cannot be scientifically proven, the essence of the ethical argument is that therapists may not simply be the neutral recipients of their patient's unearthed reports of sexual abuse—they are possible partners or provocateurs who have elicited false and exaggerated information through thorough suggestion.

In defence of the accused, an upsurge of evidence has emerged which supports the elusive, inaccurate, and malleable nature of repressed memories; that is, memories can be altered. This finding has turned (perhaps displaced) the ethical onus on to the therapist. Such studies claim that the clinician can—and often does—evoke the very sexual material he expects, especially in vulnerable patients who themselves cannot separate fantasy from reality. These charges have been based on patients' accounts of what has transpired in therapy, sworn statements during litigation, and even taped interviews of actual sessions. A new wave of malpractice lawsuits in this area is now occurring against psychotherapists, including the first courtroom challenge to clinicians who practise so-called 'recovered memory' therapy (Gross 1994).

More problematic from a therapeutic point of view, such claims are currently confirmed by clinicians' own accounts of how they proceed with abuse cases. These therapists readily admit to their persistence in probing for recalcitrant memories, particularly in instances of violent or sadistic behaviours that are believed to result in 'massive repression' (Herman and Schatzow 1987). In ardent search for hidden events, the practices may range from simple prodding to hypnosis or bioenergetic techniques. To what extent has the conscientious (and perhaps over-zealous) therapist crossed ethical lines in the name of patient advocacy? Perhaps more troublesome is the degree to which clinicians may be doing so for unexplored counter-transferential reasons (e.g. identification with victims of abuse) and covert collusion in their vindication.

THE PROMOTION OF PROPER ETHICAL PRACTICE

Personal and professional ethical development

Super-ego development is an integral part of the maturation of the psyche and forms the foundation for morality. Naturally, there are variations in the extent to which social proscriptions are internalized by the child and become an enduring voice of authority for the adult. Superimposed on the structures that govern right and wrong are differences in the myriad circumstances under which the dictums of one's conscience may be violated. As a profession, most therapists who transgress ethical boundaries are not psychopathic (Gabbard 1991); but even without serious character flaws, they may have unresolved problems that allow their moral judgement to lapse (or to be overly strict). Those with insufficient super-ego development, as manifested in repeated unscrupulous acts without remorse, cannot rely on internal mechanisms for making socially acceptable judgements; they are also most likely to manipulate external ethical rules (Karasu 1994).

Therapists who are otherwise ethical may temporarily allay anxiety or guilt by using defence mechanisms, such as denial or rationalization, in order to justify immoral behaviour (e.g. insisting that sexual intimacy is for the unloved patient's benefit).

Two levels of moral thinking are regarded as both valid and necessary in the conduct of psychotherapy: the intuitive and the critical (Hare 1991). The former refers to the clinician's instinctive ability to make proper ethical decisions that are based on deeply ingrained, intuitively available, moral principles and duties; he does not have to think twice. However, in complex situations with competing obligations or values, the last level is necessary. It refers to circumstances under which an automatic approach fails and the therapist requires outside help. Here, conscious and often consensual reality must be part of the critical decision-making process. Moral judgements may then be drawn from a range of sources: theories of ethics, professional codes, the socio-legal context, and the therapist's personal/professional identity, to which the clinician can turn in order to assist in the ethical dilemmas he is facing (Woody 1990).

Role of education in ethics of psychotherapy

Codes of ethics

The Hippocratic Oath or other codified standards for the practice of psychotherapy have primarily symbolic value as overall guides to ethical conduct. Codes are not covenants, and even the most morally scrupulous therapists will be disappointed to find that allegiance to such instruments is no guarantee of perfect ethical behaviour. Moreover, codes have profound limitations; they are often non-specific and absolute, use general terms that need to be defined or interpreted (e.g. confidentiality, patient competence, informed consent), and lack subtlety. Since they are insufficient and impractical for solving individual dilemmas, they cannot be the sole decision base in dealing with ethical problems.

Nonetheless, a code of ethics can have two important functions: (1) structuring; and (2) sensitizing (Moore 1978). Structuring has potentially preventive value and aims to hold back impulsive or unethical behaviour; sensitizing has primarily educative value and aims to raise moral consciousness. The role of codes for punitive purposes is considered a misuse, although the legal profession sometimes applies them in this fashion. In particular, they should not be used as a vehicle for revenge, vindication, or private gain.

Peer review

The promotion of ethical practice is attempted not only through the establishment of codes, but through peer review. Although this tends to be utilized to deal with transgressions that have already occurred, the primary purpose of a peer review process should be education, not control (Newman and Luft 1974). Establishing and applying professional guidelines should enhance cooperation among peers, rather than turning them against each other. But the question remains as to how much authority is, or can be, vested in peer review bodies. Two major criticisms of peer review are that: (1) the profession is unable and unwilling to police itself, even when it attempts to be disciplinary; and (2) the patient has been excluded and is poorly informed about acceptable procedures (Sullivan 1977). Therefore, the more pressing problem is less the establishment of guidelines than their enforcement. A document can always be revised, but a complicated bureaucratic and political process is not easy to alter.

Specific problems here include the voluntary nature of complaint investigations; the varied and often conflicting roles that the peer review committee member is required to act—as investigator, prosecutor, judge, and jury; absence or distortions of case reporting; fear of liability by the professional reviewers from the alleged perpetrators; and often, over-concern with confidentiality, whose priority as a principle may be used to resist investigation (Moore 1978). The bottom line, of course, is the difficulty in knowing exactly what does transpire in the confines of the therapist's office. This ambiguity is often compounded by the typical therapist, who is naturally reluctant to confront an errant colleague (who may also be a friend). Indeed, there are wide discrepancies between patient complaints or actual charges made and the professional or legal actions taken against them (Pope 1989; Strasburger *et al.* 1992). Because of these gaps, the need exists for continuing and remedial education, not only for therapists, but also in the selection, training, and evaluation of peer reviewers.

Self-exploration

On a more immediate level is the ongoing examination of the therapist's own values, attitudes, and needs. Counter-transferential responses comprise a major occupational hazard as he is not always able to maintain professional restraint or to remain objective. However, awareness of the warning signs of inappropriate or excessive feelings can prevent acting-out of those feelings. For example, the alert clinician may recognize small breaches of therapeutic rules well before boundary violations begin. Such compromises of usual practice may include extending the session for an attractive patient, revealing personal information about oneself, or making interpretations designed to please the recipient, rather than to promote insight. There may also be gradual physical progression apparent to the observant therapist—from handshake to hand squeeze, from affectionate hug to sensual embrace, or from non-sexual touching to sexual contact. Aside from these obvious cues is awareness of the excessiveness of one's emotions or fantasies. Preoccupation with thoughts and feelings of lovesickness (Twemlow and Gabbard 1989; Gabbard 1991) is perhaps the most dangerous warning signal; it is also the most frequently used justification for therapeutic boundary transgression. Continued self-exploration is one way to avoid the 'slippery slope' of misconduct (Strasburger *et al.* 1992).

RECOMMENDATIONS FOR THE FUTURE

Ethical decision-making in psychotherapy remains an imperfect process. The patient, psychotherapist, insurance auditor, hospital administrator, peer reviewer, and lawyer have all become participants in a complex morality play, and each needs to be educated in the nature of psychotherapy and its limitations. We cannot completely rely on the instinctual ethical nature of those involved nor do codified instruments automatically solve ethical problems.

In the light of the above, the profession can only assist in making recommendations that maximize the exercise of ethical choices for the future:

(1) better understanding of human nature and morality;

(2) greater exploration of the philosophical assumptions on which psychotherapy is predicated;

(3) active development of a mutual and informed partnership between therapist and patient;

(4) openness to consultation with others when ethical conflicts arise;

(5) conjoint responsibility and co-operation among therapists and their professional peers; and

(6) vigilant self-exploration and personal examination of one's values, attitudes, and behaviours, both within and outside of the therapeutic relationship.

REFERENCES

American Psychological Association (1981). Ethical principles of psychologists. *American Psychologist*, **36**, 633–8.
American Psychiatric Association (1985). *Principles of medical ethics with annotations especially applicable to psychiatry*. Washington, DC.
APA Commission on Psychotherapies (1982). *Psychotherapy research: methodological and efficacy issues*. American Psychiatric Association, Washington, DC.
Broverman, I. K., Broverman, D. M., Clarkson, F. E., *et al.* (1970). Sex-role stereotypes and clinical judgments of mental health. *Journal of Consulting and Clinical Psychology*, **34**, 1–7.
Burling, T., Lentz, E. M., and Wilson, R. N. (1956). *Give and take in hospitals: A study of human organisation*. Putnam, New York.
Castigione, A. (1947). *A history of medicine*. Knopf, New York.
Cotts, C. (1992). Paul's case. *Village Voice*, 8 September, pp. 39–44.
Deaton, R. J. S., Illingworth, P. M. L., and Bursztain, H. J. (1992). Unanswered questions about the criminalisation of therapist–patient sex. *American Journal of Psychotherapy*, **46**, 526–31.
Dubey, J. (1974). Confidentiality as a requirement of the therapist: technical necessities for absolute privilege in psychotherapy. *American Journal of Psychiatry*, **131**, 1993–6.
Frank, J. D. and Frank, J. B. (1991). *Persuasion and healing: a comparative study of psychotherapy*, (3rd edn). Johns Hopkins University Press, Baltimore.
Freudenheim, M. (1994). Companies assess psychotherapy by the numbers. *New York Times*, 12 April, pp. A1, D2.
Gabbard, G. O. (ed.) (1989). *Sexual exploitation in professional relationships*. American Psychiatric Press, Washington DC.
Gabbard, G. O. (1991). Psychodynamics of sexual boundary violations. *Psychiatric Annals*, **21**, 651–5.
Gabbard, G. O. and Pope, K. S. (1989). Sexual intimacies after termination: clinical, ethical, and legal aspects. In *Sexual exploitation in professional relationships* (ed. G. O. Gabbard), pp.115–28. American Psychiatric Press, Washington, DC.
Gartrell, N., Herman, J., and Olarte, S. (1986). Psychiatrist–patient sexual contact: results of a national survey. *American Journal of Psychiatry*, **143**, 112–31.

Goldberg, C. (1977). *Therapeutic partnership: ethical concerns in psychotherapy.* New York, Springer.

Greenson, R. (1967). *The technique and practice of psychoanalysis.* International Universities Press, New York.

Gross, J. (1994). 'Memory therapy' on trial: healing or hokum? *The New York Times*, 8 April, pp. A1, B9.

Gurevitz, H. (1977). Tarasoff: protective privilege versus public peril. *American Journal of Psychiatry*, **134**, 289–92.

Hadley, S. W. and Strupp, H. H. (1976). Contemporary views of negative effects in psychotherapy: an integrated account. *Archives of General Psychiatry*, **33**, 1291–302.

Hare, R. (1991). The philosophical basis of psychiatric ethics. In *Psychiatric ethics*, (2nd edn), (ed. S. Bloch and P. Chodoff), pp. 30–45. Oxford University Press, New York.

Herman, J. L. and Schatzow, E. (1987). Recovery and verification of memories of childhood sexual trauma. *Psychoanalytic Psychology*, **4**, 1–4.

Heyd, D. and Bloch, S. (1991). The ethics of suicide. In *Psychiatric ethics*, (ed. S. Bloch and P. Chodoff), pp. 243–264. Oxford University Press, New York.

Karasu, T. B. (1977). Psychotherapies: an overview. *American Journal of Psychiatry*, **138**, 851–63.

Karasu, T. B. (1980). General principles in psychotherapy. In *Specialised techniques in individual psychotherapy*, (eds. T. B. Karasu and L. Bellak), pp. 33–44. Brunner/Mazel, New York.

Karasu, T. B. (1994). A developmental metatheory of psychopathology. *American Journal of Psychotherapy*, **48**, 581–99.

Loftus, E. F. (1993). The reality of repressed memories. *American Psychologist*, **48**, 518–37.

Masson, J. M. (1985). *The assault on truth: Freud's suppression of the seduction theory.* Farrar, Straus and Giroux, New York.

Masters, W. H. and Johnson, J. V. (1976). Principles of the new sex therapy. *American Journal of Psychiatry*, **133**, 548–54.

Moore, R. A. (1978). Ethics in the practice of psychiatry: origins, functions, models, and reinforcement. *American Journal of Psychiatry*, **135**, 137–53.

Newman, D. E. and Luft, L. L. (1974). The peer review process: education versus control. *American Journal of Psychiatry*, **131**, 1363–6.

Person, E. (1985). The erotic transference in women and in men: differences and consequences. *Journal of the American Academy of Psychoanalysis*, **13**, 159–79.

Peterson v. *Bruen* (1990). 792 P.2d 18 (Nev. 1990).

Pope, K. S. (1989). Therapist–patient sex syndrome: a guide for attorneys and subsequent therapists to assessing damage. In *Sexual exploitation in professional relationships*, (ed. G. O. Gabbard), pp. 39–56. American Psychiatric Press, Washington, DC.

Redlich, F. and Mollica, R. (1976). Overview: Ethical issues in contemporary psychiatry. *American Journal of Psychiatry*, **133**, 125–36.

Rice, J. K. and Rice, D. G. (1973). Implications of the women's liberation movement for psychotherapy. *American Journal of Psychiatry*, **130**, 191–6.

Roth, L. H. and Meisel, A. (1977). Dangerousness, confidentiality, and the duty to warn. *American Journal of Psychiatry*, **134**, 508–11.

Schultz-Ross, R. A., Goldman, M. J., and Gutheil, T. F. (1992). The dissolution of the dyad in psychiatry: implications for the understanding of patient–therapist sexual misconduct. *American Journal of Psychotherapy*, **46**, 506–14.

Schwartz, M. F. and Masters, W. H. (1984). The Masters and Johnson treatment program for dissatisfied homosexual men. *American Journal of Psychiatry*, **141**, 173–81.

Schwitzgebel, R. L. and Schwitzgebel, R. K. (1980). *Law and psychological practice*. Wiley, New York.

Seiden, A. M. (1976). Overview: research on the psychology of women, II. Women in families, work, and psychotherapy. *American Journal of Psychiatry*, **133**, 1111–23.

Seiden, A., Benedek, E., and Wolman, C. (1974). *Survey of women's status in psychiatric education: report of the APA Task Force on Women*. Presented at the 127th annual meeting of the American Psychiatric Association, Detroit, May 6–10.

Slovenko, R. (1975). Psychotherapy and confidentiality. *Cleveland State Law Review*, **24**, 375–96.

Strasburger, L. H., Jorgenson, L., and Sutherland, P. (1992). The prevention of psychotherapist sexual misconduct: avoiding the slippery slope. *American Journal of Psychotherapy*, **46**, 544–55.

Strupp, H. (1974). Some observations on the fallacy of value-free psychotherapy and the empty organism: comments on a case study. *Journal of Abnormal Psychology*, **83**, 199–201.

Sullivan, F. W. (1977). Peer review and professional ethics. *American Journal of Psychiatry*, **134**, 186–8.

Tarasoff v. *Regents of the University of California* (1974). 118 Calif Rep 129, 529 P 2d 553.

Thompson, A. (1990). *Guide to ethical practice in psychotherapy*. Wiley, New York.

Torrey, E. F. (1974). *The death of psychiatry*. Chilton, Radnor, PA.

Twemlow, S. W. and Gabbard, G. O. (1989). The lovesick therapist. In *Sexual exploitation in professional relationships*, (ed. G. O. Gabbard), pp. 71–88. American Psychiatric Press, Washington, DC.

Washington (1989). Rev. Code Ann. Sec. 4.16.340 (1989 Supp).

Webster's Ninth New Collegiate Dictionary, (1989). Merriam-Webster, Springfield, MA.

Woody, J. D. (1990). Resolving ethical concerns in clinical practice: toward a pragmatic model. *Journal of Marital and Family Therapy*, **16**, 133–50.

RECOMMENDED READING

American Journal of Psychotherapy (1992). Special Section: Boundaries, behaviour, and sexual misconduct: current issues and the medico-legal interface, **46**, 503–55. (The contemporary relationship between psychiatry and the law in the special area of sexual boundary and behaviour violations. Obstacles and risks of today's psychotherapy practice as well as preventive measures are included.)

Bloch, S. and Chodoff, P. (ed.) (1991). *Psychiatric ethics*. Oxford University Press. (A cross-section of contemporary ethical issues in psychiatry, including conceptual chapters on the philosophical basis of psychiatric ethics, psychiatric diagnosis as an ethical problem, and the responsibility of the psychiatrist to society. Specific applications include ethics of drug treatments, suicide, involuntary commitment, and de-institutionalization.)

Gabbard, G. O. (ed.) (1989). *Sexual exploitation in professional relationships*. American Psychiatric Press, Washington, DC. (A selection of articles on the psychodynamic, ethical, legal, and rehabilitative aspects of sexual transgression, in two sections: therapist–patient relationship versus other fiduciary relationships, such as clergy–parishioner, teacher–student, and hospital staff–in-patient.)

Hundert, E. M. (1987). A model for ethical problem solving in medicine, with practical applications. *American Journal of Psychiatry*, **144**, 839–46. (A model applicable to both theoretical and practical problems in medicine. Three areas are demonstrated: personal ethical problem-solving, hospital ethics committees, and teaching of medical ethics.)

Lakin, M. (1988). *Ethical issues in the psychotherapies*. Oxford University Press. (Everyday practice with emphasis on ideologies and values, and dilemmas of different modalities, for example, individual, marital, family, group, organizational.)

Lakin, M. (1991). *Coping with ethical dilemmas in psychotherapy*. Pergamon, Elmsford, NY. (Discusses ethics in everyday psychotherapy practice, including cross-cultural and gender value conflicts; demonstrates importance of supervision for teaching, modelling, and development of ethical awareness.)

Loftus, E. F. (1993). The reality of repressed memories. *American Psychologist*, **48**, 518–37. (Scholarly review of the phenomenon of repression in psychotherapy in relation to contemporary claims of childhood sexual abuse. Addresses clinical, ethical, and legal implications by exploring the accuracy and authenticity of early memories, the judicial system's response to adult allegations of past trauma, and the therapist's role in memory retrieval and treatment.)

Rosenbaum, M. (ed.) (1982). *Ethics and values in psychotherapy*. Free Press, New York. (Philosophical and practical issues in psychotherapy ethics, covering special problems in different modalities, for example, family therapy.)

Thompson, A. (1983). *Ethical concerns in psychotherapy and their legal ramifications*. University Press of America, New York. (A compendium of illustrative cases and legal commentaries on different ethical issues, from onset of therapy to 'policing' the profession.)

Thompson, A. (1990). *Guide to ethical practice in psychotherapy*. Wiley, New York. (Organized according to six major ethical principles that are honoured and breached in psychotherapy: autonomy, fidelity, justice, benificence, non-maleficence, and self-interest.)

Woody, J. D. (1990). Resolving ethical concerns in clinical practice: towards a pragmatic model. *Journal of Marital and Family Therapy*, **16**, 133–50. (Five decision bases proposed for resolving and preventing ethical concerns and dilemmas in clinical practice.)

Index